Usage of this Ma

This manual shows essential, but often forgotten, dy
in the Yoga postures. Conscientious application of th
maximum results from your time and effort.

To get a clear idea of what is involved in the study of Yoga, read the first dozen pages carefully and review them occasionally. Doing one program per year offers a safe and easy way to approach what will hopefully be a lifetime of yoga. That means for the first year you need only spend a fleeting 10 minutes a day. Done conscientiously, this will naturally lead you to where you truly want to be. That is the long term result that concerns us most here. After you have established your long term practice, be sure to review the particulars of each postures you are doing, at least every decade (or sooner), to spot what will have certainly lapsed over time.

At some point, photocopy the diagrams of either the program or cycle you are developing, and arrange them in a binder in the order in which you practice them. This puts the information at your fingertips. It helps a lot not having to stop and thumb through the book (and cool down) to find useful tips. Also, video yourself a few times to expose your 'blind spots' (see what you're missing).

Dedication

I dedicate this manual to the Bhagavad Gita, Tao Te Ching and to other ancient scriptures. These provide a foundation in wisdom that makes Hata Yoga more than just contortionist gymnastics. I deeply appreciate the sound practical approach to Hatha Yoga that the Iyengars (B.K.S., Prashant and Gita) gave me. I thank Ingela Abbott, my ex-wife, for her early support and for the artistic grace she gave to the illustrations. I am grateful to my wife Leslie for help throughout, from the little booklet version of 1980 to this final product, and finally to my sons, Luke and Kyle, for giving me reason to finally finish this book.

Table of Contents

Principles

(from an older and perhaps wiser point of view)

I wrote this Yoga manual in 1979. Now, 30 years later, it still holds up well. I've decided to leave the original introductory pages mostly as is, especially *PRINCIPLES (from a younger point of view)*. These reflect my youthful belief in *free will* : that anything is possible if I set my mind to it. Naturally, it reads a bit strident, naively so from my point of view today. Yet, its message may offer a useful perspective.

Ideal Free Will

Soon after I finished the manual, I began to question my faith in free will*, and I began earnestly searching for evidence of it. So far, I've found nothing in human behavior that can not be explained by a simpler motivation—the biological push-pull force of need/fear. In the end, free will appears to be a case of wishful thinking more than fact. It seems that I just *needed* to believe in free will. Why?

Conflicting needs (or fears) was the problem, and free will promised a solution. If, as it now appears, free will is no more than a promise, what can I do? Ironically, I've found hope lies in knowing that the strongest need (or fear) I feel at the moment determines what I do (or don't do). Paradoxically, this makes 'free will' and need/fear almost synonymous, i.e., need and fear determine what I want, and what I worry about. Need and fear, wanting and worrying are as interdependent as muscle and bone.

Actual Free Will

Happily, the resolution of conflicting needs (or fears) depends largely upon me being mindful of what I *truly* want of life. And what is that? Honestly, I've always known what I want deep down. We all have (and do), intuitively anyway. It is just that short-term desires and worries keep distracting us. We forget again and again, turning over one new leaf after another as we wander and stumble down life's very short road.

* http://centertao.org/essays/core-issues-of-human-nature/free-will

Prioritizing desires counteracts this distraction by diminishing the impact of desire (and worry) on us. In doing this, we are effectively desiring not to desire. As the *Tao Te Ching* puts it: "*Therefore the sage desires not to desire, and does not value goods which are hard to come by*"... (64).

Watch Your Self

If I had to sum up the secret of yoga, I'd say it all comes down to watchfulness—or as Buddha said, *Right Mindfulness, Right Attentiveness, Right Concentration.* In a yoga posture, this means watching your body, mind, and emotion moment to moment. Are you pushing too hard, (too 'Ha'), or taking it too easy (too 'Tha')? All you need do is watch for these lapses from the 'middle path', and go the other way... towards balance.

Watching oneself honestly couldn't be easier or more straightforward. This is a level playing field, perhaps the only one in life—no knowledge, skill, teaching, or innate talent is required. And yet, as the *Tao Te Ching* says, *"Our words are very easy to understand and very easy to put into practice, yet no one in the world can understand them or put them into practice"...* (Ch.70). Okay, that may be an over-statement, but not by much. Living in watchful self-honesty is most difficult.

Why? Because every innate advantage we have has its downside. I can't emphasize this enough; every plus we enjoy has a minus we suffer. Worse yet, what we *think* is so gets in the way of seeing what is actually so. We fool ourselves. As the *Tao Te Ching* puts it, *"To know yet to think that one does not know is best; Not to know yet to think that one knows will lead to difficulty."*... (Ch. 71).

Balance

Individually, we are on both sides of balance's happy medium—over-doing some areas, under-doing other areas. Clearly, balance lies in under-doing the former and over-doing the later. And fortunately, despite fears to the contrary, there's little chance of overcompensating in either direction. Why?

An iceberg makes a good metaphor. Its tip is like our more fickle outer nature. The ways we under-do or over-do life are actually symptomatic of our more primal inner nature. That means, unlike the iceberg's tip, our inner nature changes little. Sure, we may *think* we change, but that's just the tip of the iceberg talking. Like free will, the ideal of true change is more likely a case of wishful thinking. Getting to know and accept our inner, 'original' nature is the shortest path to balance.

Is it Karma?

Our primal nature is like an iceberg below the water line, massive and unseen. As it bobs and tilts one direction, we react by 'over-doing' or 'under-doing' in the opposite direction to counterbalance. Deeper down our primal nature may itself be counterbalancing still deeper currents. Who knows—it's a little murky down there.

This whole balancing process may represent a kernel of truth in the myth of Karma—not a cause and effect chain of Karmic past and future, but of 'karmic' layers of cause and effect... moment to moment. This is where balance lives, without memory, past or future. Only now!

One practical consequence of seeing life this way is that you soon realize all your perceptions and actions are merely reflections of yourself. In other words, what you perceive or do 'out there' is really symptomatic of your own needs/fears (a.k.a. loves/hates) deep down 'in here' right now.

Self-honesty floods awareness; the judge becomes the judged. Judging books by their covers becomes increasingly difficult when you realize that you are just perceiving symptoms of a deep, less-definable other side. Such a blurring of distinction (*"mysterious sameness"* as the Tao Te Ching puts it) can really help you avoid being knocked off balance by self-serving judgments and biases.

Thinking beats the drum

Of human emotions, desire is the one with which all religions take issue. As the Tao Te Ching puts it, *"There is no crime greater than having too many desires; There is no disaster greater than not being content"...* (46)

However, I say desire is not the real problem, per se. Viewed more closely, desire seems to be a amalgamation of instinctive emotion ('gut' need) and thinking. Without that thinking side, we'd be moved by spontaneous need just like all other animals. Need (and its source spring, fear) is the driving force behind all action. Without it we're dead—literally. It is the thinking side of desire we could (and should) have misgivings about. Thinking beats the drum of emotion, easily making mountains out of molehills (of need and fear).

Just look at the world: From political and religious extremists at one end, down to the little neurotic quirks, opinions and biases that are common to everyone at the other end. All illustrate the consequences of overly trusting that what we think is true. However, when we take thought with a grain of salt, it becomes easier to calm down and preserve emotional equilibrium.

But, who am I kidding? This is a tough nut to crack. Those primal emotions (need and fear) drive thinking. To make matters worse, thinking feeds back into and reinforces emotion. It is a vicious cycle. Still, contemporaneously knowing this is going on *as I think* helps me distrust thinking, even as I'm thinking. This lack of faith in thought weakens its ability to feed into and re-enforce emotion.

Civilization's price tag

One of the primary functions of civilization is providing the means to achieve our goals and satisfy our desires. To meet this end, civilization must side-step nature's wild ruthless side—a side which happens to help keep life balanced. It's not surprising that our nearly obsessive avoidance of nature's uncomfortable side increases the difficulty of maintaining balance. No wonder we easily swing from one extreme to the other. Civilization's endless blind pursuit of safety and comfort comes with unforeseen, unwanted, and unpleasant consequences. We only think we've conquered nature; the negative consequences prove otherwise.

I have a motto to help me counteract civilization's safety and comfort bias and keep me more grounded: "Short term pain, [leads to] long term pleasure. Short term pleasure, [leads to] long term pain". Civilization is biased towards the later. Balance lies in accepting the former. That is the principle essence of yoga for me—balance.

The Spirit of Yoga

Through these Principles I've tried to convey the *spirit of yoga*. Yoga done amid this spirit is truly yoga no matter how stiff, weak, or far from the ideal form you are.

Conversely, yoga done without this spirit is not yoga... no matter how much it looks like yoga. It is merely exercise, which isn't bad; it's just not yoga. Naturally, no one else will know. Only you can know when you are too 'Ha', or too 'Tha'. Only you can fear your imbalance and feel the need to tilt yourself in the other direction—towards balance and what you truly want.

PRINCIPLES

(from a younger point of view)

All living things strive for homeostasis. This is the state of physiological and psychological equilibrium produced by a balancing of the life process. The Yogi realizes this is a cornerstone of contentment. This involves having both good health and an ability to avoid the turmoil of compulsive emotions which inevitably cause confusion, anxiety, stress, and depression.

Beyond this, the Yogi yearns for a deep and broad awareness of life. As this awakens, his main objective is maintaining this awareness under all conditions possible. Clearly though, to achieve and sustain this quality of perception, the mind must be free of its over-reactive nature. Indeed, how can the mind be aware of the subtle while it is being continually agitated by emotions of anger, fear, and compulsive desire?

Sound physical health aids in the process of increasing awareness and control. Consciousness, manifested through the nervous system, is influenced by the vitality of the other body systems. Unfortunately, modern living causes atrophy of the original health you were born with. The natural animal vitality as seen in the wilderness begins disappearing in the human even by the time he starts school.

Significant recovery of original vitality depends upon the efficient functioning of each body system. This depends upon one fundamental evolutionary law:

Development follows the utilization of potential. For example, increasing use of a weak heart through exercise develops micro-circulation in this muscle. This helps keep it disease-free. In Hatha Yoga, better health is achieved by challenging all weaknesses. This increases the efficiency of all major and "minor" parts of the body.

The body systems are intimately interconnected, so even subtle changes in one area eventually affect the whole body. With this in mind, observe below what happens physiologically through Hatha Yoga.

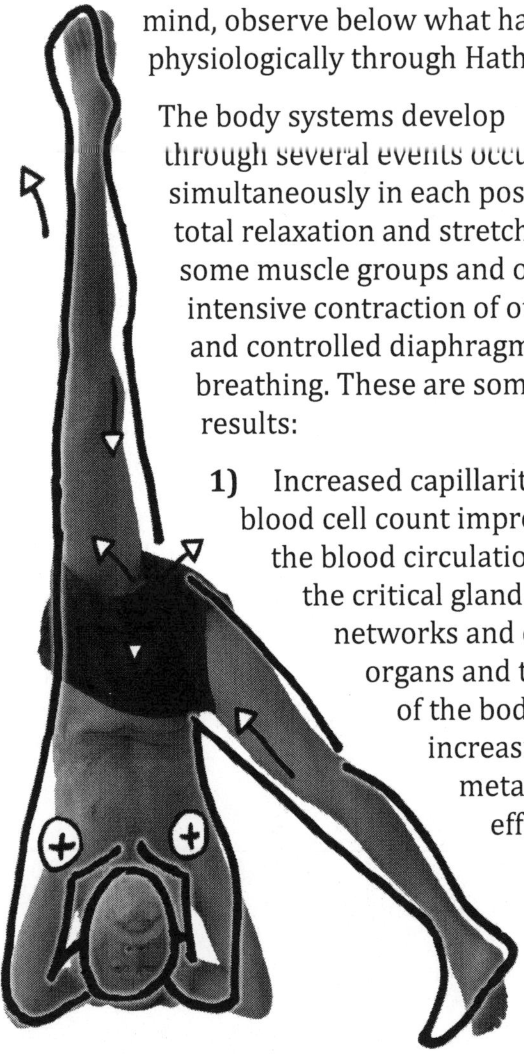

The body systems develop through several events occurring simultaneously in each posture: A total relaxation and stretching of some muscle groups and organs, intensive contraction of others, and controlled diaphragmic breathing. These are some of the results:

1) Increased capillarity and blood cell count improves the blood circulation in the critical glands, nerve networks and other organs and tissues of the body, thus increasing metabolic efficiency.

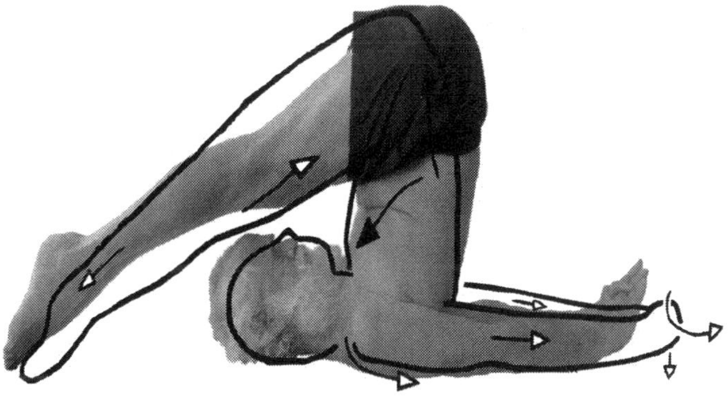

2) A toned endocrine and nervous system produces a more responsive feedback loop for the various body functions.

The body's physical and mental harmony relies on the efficient functioning of this loop and its associated system, circulation.

3) A massaged lymphatic system drains the body of dead cells and toxins, and improves inter-cellular circulation and absorption of body nutrients.

4) A massaged digestive system speeds up and improves nutrition absorption and waste elimination in the intestines, thus helping to avoid illnesses of the digestive tract.

5) A toned, strong, and limber muscular system gives you a comfortable, well-functioning body for the rest of your life.

In addition, each posture is a physical "mantra" that, through watchful practice, pulls the mind into a meditative state. This aligns billions of cortical synapses into better integrated neural matrixes which facilitates memory, concentration, relaxation, and even depth of awareness.

The unique thing about Hatha Yoga is the condition under which this meditation takes place. To sit calmly and meditate is one thing; to remain calm and meditate even under difficult active conditions is a unique and valuable kind of meditation.

Developing psychological health depends on the same evolutionary law governing physiological health. In Hatha Yoga, both physical and mental powers are developed simultaneously, and assist each other in the process. The meaning of Hatha Yoga tells us why.

Hatha is actually two words, Ha and Tha. **Ha** (sun) is work, the "burning fire" of the body radiating energy, and **Tha** (moon) is the reflective quality of mind; the deepest root of awareness that watches. **Yoga** means a merging or joining. So this is the Yoga of Ha and Tha; the union of the reflective, still mind and the creative, active body.

The mind is always agitated to some degree, especially when confronting difficulty. In Hatha Yoga you go to your physical limits. This demand for perfection in action brings you to your mental and emotional limits. Thus you are brought head on into the usual emotional reactions which disturb daily life, i.e. compulsive expectations, frustration, insecurity, and confusion. These are those reactive psychological states that upset homeostasis, and hinder contentment.

In Hatha Yoga, you voluntarily face up to, and gradually deal with these reactions. Your objective is to work hard while maintaining the subtlest awareness: to watch but not get emotionally dragged into the battle of life. This challenge brings all the major and minor powers of the mind into play.

Hatha Yoga deliberately sets up a situation in which you can discover, use, and (over time) strengthen these aspects of self-harmony: reason, vitality, patience, carefulness, attention, and a peaceful sense of "self-surrender".

These powers help you keep perspective which calms restless desires and destructive reactions. This liberation of the mind, along with good health, helps bring deeper contentment within reach.

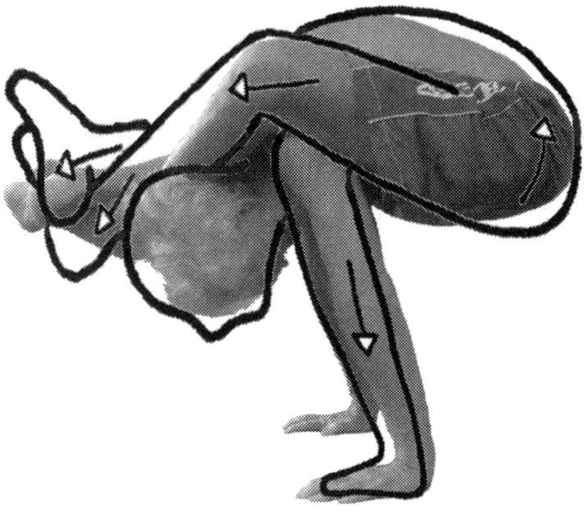

"Do thy work in the peace of Yoga and, free from compulsive desires, be not moved in success or in failure. Yoga is evenness of mind - a peace that is ever the same".
Bhagavad Gita 2-48

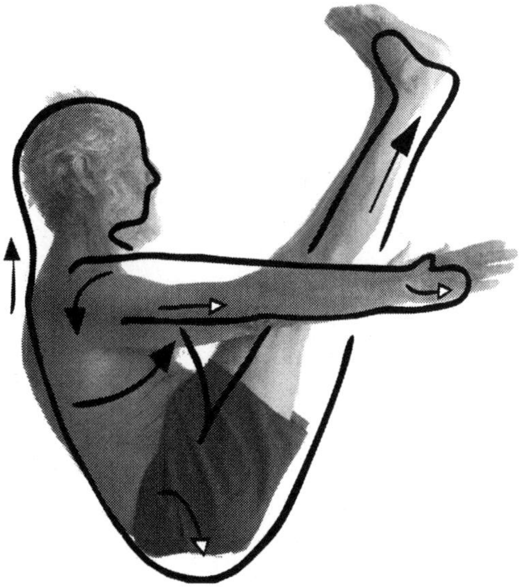

PRACTICE

To develop vitality, you must use it. Therefore, direct your 'energy flow' from toes to fingers. Constantly challenge the weak and dull areas of the body, emotions, and mind. Let the life force surge through you. Without expecting perfection, work with perfection. Sweat!

To develop a watchful mind you must surrender and devote yourself to every moment of every activity. Live in the fire of the senses and watch the nature of activity and the attitude behind it. Notice the quality. What is in the activity that "shouldn't be", and what isn't in the activity that "should be". Finally, let go of thoughts and feel the silence and stillness. Watch!

Here are more points that help you attain a balanced use of mind and body. Development depends on the extent to which you remember and use them.

Do You:

1) Practice daily and sufficiently.

2) Extend spine from sacral to cervical.

3) Extend the base of the neck (the root of watchfulness).

4) Extend the ribs and raise the sternum.

5) Roll the shoulders back and down.

6) Contract or open the buttocks as required.

7) Straighten and lock the arms and legs as required.

8) Keep beauty and symmetry in the form.

9) Completely relax facial muscles; jaw, around eyes and mouth, forehead, throat, tongue, temples, and any part of the limbs or trunk not working for the posture.

10) Keep the mouth shut with the teeth just lightly touching.

11) Keep the eyes open with the gaze steady but not strained.

12) Keep your gaze at nose level (usually), and never cross-eyed.

13) Hold postures for a set time, 15-60 seconds (6 - 18 breaths).

14) Maintain as even a diaphragmatic breathing as possible under the conditions and avoid holding the breath.

15) On the exhalation, extend and move into the posture.

16) On the inhalation, return from the extension.

17) Breathe through the nostrils and avoid grunting.

18) Avoid cheating in the postures to make them easier.

19) Remember that if a posture is easy or boring, it is being done wrong.

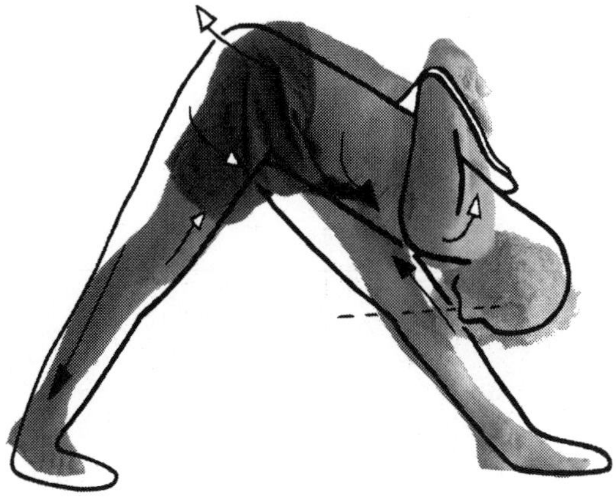

20) Remember that body heat is proportional to challenge.

21) Watch for, challenge, and patiently extend your limits without overworking them.

22) Apply the most effort/time to your weakest areas.

23) Avoid ALL rushing. Take deliberate care in activity and in attitude.

24) Use long, even exhalations to deepen the extension. This is especially true fore painful postures.

25) Use appropriate effort, i.e., strive decrease involuntary actions and reactions and increase voluntary ones.

Many of the points listed above could be practiced in ALL your activity throughout the day. Look carefully at your own life actions and attitudes.

How do you sit, stand, or walk? Do you lean against things? Why? How do you eat, put on shoes, wash the dishes, brush teeth, deal with people, or get out of bed? Why do you sleep too much or too little? Why aren't you always honest? Do you maximize consumption of fresh vegetables, and fruit, and moderate your consumption of grain, meat and dairy?

How do you deal with success and failure? Do you expect things of others, while you blindly (or knowingly) repeat essentially the same "sins"? Are you irritated (a subtle anger) by the faults of others or by unpleasant events? Why? Is your mind flitting about on trivia? Are you a pawn in the grip of compulsive desire and worry? Do you let endless petty fears dictate your life?

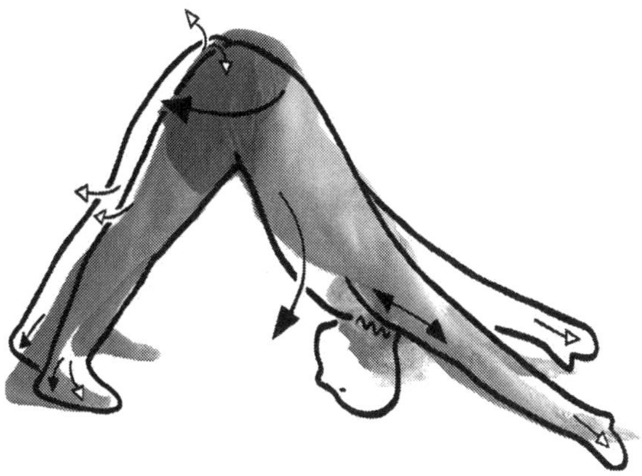

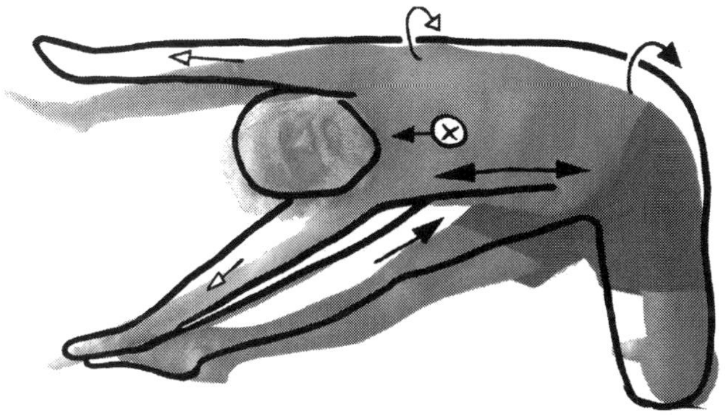

Why aren't all these aspects of your life guided by watchfulness to develop a more appropriate and balanced response? There can be no real contentment or fulfillment in life with this left unattended.

The degree of self-balance you achieve in this life hinges on watchfulness. Watchfulness enables you to notice the seeds of compulsive reactions, which helps you avoid subsequent over-reaction. This active but non-attached attention can and should be practiced throughout the day, moment to moment, in the most "boring" and mundane to the most "important" and stimulating matters. Only then can it become a significant force in your life.

> *"A harmony in eating and resting, in sleeping and keeping awake. A perfection in all that one does. This is the Yoga that gives peace from all pain",* Bhagavad Gita 6-17

Hints and Precautions

1) It is wise to begin Yoga with a realization that years of physical and mental neglect cannot be overcome by a few months or even a few years of Yoga practice — especially if not done conscientiously. In Yoga, you work step by step with daily effort, dealing with the deep causes of your "problem" and not just with the relief of symptoms.

2) Practicing the postures in the early morning when the body and mind are fresh and the determination is strong will do much to set the whole day going well. In addition, the postures are best done when the bowels, bladder, and stomach are empty, which is more likely before breakfast. Otherwise the postures can be done from 2-6 hours after a meal, depending on what and how much you have eaten and the type of postures you do.

3) People with high blood pressure may have to take precautions in the inverted postures. Ask your doctor. Women perhaps shouldn't do the inverted postures during menstruation. No one should do postures during fever, headache (severe), or with other acute symptoms.

4) The graph (next page) is a tool for directing your forgetful and scattered mind. It can work as a mirror to show you how much your daily life reflects the actions and attitudes which you feel contribute to self-balance.

It reminds you of your priorities and allows you to keep a record of practice which cuts down on self-deception. It helps you begin to see yourself in a truer perspective. Without that, you end up repeating the same old straying from what you truly want of life.

You can change the five aspects I list there to anything you believe to be important for your life. Some miscellaneous factors to keep track of might be: posture, brushing teeth, doing responsibilities, speech, smoking and eating habits, being too tidy or too sloppy, being too frank or too deceptive, being too lazy or overworking, being too friendly or too reserved, etc. The idea is not to 'change' any of these. Merely being aware of them is enough; true change happens naturally.

The graph area with the numbers 1-5 allows you to plot an in-line graph. After a few months you'll have a good indication of the "flow" of your life.

5) Daily practice is vital for Yoga to be effective. Beginners during the first year should spend at least 10 minutes a day on their home practice. Those who wish to realize the full potential of Hatha Yoga must work towards the advanced postures. As you do this, your practice will gradually increase to about an hour a day. If this seems a bit much, think of all the "wasted" moments of the day, i.e., idle talk, drifting thoughts, indecision, procrastination, trivia.

Yoga can transform such dead-and-gone-before-you-know-it moments into awakened ones. In fact, due to increases in overall life efficiency, you will end up with more time than you had before.

6) Initially you will have difficulty getting into and holding some of the postures. Try some of the "impossible ones" each day as best you can. They are certain to come in time. Don't expect results, just work with full energy and be patient. Working with full energy, however, doesn't mean over-exerting yourself! Take it easy in the beginning. Try easier variations (Var:) first.

To avoid injury, always be wary of sharp, acute pain. Back off if you feel that. Good pain is sweat pain, the soft smooth agony / ecstasy of hard work. Speaking of work, you can browse through the all the posture illustrations and try ones that look like they'd be just plain old work. No "proper" sequence is necessary. Do what suits your body at the time. As the body changes (flexibility, strength, or weight) you'll adjust your practice to suit.

7) Scriptures can help cultivate how to approach Hatha Yoga to achieve truly 'yogic' results. Study a verse from the teachings of the Bhagavad Gita, Buddha, the Tao Te Ching, Christ, etc., every few days. Reflect on it during your Yoga practice and throughout the rest of the day in all activity. Reflecting does not necessarily mean verbatim repetition. If possible, just recall the feeling the verse gave.

In reading, try to see through the mystical, simplistic, or rigid language peculiar to each

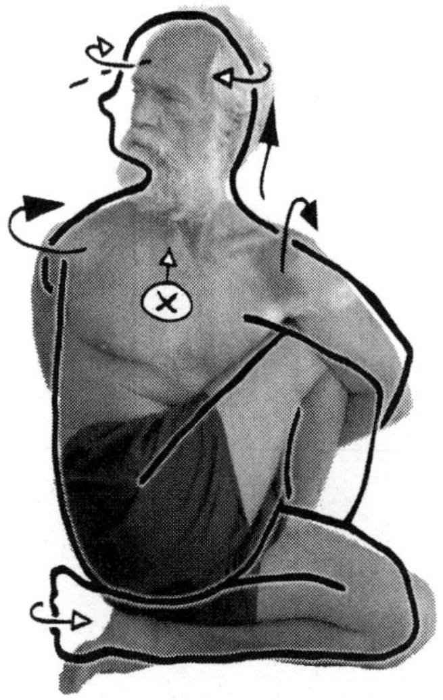

	S	M	T	W	T	F	S	S	M	T	W	T	F	S	S	M	T	W	T	F	S	S	M	T	W	T	F	S
Yoga																												
Scripture																												
Diet																												
Work																												
Contentment																												

1																												
2																												
3																												
4																												
5																												

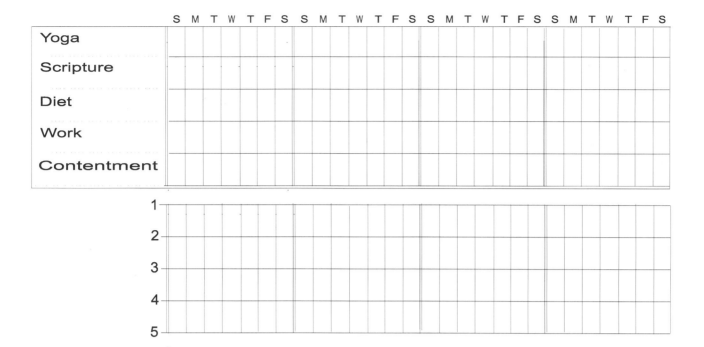

Scripture. On the other hand, avoid rushing through and dismissing too much as irrelevant. There is often a more profound meaning to discover when reading between the lines.

In a sense, this means interpreting the passage in such a way that "its" message makes you feel good. Think of scripture as a mirror of your own mind, instead of a prescription for what you 'should do' or proscription for what you 'shouldn't do'.

Mascaro's translation of the ***Bhagavad Gita*** (published by Penguin Classics) is one of the clearest available. The ***Tao Te Ching*** by D.C. Lau (Penguin Classics) is one of the more faithful translations of the original Chinese.

8) By comparing the nutritional content of the basic foods (see next page), you can see that fresh vegetables are the only foods which contain sufficient, and indeed abundant amounts of the known substances the human body needs, without giving excessive calories, proteins or fats which, in large quantities, can be detrimental to health in the long run.

Therefore it is wise to eat as much of these as possible or practical and then to fill out the rest of your diet with fruit, grain, nuts, beans, and/or animal products.

9) For help in learning how to move into or out of the Yoga postures, take a Hatha Yoga class from a competent teacher and/or refer to B.K.S, Iyengars' most excellent book - ***Light on Yoga.***

10) The basics of Pranayama are learned naturally, in due course, through Hatha Yoga practice. Insights into the principles of breath harmony are found in the scriptures.

11) The length of time spent on any of the various techniques of formal meditation is not nearly as useful as bringing meditation (watchfulness) into every aspect of your daily life.

Insight on this constant meditation is found in the scriptures. For example see - ***Bhagavad Gita*** 4-18, 6-24, 15-9 ; ***Tao Te Ching*** Ch.16; Matthew 24-42, 26-41 (the ***Bible***); and ***Buddha's Four Noble Truths*** (see page 175).

ILLUSTRATIONS

The dynamics of each posture, as indicated in these illustrations, are best learned gradually. In the beginning, concentrate on the large black arrows. After you feel you are applying those, begin working on the small white arrows. Finally, search the posture and see if you can come up with some 'small white arrows' of your own.

Food Type \ Daily Need	Calorie 2000	Protien 40-g.	Fat 2-g.	Calcium 0.5-g.	Iron 10-mg.	Vit. A 700-u	Vit. C 75-mg.	Vit. B1 1.2-mg.	Vit. B2 1.7-mg.	Niacin 18-mg.
0.5-Kg Meat	2000	150-g.	150-g.	1.0-g.	40-mg.	150-u.	----	1.5-mg.	1.5-mg.	30-mg.
0.7-Kg Grains	2000	70-g.	21-g.	0.2-g.	21-mg.	-----	-----	2.1-mg.	0.8-mg.	21-mg.
4.0-Kg Green Veg.	2000	160-g.	2-g.	20.0-g.	1000-mg.	24000-u.	6000-mg.	3.2-mg.	10.0-mg.	40-mg.

(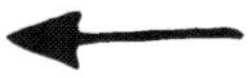) Area of **principle** concern*

(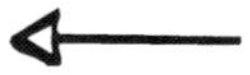) Area of **perfecting** concern

(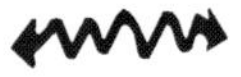) Total **relaxation**

(⊗) Thrusting **out** of the page

(⊙) Thrusting **in** to the page

(*Var:*) Variation for beginners.

The holding time is indicated for each posture (60s., 5min., etc.). Of course you may stay longer or shorter than this time. Listen to your body; it will tell you.

Most of the postures from 1 - 48 are covered in detail in the Step By Step Lessons, beginning on page 177. If a posture is covered in those lessons, its page number is given on its full page illustration.

Don't be too concerned if you don't understand what a particular arrow is trying to show. Just watch and explore your body in that area. Be sensitive to it and you will eventually find out. Some of these "energy" areas are not really possible to feel until after some years of practice.

Program Overview

Advancement to each higher program depends mostly on how much time, interest and effort you put into your practice. Technique, strength and flexibility are much less important. These come naturally, in due course, with conscientious work.

Programs 1 - 3 require 10-30 minutes to run through once you know what you're doing. Taking on new postures one by one gradually keeps you in that content, 'you know what you're doing' realm. As the Tao Te Ching says, *There is no disaster greater than not being content.*

Programs 4 onward can require about 60 minutes to run through. The postures become more challenging, but learning just one or two new ones a month will keep it manageable. As Program 4 has 27 new postures, you will spend a year or two on it before going on to Program 5. With steady practice then, you may reach Program 8 in eight years. But who cares? After all, this is a lifetime journey; walk it step by step!

When you can do the majority of the postures in a particular program fairly well, you can incorporate new postures from the next program into your daily practice. When starting a new posture, do it after a similar but easier posture which you already do. To know where you should include a new posture, study the routine from the next program to see where this new posture is done relative to the postures you have been doing.

Step By Step Lessons (Page 177)

These are a series of detailed lessons on most of the postures in Programs 1-3. Everyone, from beginners to the more advanced should at least take a look at these, especially if you are learning the postures on your own.

'Do It Yourself' Program

Note: The following several pages reflects my now 'older point of view'.

No matter what program you are on, it can be very useful to read ahead and study the instructions given for the more advanced postures. Much of what is said about these

* Only Programs 1-3 have this black arrow. After that you must determine the "concern".

postures also applies to the basic postures you will be working on.

In fact, there is nothing *truly* special about posture placement in the programs. I can easily see other ways to arrange them. Each person is different physically, emotionally, and mentally. Thus, feel free to change the sequences to suit your particular needs. If done with careful consideration there is no danger.

Done recklessly, you could well regret it. For example, when first trying out one of the advanced head stands, I began goofing off and fell. I 'tweeked' my neck, and took over ten years to fully recover. Don't goof around. Pay attention and all will be well.

Finally, keep track of self-discovery by sketching in any dynamics you feel missing, or annotate the arrows already shown. If you feel it's an essential tell me so I can incorporate it in the next edition. I don't know what I missed, but I'm sure I missed 'it'. Find 'it' and let me know

Getting Old And A Little Feeble Are We?

Well I sure am. The older I get the more quickly the years fly by, and the more real physical decline becomes. So far, arthritis is my only big issue. Were it not for Yoga, I'd be in such worse shape. As always, I strive to come right up to my edge, but now I must be more watchful than ever to avoid going over the edge.

More Unsolicited Advice

The Ideal Journey

Incorporate the principles conveyed in all the postures to your daily activities throughout the day, in every way, according to ability. This is the *ideal* long term objective.

That said, be wary of the ideal. Real life is what you actually do, the ideal is merely where you want to go. Whether you 'arrive' or not doesn't matter. Indeed, thoughts of 'arrival' get in the way of the day-to-day, step -by-step journey. As the ***Tao Te Ching*** puts it, *A journey of a thousand miles starts from beneath one's feet.*

The Feet and Shoes

Speaking of feet. One of the worst aspects of modernity is the ubiquitous use of shoes. The feet "die". Don't believe me? Just try wearing stiff thick gloves throughout the day, in every activity. The resulting loss of tactile stimulation from the environment is profound. The same is true for the feet, but we don't tend to notice this because we are habituated to shoes, almost from birth.

This loss of tactile stimulation has a real, if subtle, effect on balance. As one gets older, loss of balance becomes a serious issue. Lose the shoes and live longer, I say.

Doing The Posture The Proper Way

There is no truly "proper way" in regards to how a yoga posture looks. In yoga, watchful self-honesty is the only "proper way".

The illustrations show you an ideal to aim for, and not where you must actually be. Eventually (perhaps years from now), you may be able to match the illustration. At that point, you'll just have to figure out a way to put the ideal just beyond your reach.

For example: The photo (next page) is of my son Luke and I doing Ustrasana, a back-bend. He is fully extended so the advanced back-bends are the *ideal just beyond his reach*. On the other hand, I have my hands full. Honestly, I'm also less inclined to develop back-bends. I regard them the least useful ('natural') direction of movement in the wild. However, for the pure Yoga of it, they are truly what I need to work on most (obviously). The stiffer you are, the "easier" yoga is, because the '*ideal just beyond your reach*' is obvious. As flexibility increases it is easier to coast and just 'look good', without actually doing Hatha Yoga.

Feeling Hopelessly Stiff Or Weak?

Watchfulness is the standard for success, *not how the posture looks*. Eventually you will enjoy a "pseudo-yogic" success as improving strength, flexibility, and balance allow your postures to look 'good'. That's the icing on the cake. Truth is, success and failure must coexist in each

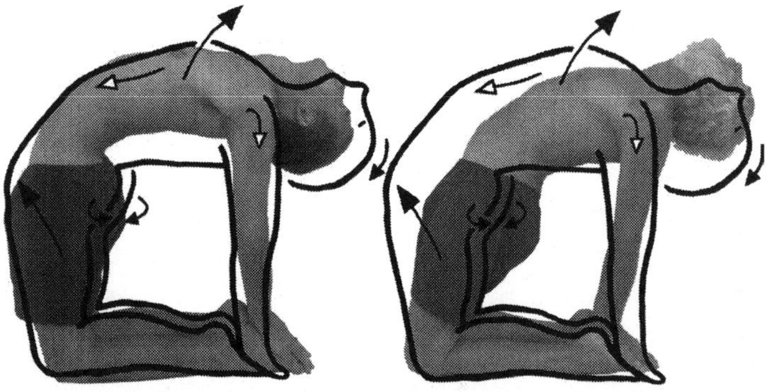

moment. Yoga is a dynamic process where you exist at the limit of your strength (success) and weakness (failure) each watchful moment. It is not how skillful you are that counts in yoga. It is how self-honest and watchful you are. Only then are you able to balance success and failure.

Again, These Are The Essentials

1) Watch what you are doing carefully.

2) Do what you can, not pushing too hard or slacking off.

3) As you become able to do what you can, gradually extend what you are doing toward the 'ideal' as depicted in the drawings. This can take decades! This may be your current stumbling block. The trick is to remember that this is a lifelong practice. Simply doing what you can is all you need do. Compromise any way necessary to adapt the posture to your particular bodily circumstance.

Taking a long-term view is difficult. We naturally look to 'fix' things 'now'. In truth, time pretty much takes care of everything. All we need do is 'show up', work and be attentive. Do that and you can't fail!

Ha Ha, Tha Tha, and the Balanced Between

Yoga, like life, follows a natural course. First comes the challenge of facing down fear: fear of hard work, pain, and failure of meeting your expectations. There is also the fear of embarrassment and censure, either in your own eyes or in the eyes of others. This initial exercise phase ('Ha') is the essential beginning step. It can be a hurdle. Next, you integrate the more subtle, spiritual 'Tha' into this base. This 'Tha' is the watchful, mindful, careful side of the Hatha Yoga coin. For some, it is easy to keep slogging away, like a bull in a China shop, on the 'Ha' side. Others get bogged down on the spiritual 'Tha' side, avoid jumping in, and instead passively watch life go by. Balance is the key.

I regard the ***Bhagavad Gita*** as *the* guide on yoga. One reason I stopped teaching was that many wanted to learn yoga as a body exercise instead of as spiritual practice. It boiled down to being gymnastics instead of 'Ha Tha' meditation. Folks doing yoga for 'body training' were overly on the 'ha' side of balance. Although, by the same token, those doing yoga as a 'spiritual' practice tend to be overly on the 'tha' side of balance. Neither were very inclined to stretch to the other side toward balance, *at least not by anything I'd say or do*. I imagine balance comes to each of us over time naturally, if it comes at all.

I find we all tend to fall on either side of the 'happy medium'. We either push too hard (yang) or slack off soft (yin). Watch where you are in the moment and either 'relax' or 'work'. That is the essence of 'Ha' 'Tha' Yoga.

You are on the right path if you can integrate physical work (action) and spiritual rest (attentiveness) into a balanced practice. This is the only way to get the maximum benefit for body, emotion, and mind.

Yoga Classes Vs. A Private Practice

Doing yoga with other people has great benefit. It is both a social joy and a way to gain insight into your own practice by observing others. One caution though: Take the opinions you hear with a grain of salt. I find 'the why' behind what people say far more revealing than 'the what'.

Doing yoga with others is the only way many people can do it at all. A private personal daily practice is difficult. Over the years I've advised people wanting this to just do a posture or two daily. This will grow into an optimum practice naturally. Who cares whether this takes years. No matter! Interestingly, I've never known anyone who could do that. It seems we are innately driven to do "all or nothing". I expect this "all or nothing" presents one of the greatest barriers to a balanced approach.

Social instincts are powerful forces (e.g., the pressure to show up, keep up, compete, avoid shame). These emotions keep our nose to the grindstone in a group practice. However, private practice lacks most of this. Absent these social forces, you alone are the witness of your life. Then your yoga (and life) really come down to the essence... *what do you truly want out of life?*

Tat Tvam Asi

Tat Tvam Asi is an ancient Hindu spiritual "motto". It means "that thou art". This speaks to the oneness of all. I see something else between the lines though in the word order: 'that'

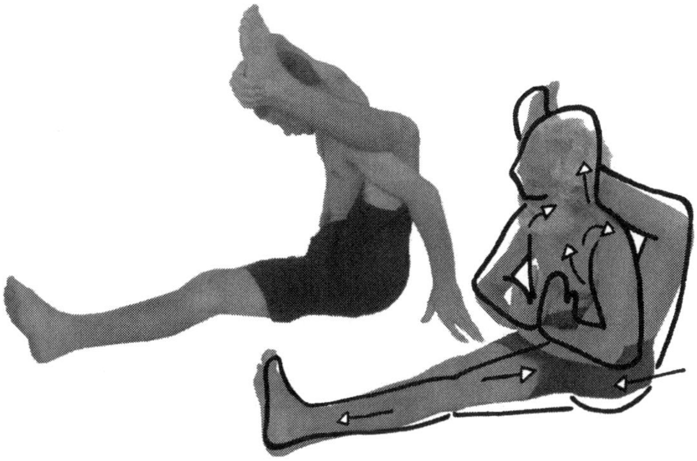

(otherness) is primary, the 'thou' (yourself) is secondary. Placing 'that' before 'thou' is humbling, and one key to honestly know what you *truly want of life.*

Reaching For The Ideal Just Beyond Reach

My wife's sister asked her awhile back, "Why does he put his head behind his neck (photo above)? That's weird". The reason I do is because my limit exists there—the *ideal just beyond reach.* I must go to my limit to work in the 'Ha Tha' zone. Only there can I experience 'grace under fire'. Both son Luke and I are at our limit; we are experiencing exactly the same yogic reality despite the different and superficial 'look' of it.

By the way, I may be more innately flexible in bending forward, while Luke is more innately flexible in bending backward. Also, I've not done the advanced back-bends for 30 years, so I've lost some previous, hard-won flexibility. Now is a perfect time for me to resume doing them; advanced back-bends can give me an *ideal truly beyond my reach!*

Video Yourself

One very useful 21st century advance is the ability of anyone to video their yoga practice. Doing this sporadically can reveal your 'blind spots', i.e., general errors and ways you may be cheating yourself.

Alas, The Word 'Limit' Limits

The difficulty with the word limit, and words in general, is the emotional bias they impart. Expectations (desire, want, crave, wish) of achieving an ideal, like "reaching my limit", becomes your Achilles' heel. Instead of thinking about limit in terms of 'strength limits', view it in terms of 'weakness limits'. You'll never have trouble reaching your 'weakness limit'; it is the foundation. As the Tao Te Ching puts it, "*Turning back is how the way moves; Weakness is the means the way employs.*" When you feel lazy and just lie in bed, you are at your 'weakness limit'. When you're working with maximum effort, you are at your 'weakness limit'. You can't lose when *weakness* becomes your ideal.

Don't let thoughts, names or words, trap you! Words and thoughts easily mislead. Because we trust what we think is true, we don't realize it until we reach a truly dead end. Be wary of how thought bubbles up from, and serve to rationalize, emotion. Again:

> *To know yet to think that one does not know is best; Not to know yet to think that one knows will lead to difficulty.*
>
> *It is by being alive to difficulty that one can avoid it. The sage meets with no difficulty. It is because he is alive to it that he meets with no difficulty.* - Tao Te Ching

中道
CenterTao.org

Program 1

The postures are arrange left to right, top to bottom.

This is the *posture number.* It is the number at the top of each posture's page.

3

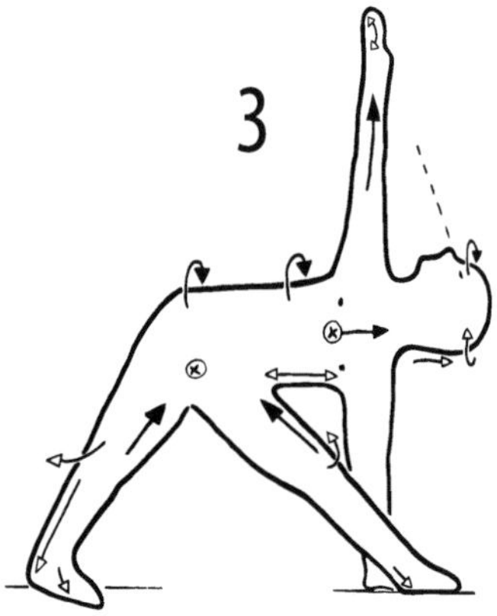

Utthita Trikonasana

6

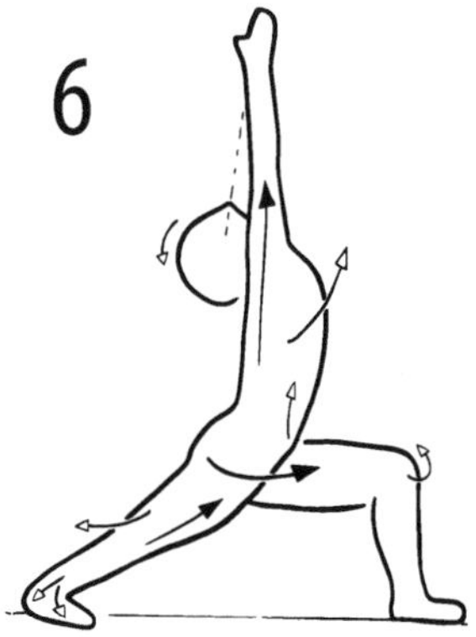

Virabhadrasana I

18

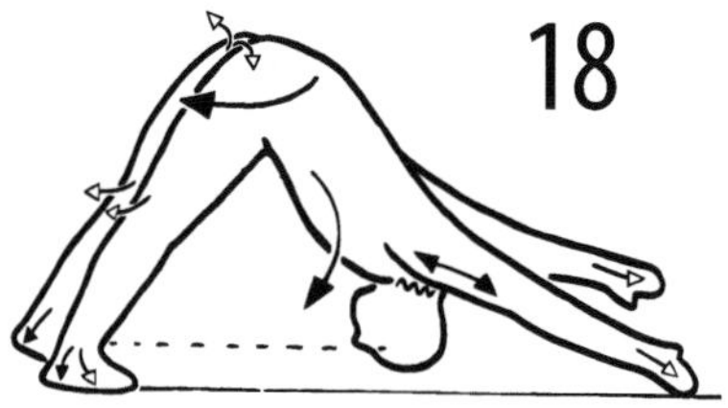

Adho Mukha Svanasana

19

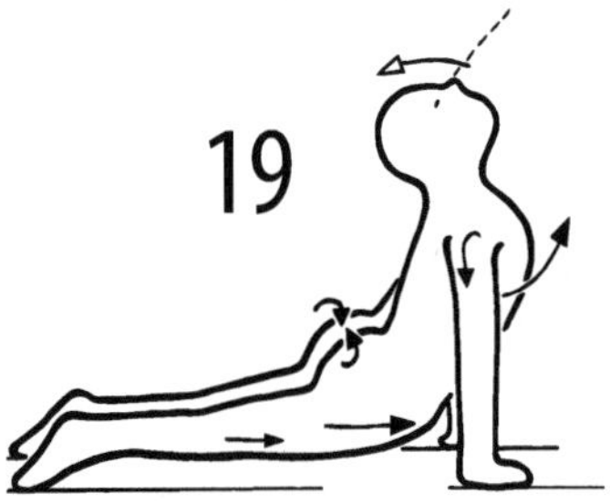

Urdhva Mukha Svanasana

23

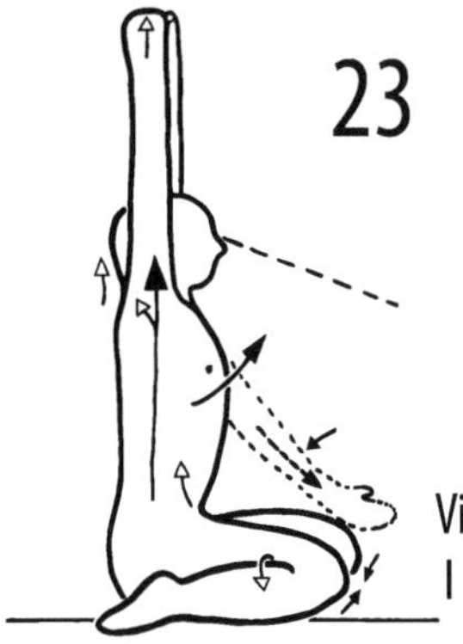

Virasana I & II

16

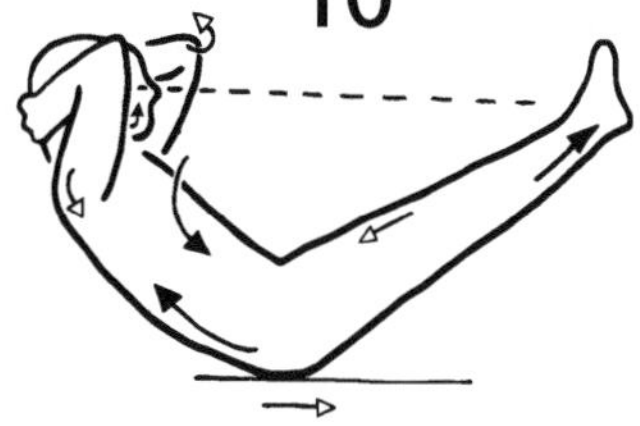

Ardha Navasana

17

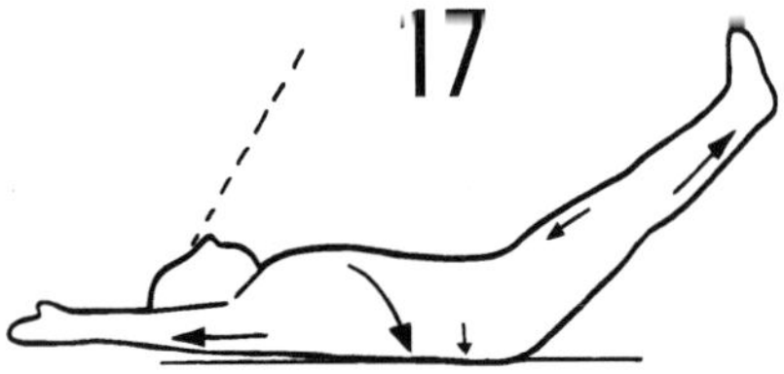

Urdhva Prasarita Padasana

26

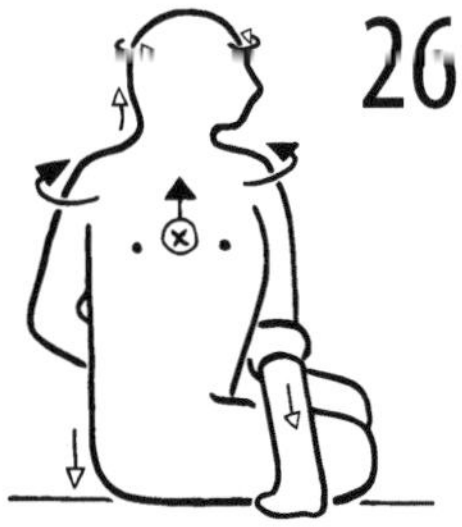

Bharadvajasana I

13

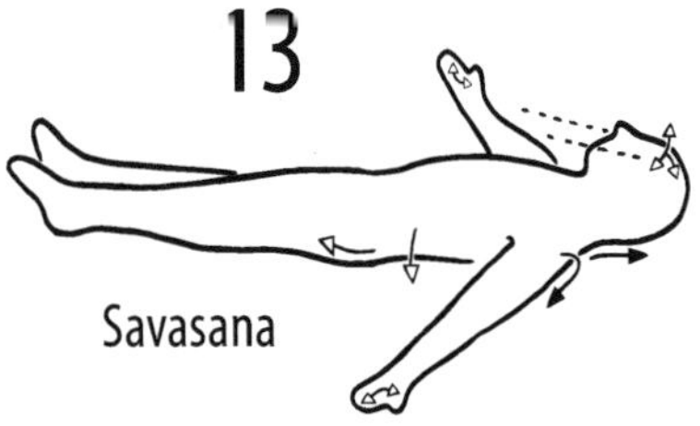

Savasana

<u>TIPS:</u> Watching your body is *the secret* of yoga. So simply mimicking the drawings in a relaxed watchful way works well. Watching is best; thinking is problematic, so save that and the details for later. For the details (and for easier variations) turn to the *posture number* page (the number by the postures) every now and then to recall what you're aiming for. Also, review the introductory pages. Having a 'gut' sense of these principles will be your best yoga teacher in the long run. For more detailed steps study the ***Step By Step Lessons***, page 177.

Most yoga postures are done twice. First turn, twist or bend the body in one direction, then repeat the posture in the other direction. One side will often be stronger (or more flexible) than the other. One long term goal / benefit of yoga is bringing the 'weak' side into balance with the 'strong' side. By the way, do skip any that are painful. You'll grow into them over time.

Please adapt to suit your own style and need. Remember, these illustrations show you the ideal you are aiming for. It will be years, if ever, before you reach that. The quality of yoga is not determined by how closely you match the ideal, but rather by the moment to moment nature of your practice, i.e, careful, attentive, self honest, persevering, timely, patient... In a word, watchful.

When you understand how to do the postures in Program 1 fairly well, begin adding postures from Program 2 into your daily routine.

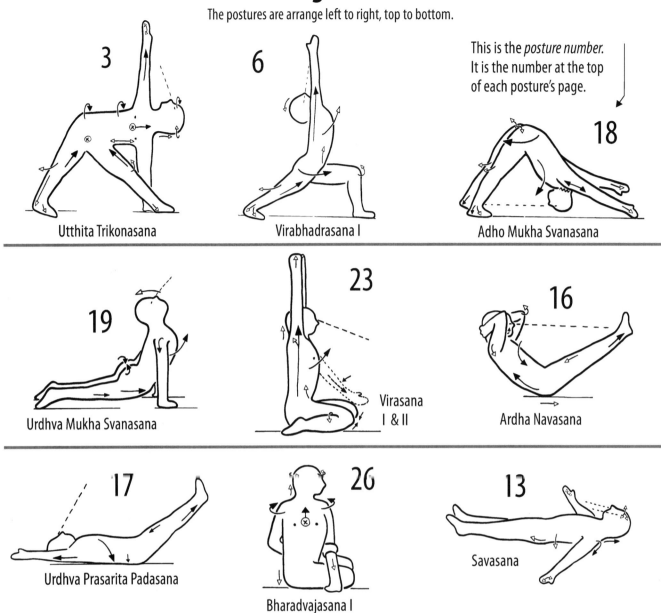

Program 2: First Day

3

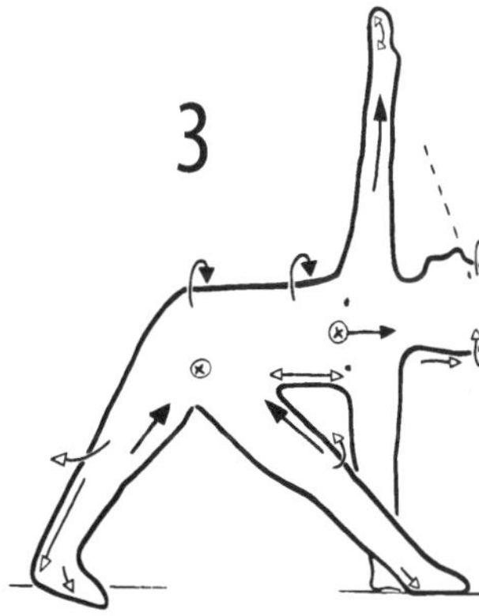

Utthita Trikonasana

4

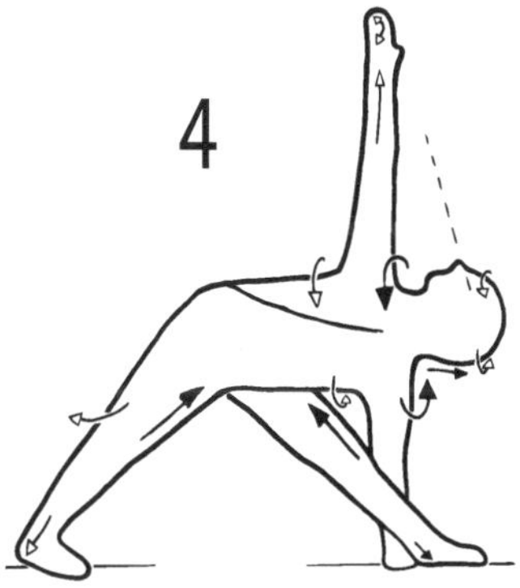

Parivrtta Trikonasana

5

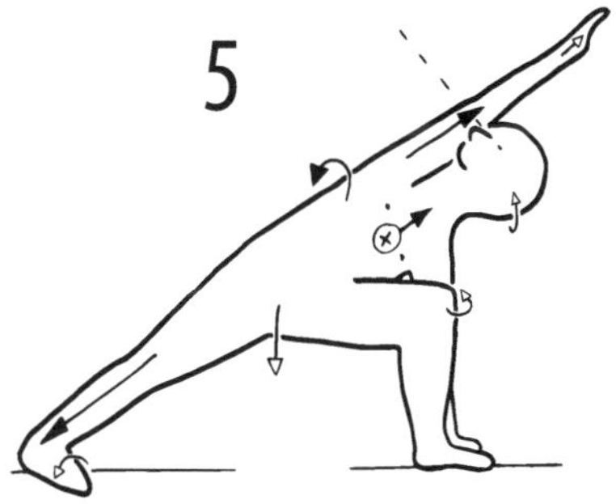

Utthita Parsvakonasana

6

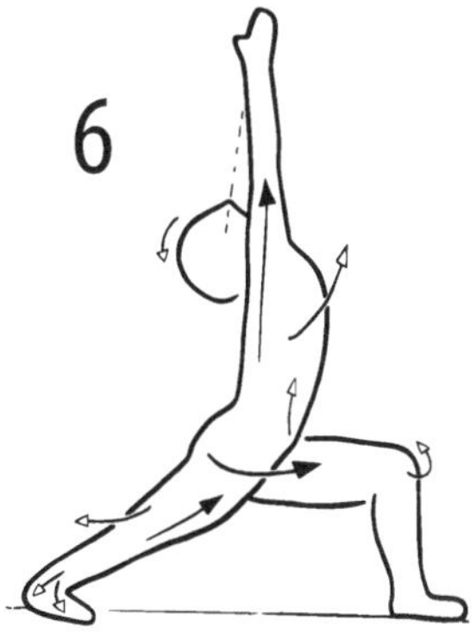

Virabhadrasana I

7

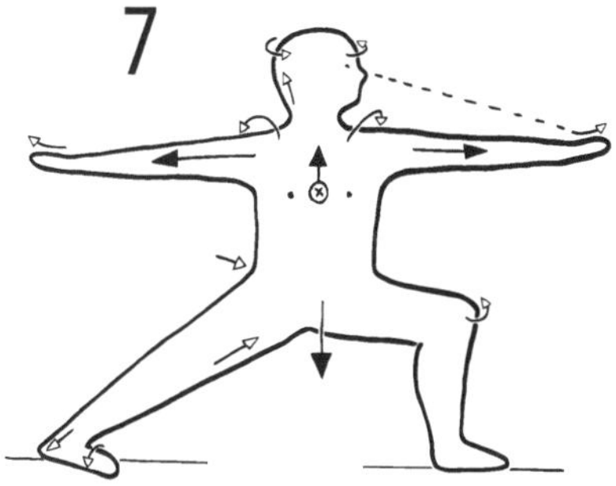

Virabhadrasana II

8

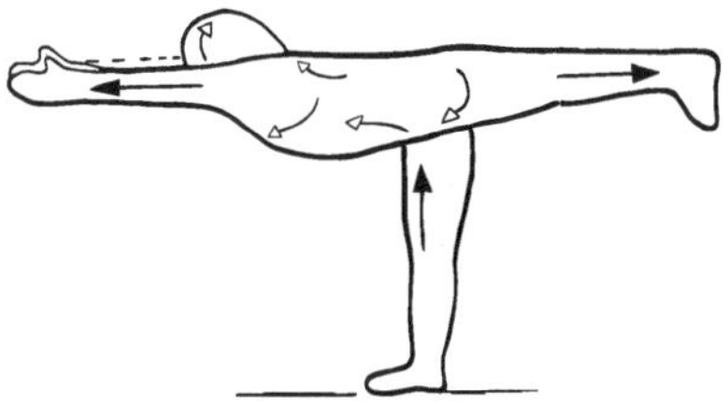

Virabhadrasana III

9

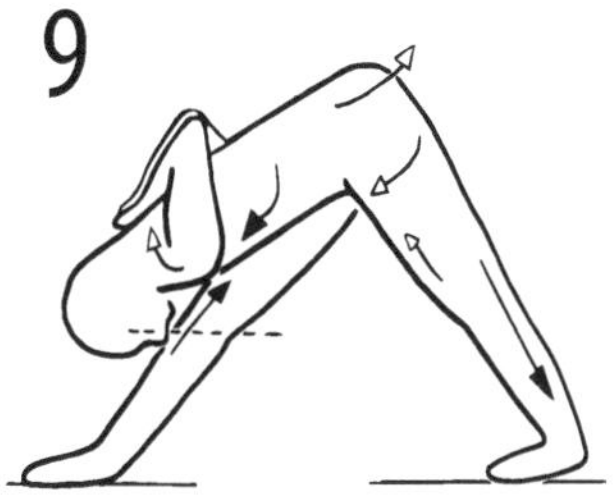

Parsvottanasana

10

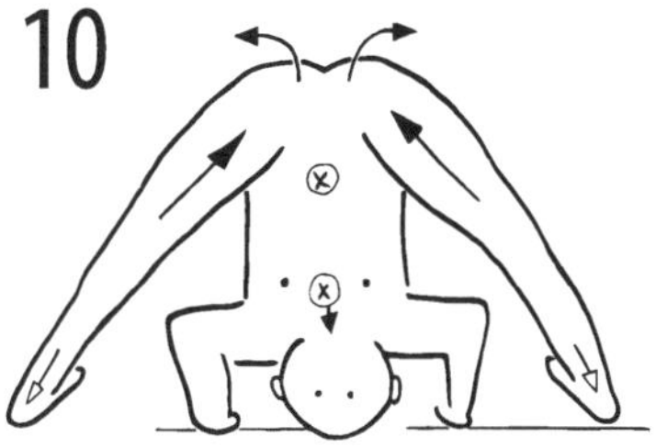

Prasarita Padottanasana

11

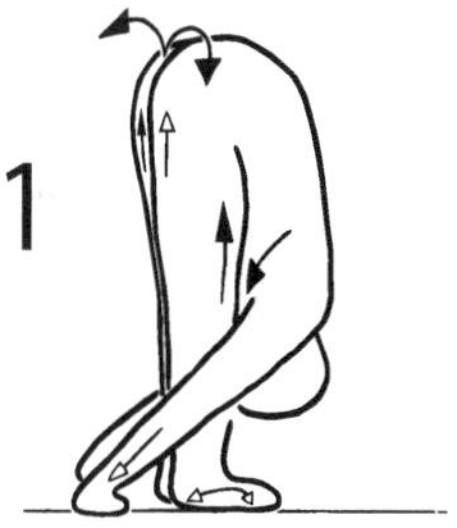

Uttanasana

12

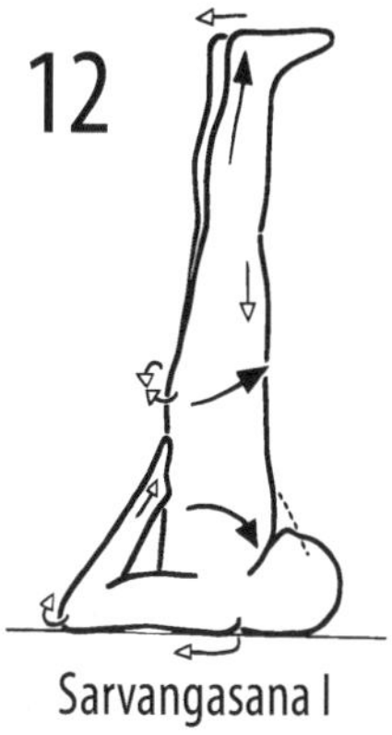

Sarvangasana I

13

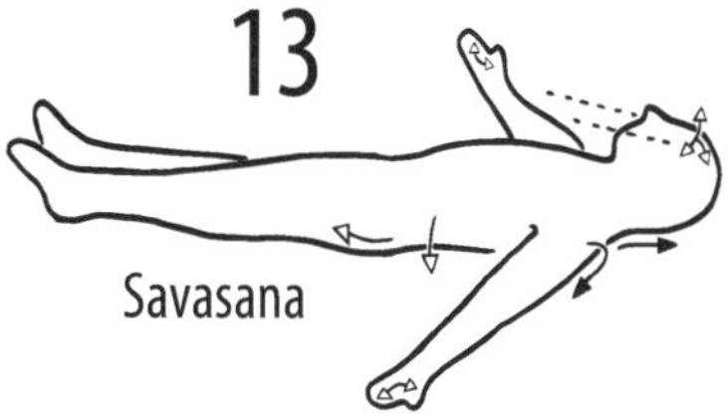

Savasana

TIPS

Begin Program 2 once you feel secure doing Program 1. You can also just keep doing Program 1, adding postures from 2 as you are able.

It is not necessary that you 'master' the postures in a program before going on to the next program, or even that you do all of them before going on. Some postures can take much longer - years - than others, depending on the person (body type, innate strengths and weaknesses, 'luck'). Also, what's the hurry? Proceed at your own pace.

In truth, you can remain on any Program for as long as you like before taking on more postures. If yoga is a lifetime gift you are giving yourself, there is no rush. Take a lifetime to give it, but do continue to give. A steady gradual giving of yoga to your body and mind wins the day.

Program 2: Second Day

(or combine with First Day postures for a more intense daily routine)

18

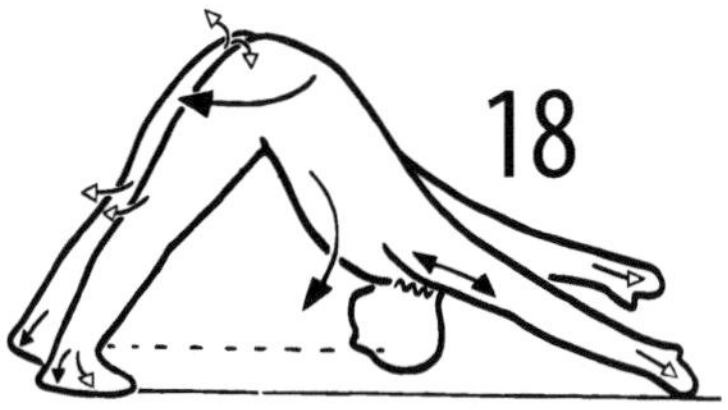

Adho Mukha Svanasana

19

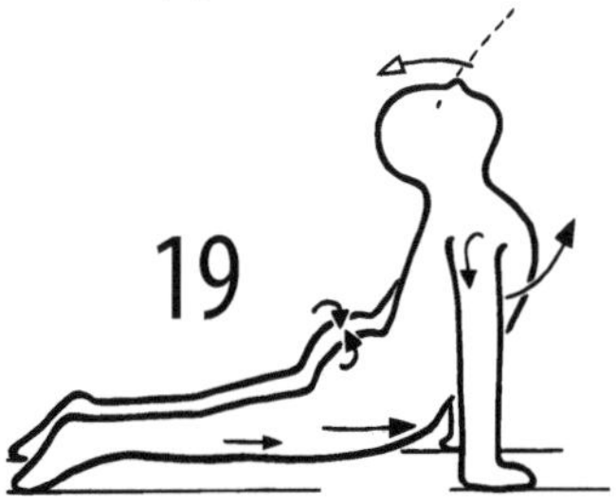

Urdhva Mukha Svanasana

20

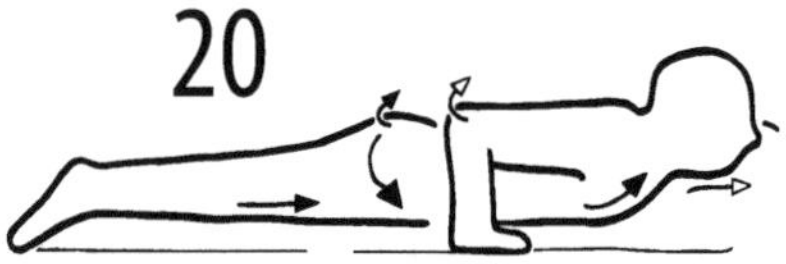

Chaturanga Dandasana & Nakrasana

21

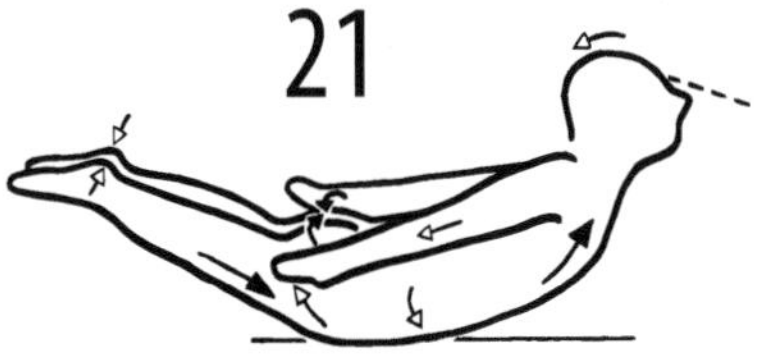

Salabhasana

22

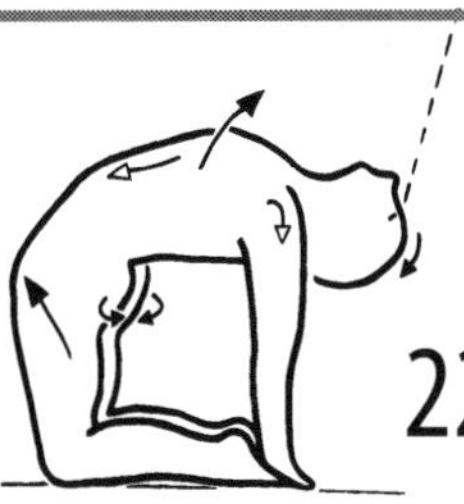

Ustrasana

23

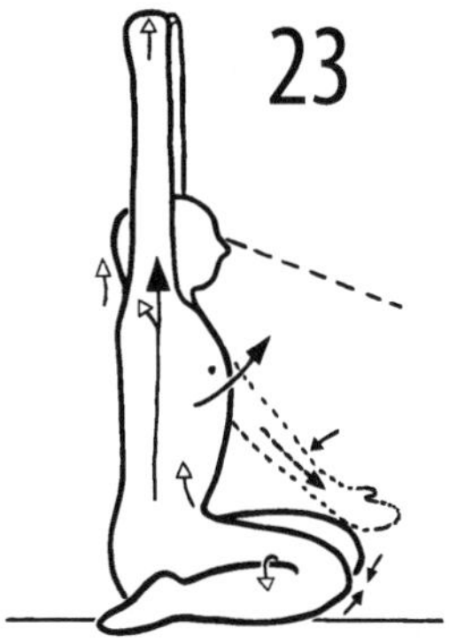

Virasana I & II

24

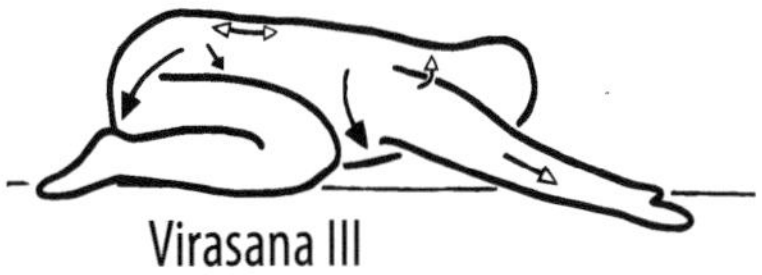

Virasana III

25

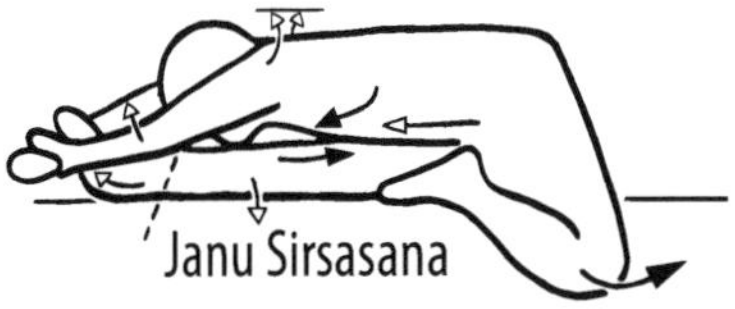

Janu Sirsasana

15

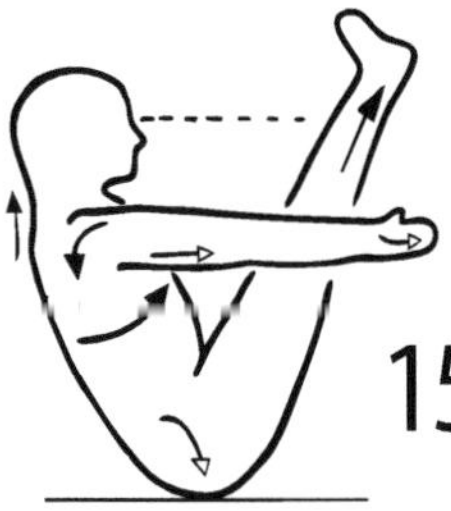

Paripoorna Navasana

16

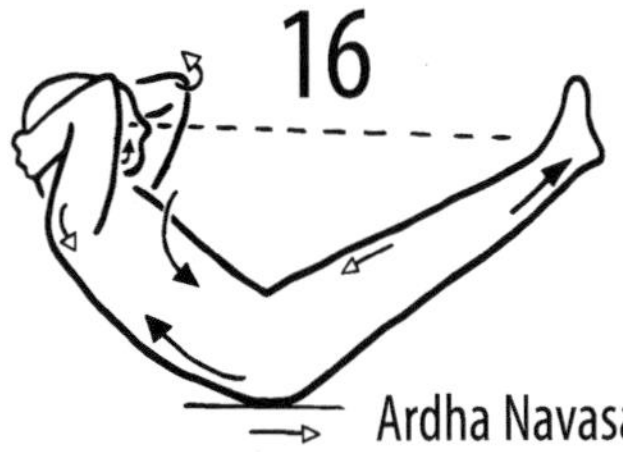

Ardha Navasana

17

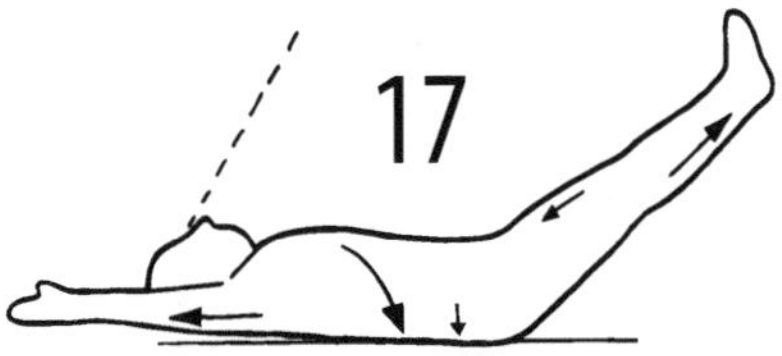

Urdhva Prasarita Padasana

26

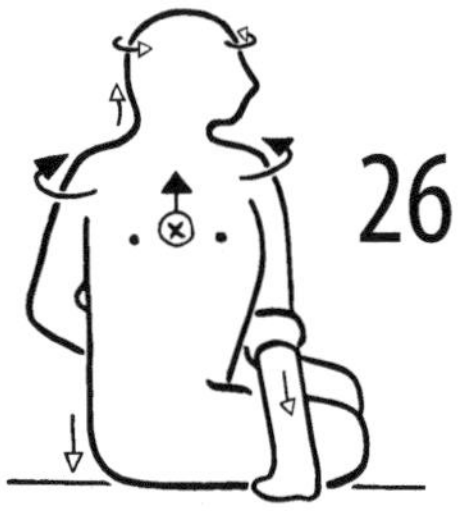

Bharadvajasana I

12

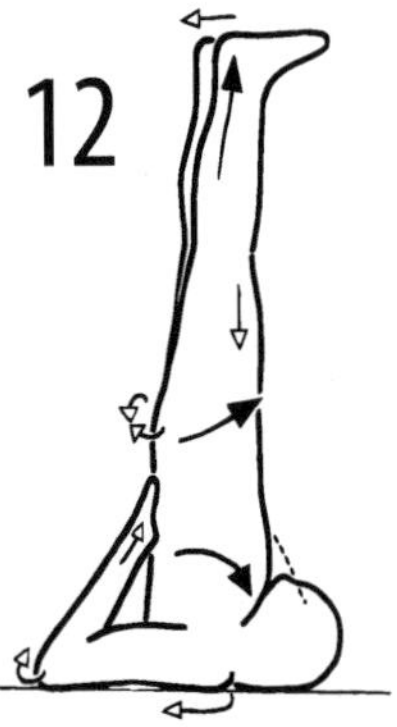

Sarvangasana I

13

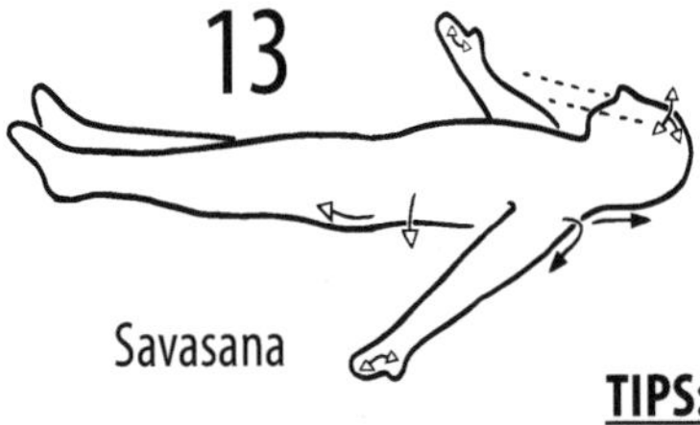

Savasana

TIPS:

Feel tree to try out doing the postures in a different order. Now a days, for example, I do posture #12 first. Then I do #18, through #26, and then #15 through #17. 'Listen' to your body; it may feel another order feels better.

Again, I must emphasis how the quality of your yoga practice lies not in how flexible or strong you are, but by how conscientious your work and rest (Ha and Tha). Gymnasts and contortionist may easily do these postures (as a sport, or for show), and yet not be doing yoga. The postures are simply a means of self discovery; finding self harmony (balance) is the destination. We are innately drawn to 'judge books by their covers' and 'look good', so it is easy to overlook this deep, subtle, true side of yoga.

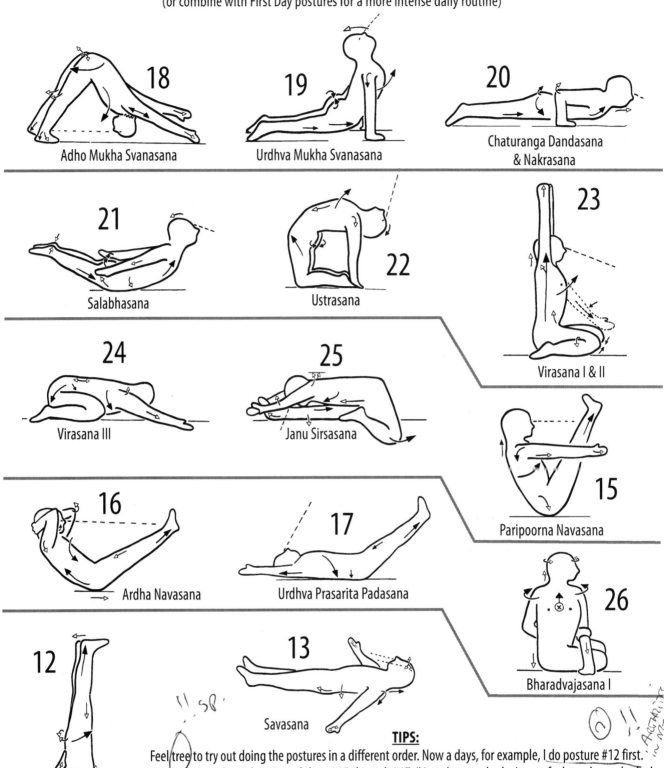

Tadasana

tada = mountain, asana = posture

(see Lesson Index, page 177)

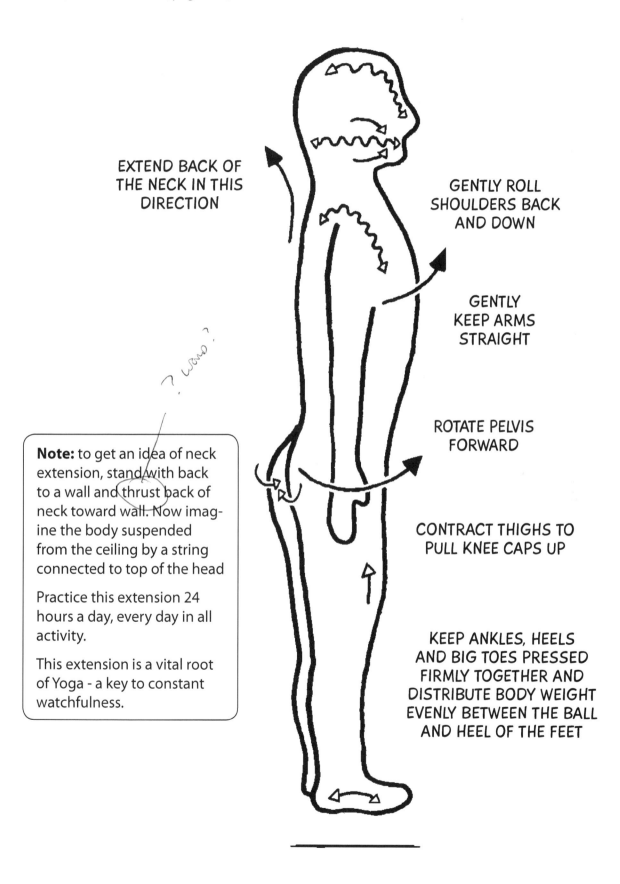

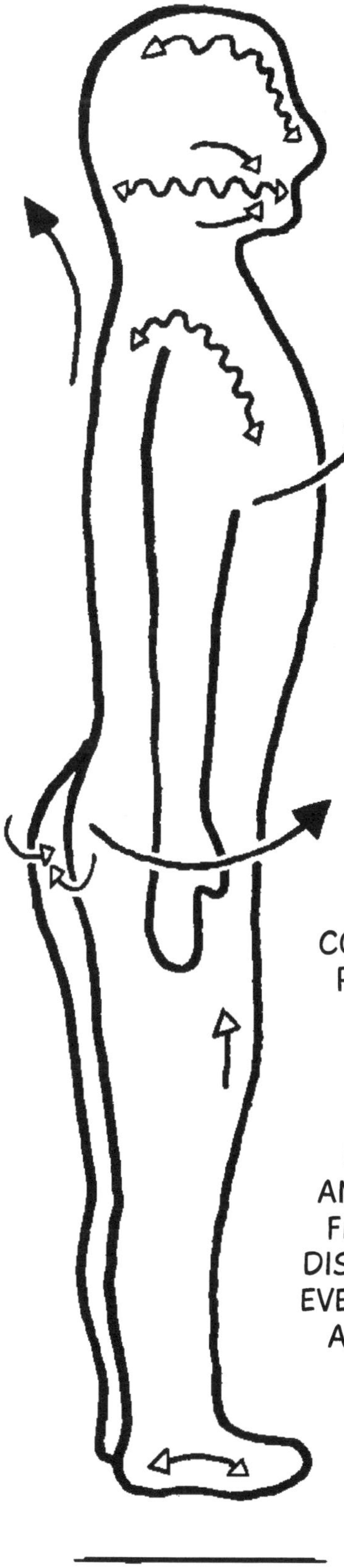
EXTEND BACK OF THE NECK IN THIS DIRECTION
GENTLY ROLL SHOULDERS BACK AND DOWN
GENTLY KEEP ARMS STRAIGHT
ROTATE PELVIS FORWARD
CONTRACT THIGHS TO PULL KNEE CAPS UP
KEEP ANKLES, HEELS AND BIG TOES PRESSED FIRMLY TOGETHER AND DISTRIBUTE BODY WEIGHT EVENLY BETWEEN THE BALL AND HEEL OF THE FEET

Note: to get an idea of neck extension, stand with back to a wall and thrust back of neck toward wall. Now imagine the body suspended from the ceiling by a string connected to top of the head

Practice this extension 24 hours a day, every day in all activity.

This extension is a vital root of Yoga - a key to constant watchfulness.

Walk, Walk-Run, Run (2)

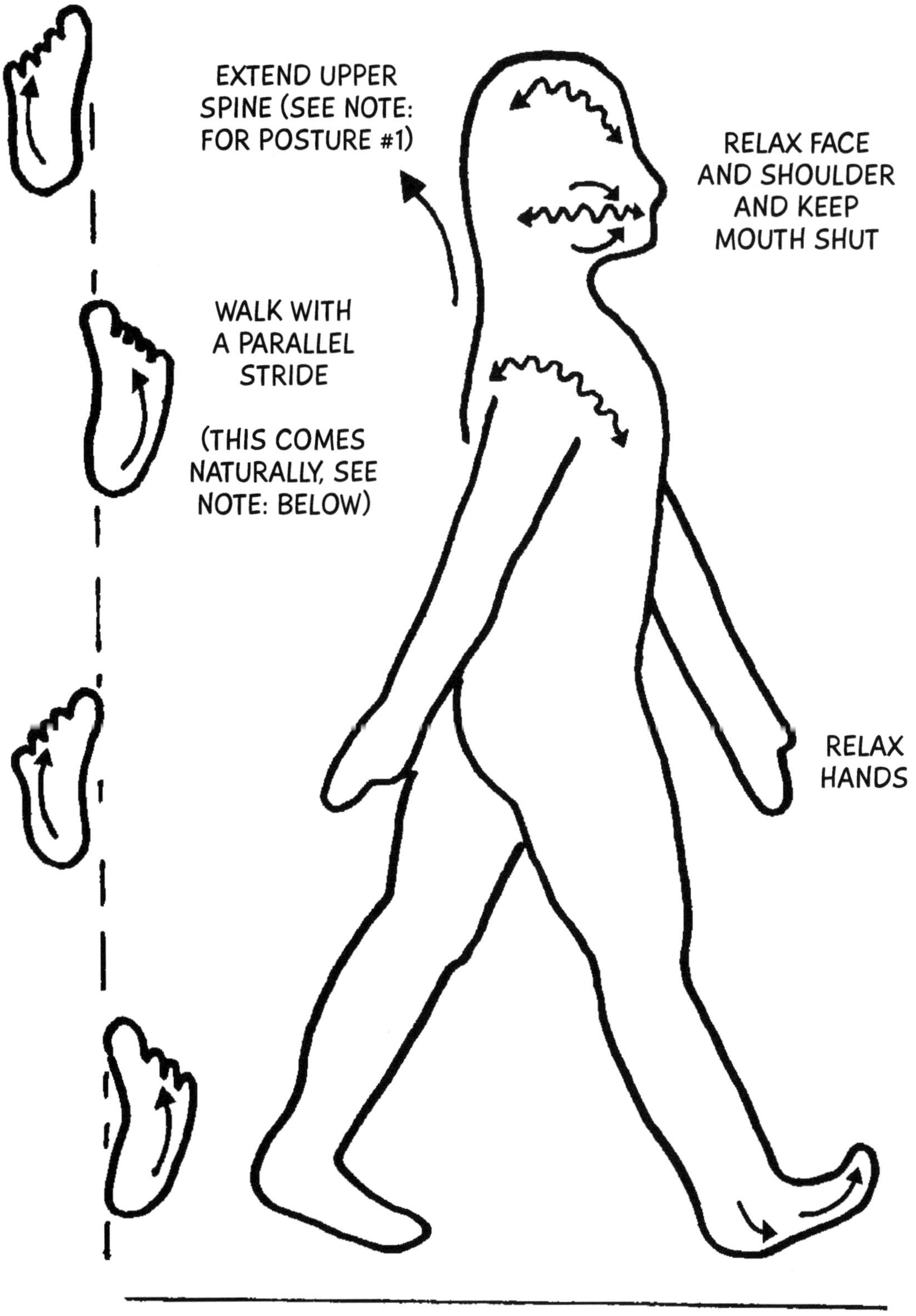
EXTEND UPPER SPINE (SEE NOTE: FOR POSTURE #1)
RELAX FACE AND SHOULDER AND KEEP MOUTH SHUT
WALK WITH A PARALLEL STRIDE
(THIS COMES NATURALLY, SEE NOTE: BELOW)
RELAX HANDS

Note: This shows some general principles to consider. For example, the heel touches the floor first, then the outer sole, then the ball of the foot, then the outer toes and finally the big toe, but almost simultaneously when barefoot.

Utthita Trikonasana 20-60s (3)

extended three angle

(see Lesson Index, page 177)

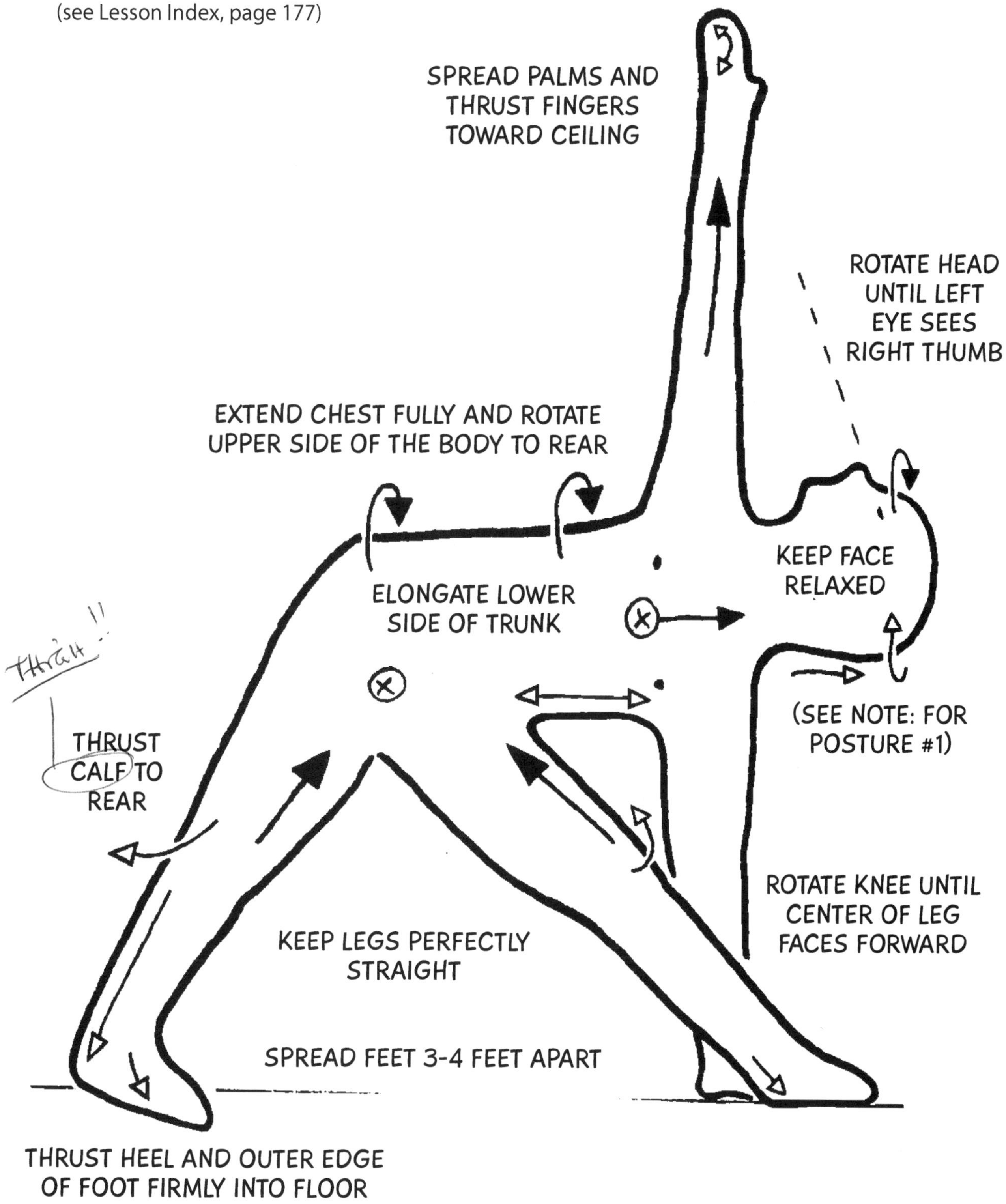
SPREAD PALMS AND THRUST FINGERS TOWARD CEILING
ROTATE HEAD UNTIL LEFT EYE SEES RIGHT THUMB
EXTEND CHEST FULLY AND ROTATE UPPER SIDE OF THE BODY TO REAR
KEEP FACE RELAXED
ELONGATE LOWER SIDE OF TRUNK
(SEE NOTE: FOR POSTURE #1)
THRUST CALF TO REAR
ROTATE KNEE UNTIL CENTER OF LEG FACES FORWARD
KEEP LEGS PERFECTLY STRAIGHT
SPREAD FEET 3-4 FEET APART
THRUST HEEL AND OUTER EDGE OF FOOT FIRMLY INTO FLOOR

Var: you may grasp the ankle or shin bone instead of placing it on the floor. Contracting the thigh muscle to 'pull up the knee caps' and reaching for the ceiling are the essentials.

Parivrtta Trikonasana 20-60s (4)

revolved three angle

(see Lesson Index, page 177)

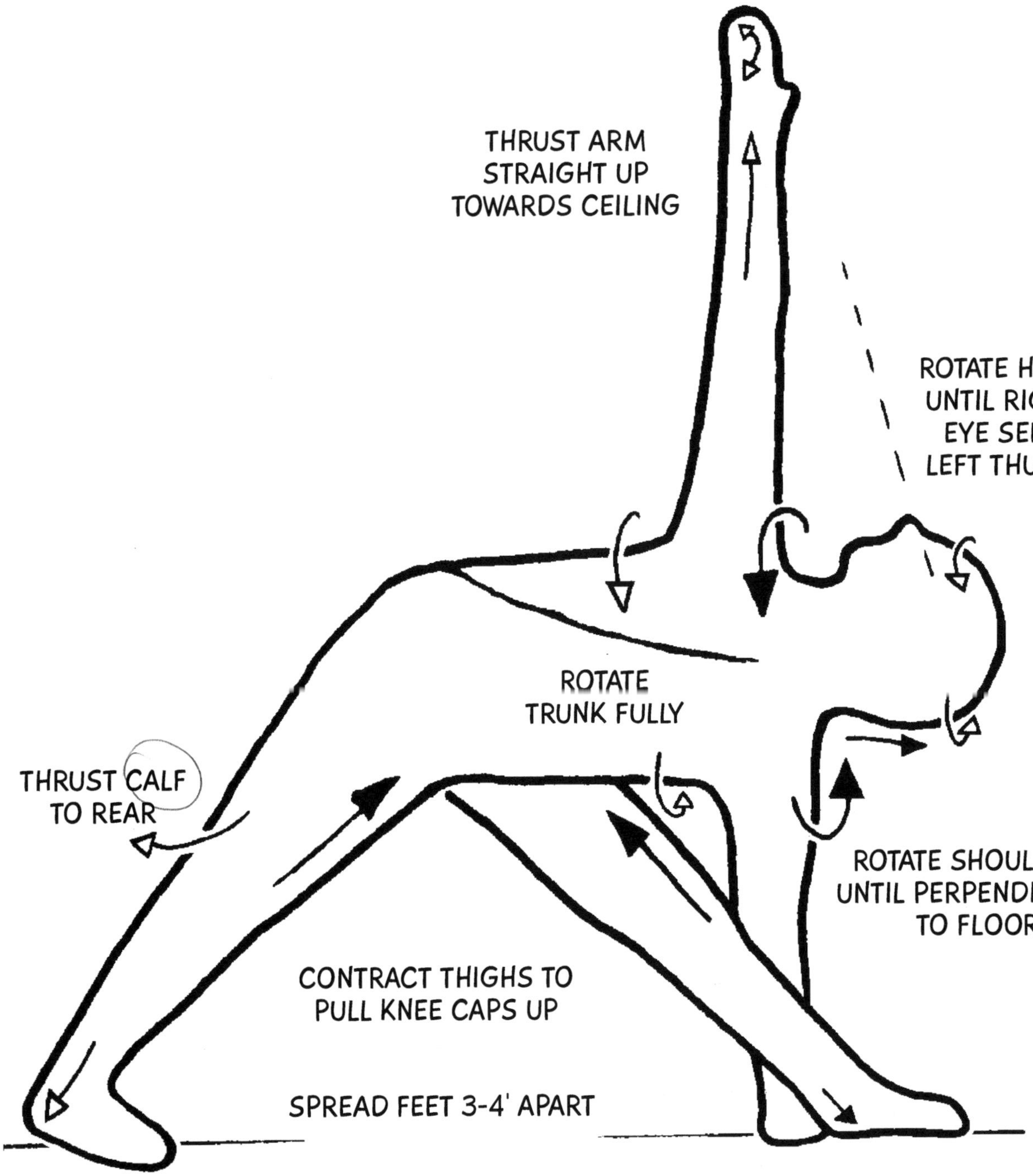
THRUST ARM
STRAIGHT UP
TOWARDS CEILING
ROTATE HEAD
UNTIL RIGHT
EYE SEES
LEFT THUMB
ROTATE
TRUNK FULLY
THRUST CALF
TO REAR
ROTATE SHOULDERS
UNTIL PERPENDICULAR
TO FLOOR
CONTRACT THIGHS TO
PULL KNEE CAPS UP
SPREAD FEET 3-4' APART

Note: you can place the rear foot firmly against a wall to help you stabilize the balance. Reach for the 'stars'.

Again, for help in learning how to move into or out of the Yoga postures, take a Hatha Yoga class from a competent teacher and/or refer to B.K.S. Iyengar's most excellent book, *Light on Yoga*.

Utthita Parsvakonasana 20-60s (5)

extended side angle

(see Lesson Index, page 177)

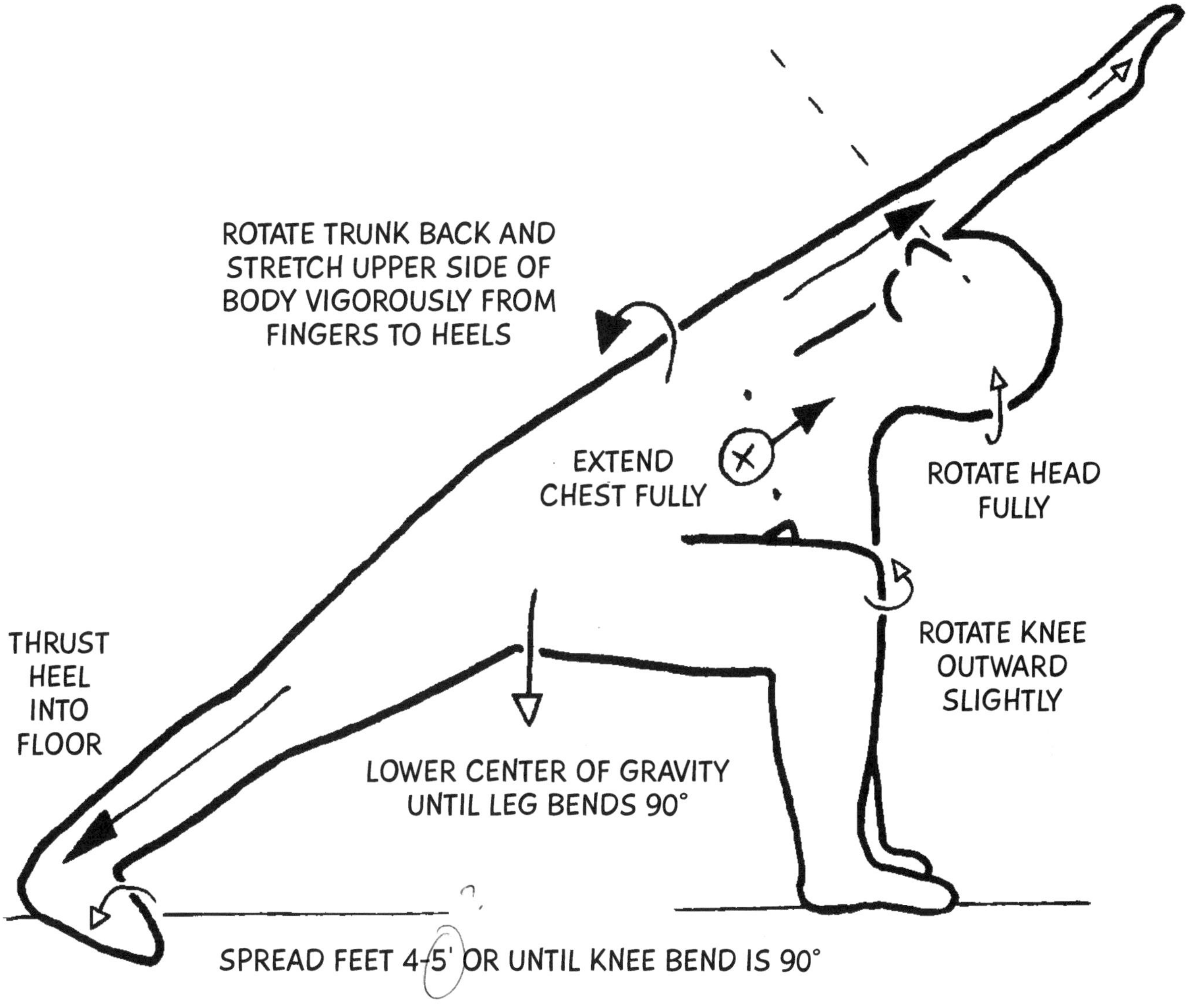
ROTATE TRUNK BACK AND STRETCH UPPER SIDE OF BODY VIGOROUSLY FROM FINGERS TO HEELS
EXTEND CHEST FULLY
ROTATE HEAD FULLY
ROTATE KNEE OUTWARD SLIGHTLY
THRUST HEEL INTO FLOOR
LOWER CENTER OF GRAVITY UNTIL LEG BENDS 90°
SPREAD FEET 4-5' OR UNTIL KNEE BEND IS 90°

Var: If you need to, rest the upper arm along the upper side of the trunk instead of extending it outward.

Note: For added stretch, do this posture with the lower arm placed in front of the bent knee instead of behind it. Feel you're being stretched apart by two giants, one grabbing your foot, one grabbing your arm.

Virabhadrasana I 20-30s (6)

a powerful Indian hero-warrior

(see Lesson Index, page 177)

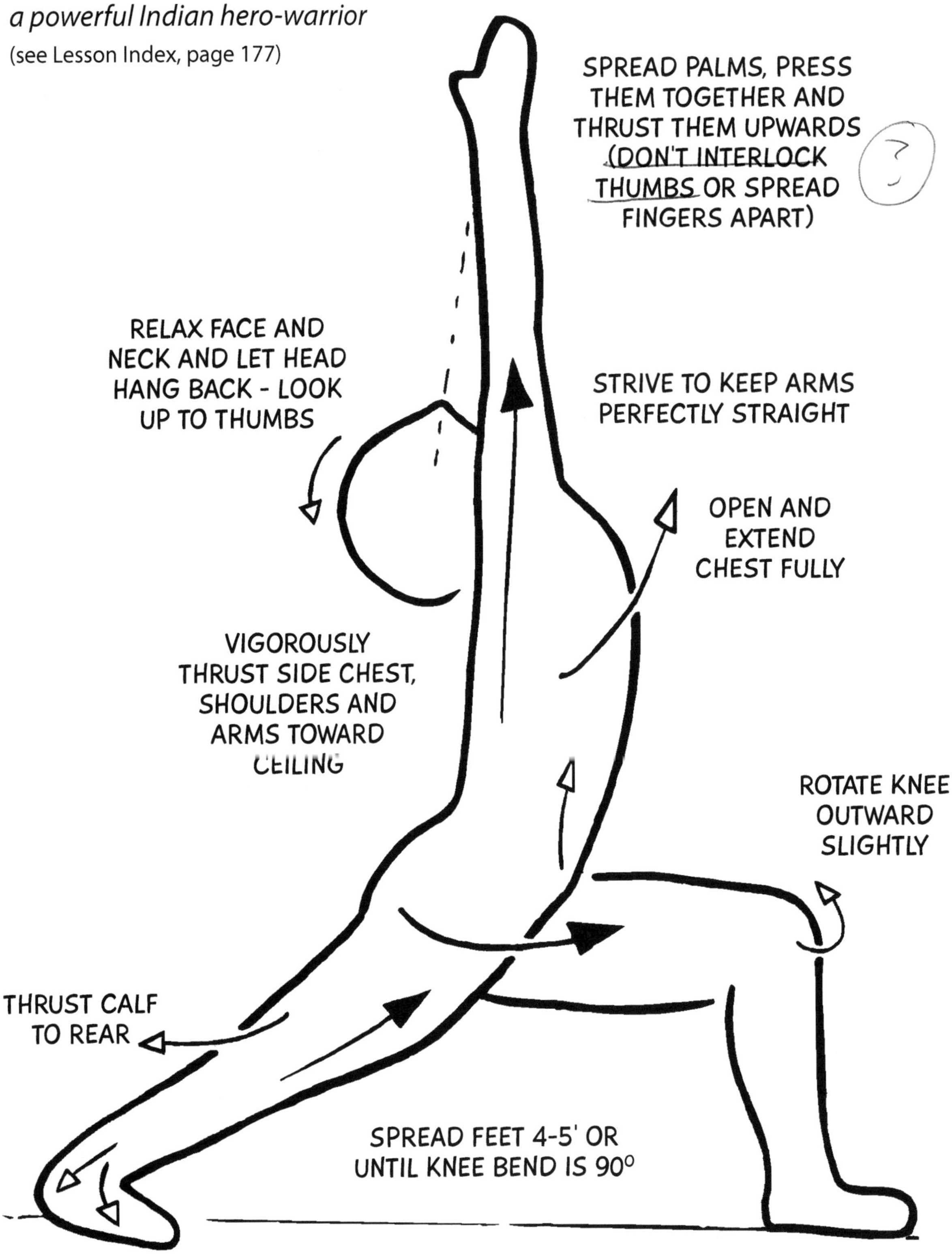
SPREAD PALMS, PRESS THEM TOGETHER AND THRUST THEM UPWARDS (DON'T INTERLOCK THUMBS OR SPREAD FINGERS APART)
RELAX FACE AND NECK AND LET HEAD HANG BACK - LOOK UP TO THUMBS
STRIVE TO KEEP ARMS PERFECTLY STRAIGHT
OPEN AND EXTEND CHEST FULLY
VIGOROUSLY THRUST SIDE CHEST, SHOULDERS AND ARMS TOWARD CEILING
ROTATE KNEE OUTWARD SLIGHTLY
THRUST CALF TO REAR
SPREAD FEET 4-5' OR UNTIL KNEE BEND IS 90°

Var: Place the hands on the hips and concentrate on rotating the pelvis. Also, you may separate the palms 12" or so and then thrust them upward.

Note: You're reaching up to touch the sky; you're rotating forward and sinking down into the earth.

Virabhadrasana II 20-30s (7)

a powerful Indian hero-warrior

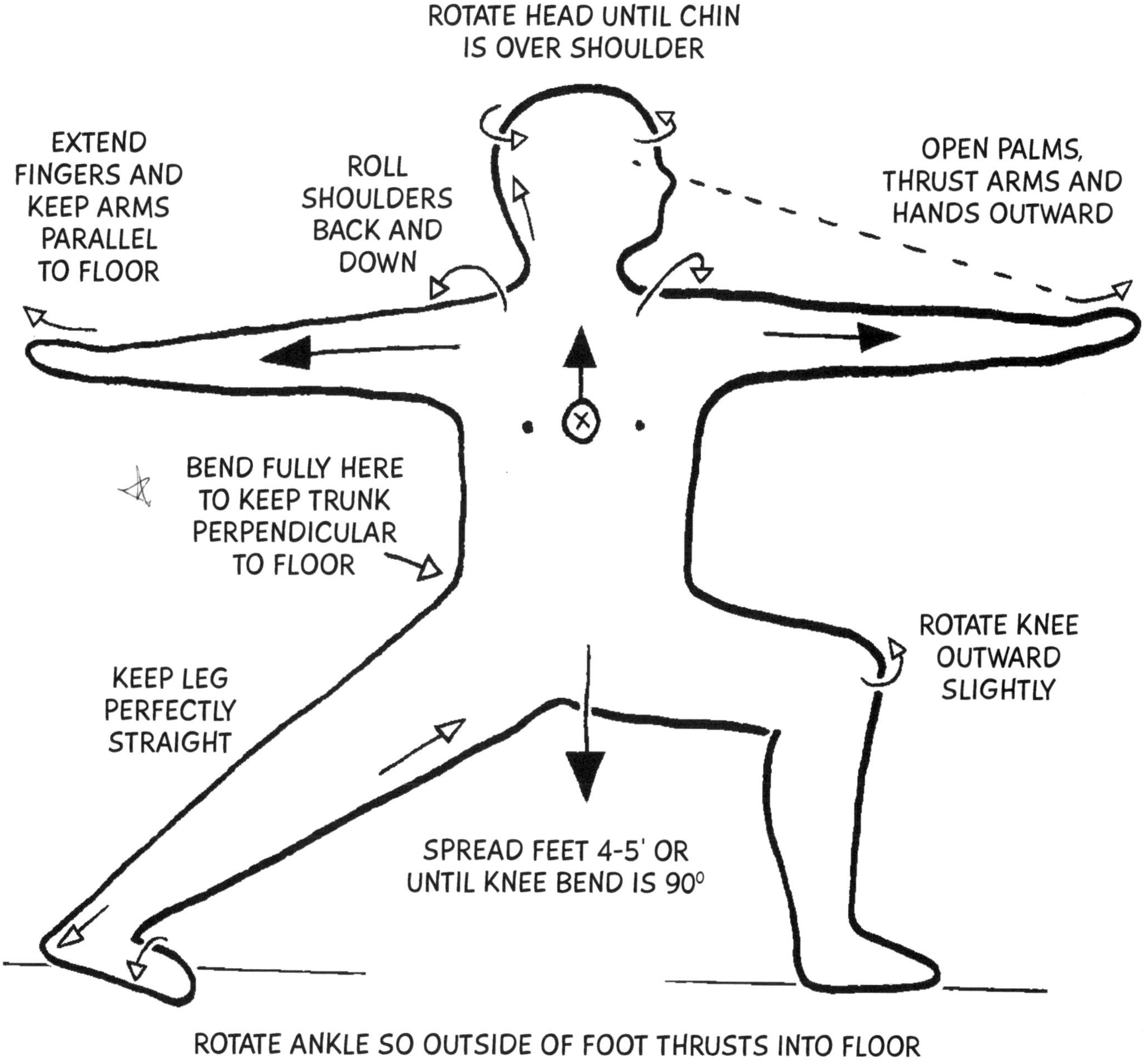

ROTATE HEAD UNTIL CHIN IS OVER SHOULDER
EXTEND FINGERS AND KEEP ARMS PARALLEL TO FLOOR
ROLL SHOULDERS BACK AND DOWN
OPEN PALMS, THRUST ARMS AND HANDS OUTWARD
BEND FULLY HERE TO KEEP TRUNK PERPENDICULAR TO FLOOR
ROTATE KNEE OUTWARD SLIGHTLY
KEEP LEG PERFECTLY STRAIGHT
SPREAD FEET 4-5' OR UNTIL KNEE BEND IS 90°
ROTATE ANKLE SO OUTSIDE OF FOOT THRUSTS INTO FLOOR

Note: In this and other postures, never use strained exhalations. Breathe fully from the diaphragm and keep the chest 'proud', extending it fully. You allow the diaphragm to relax naturally, while still keeping chest fully extended.

Virabhadrasana III 20-30s (8)

a powerful Indian hero-warrior

(see Lesson Index, page 177)

Var: place the hands on the hips and concentrate on balance while lifting the trunk and leg upward. You can also use the hands to hold on to something to help with the balance in the beginning, if you really need to. Hold hands apart at shoulder width, but do keep the arms extended.

Later, focus on vigorously reaching out to 'touch' the wall as you lift the arms and bring the palms together until they touch.

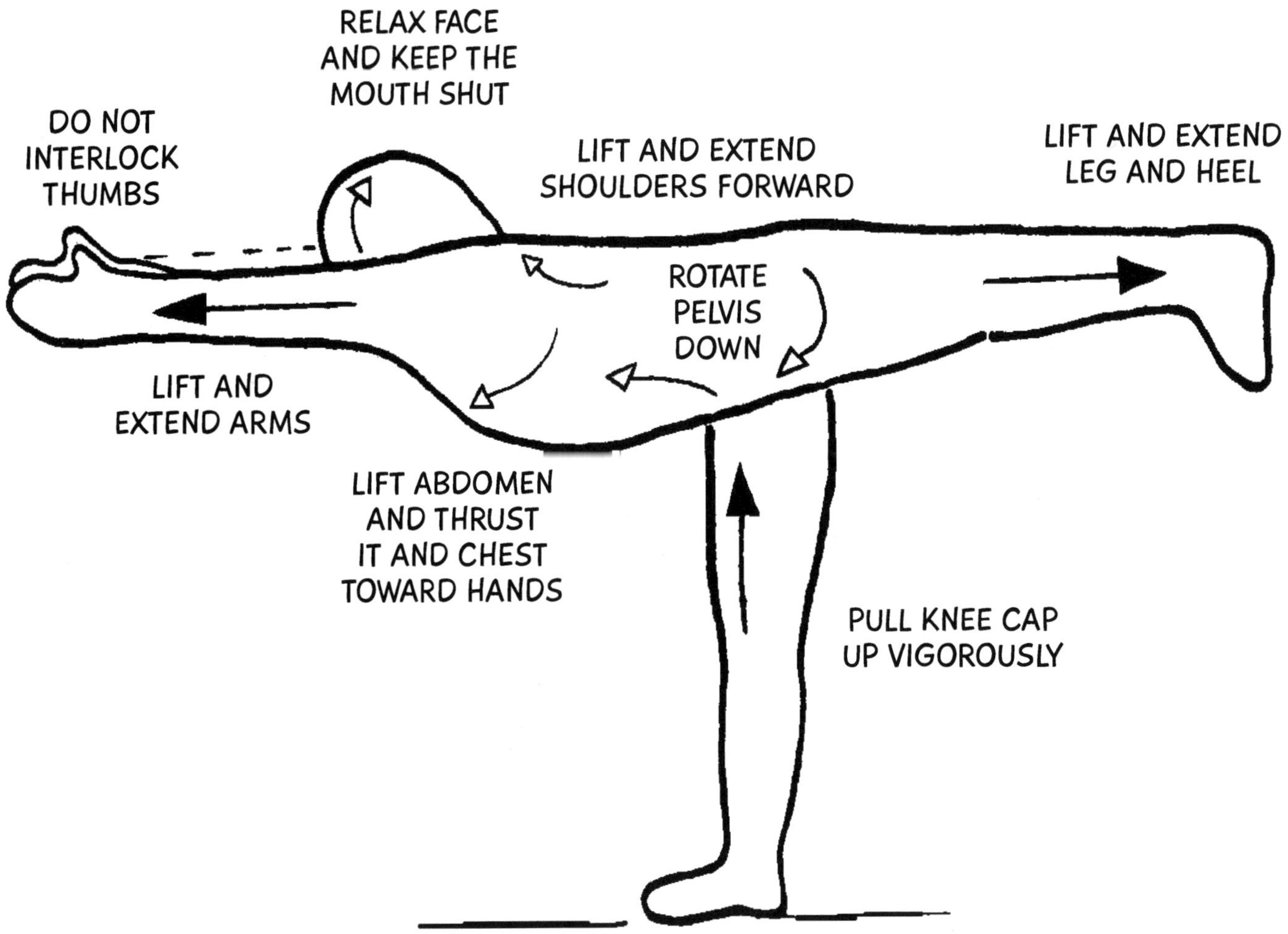
RELAX FACE AND KEEP THE MOUTH SHUT
DO NOT INTERLOCK THUMBS
LIFT AND EXTEND SHOULDERS FORWARD
LIFT AND EXTEND LEG AND HEEL
ROTATE PELVIS DOWN
LIFT AND EXTEND ARMS
LIFT ABDOMEN AND THRUST IT AND CHEST TOWARD HANDS
PULL KNEE CAP UP VIGOROUSLY

Note: Where you balance on one leg, concentrate primarily on keeping this lower leg perfectly straight by pulling the knee caps upward vigorously. Also keeping the ankle firm and feeling it rooted to the floor will increase stability and balance greatly.

Savasana 5-20min (13)

corpse

(see Lesson Index, page 177)

Note: arrange body in this manner and then relax totally. Feel each part of body as heavy as clay sinking into the floor. With each exhalation imagine yourself exhaling all thoughts, emotions, and even your very body, untill all is empty and silent and you are no more. Feel now the eternal nature of creation.

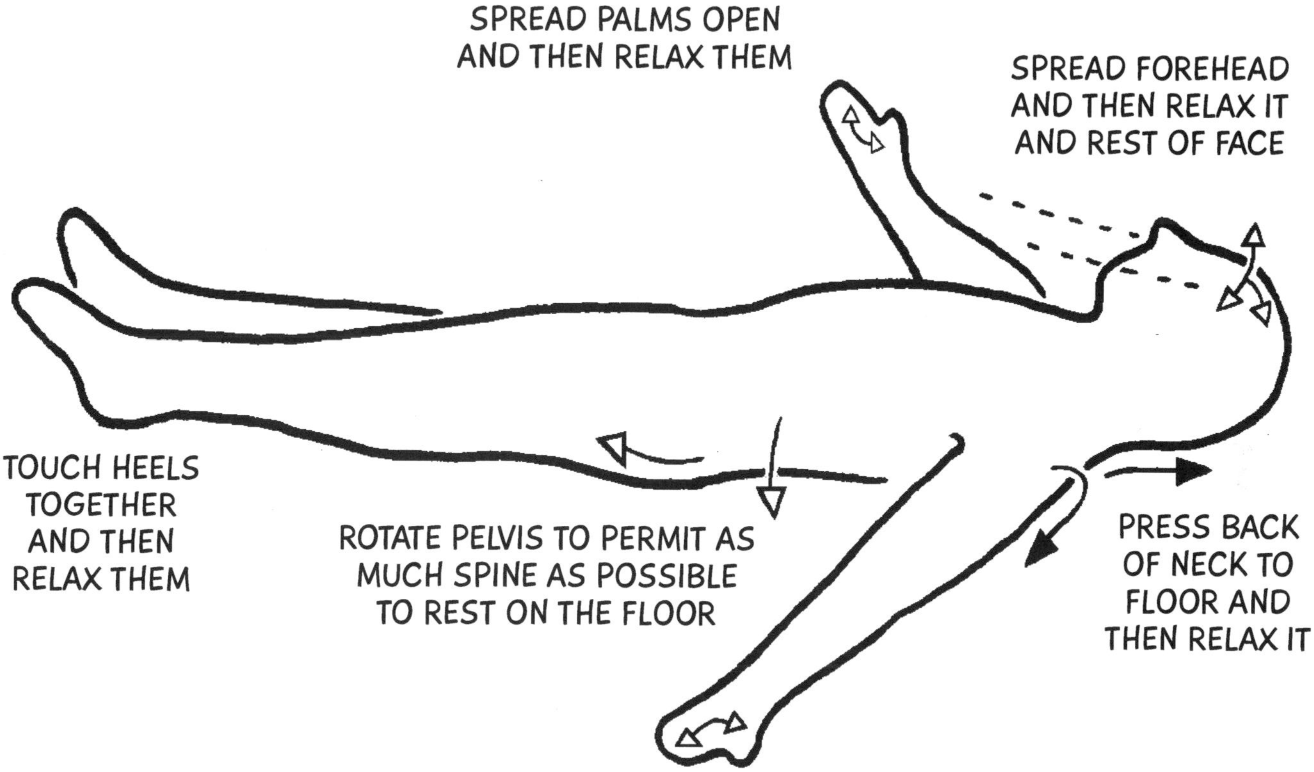
SPREAD PALMS OPEN
AND THEN RELAX THEM
SPREAD FOREHEAD
AND THEN RELAX IT
AND REST OF FACE
TOUCH HEELS
TOGETHER
AND THEN
RELAX THEM
ROTATE PELVIS TO PERMIT AS
MUCH SPINE AS POSSIBLE
TO REST ON THE FLOOR
PRESS BACK
OF NECK TO
FLOOR AND
THEN RELAX IT

Note: breathing in this posture is gentle and even using just the diaphragm. The chest remains perfectly relaxed. Don't try to slow your breathing rate - just breath naturally and feel stillness throughout the entire body, emotion and mind.

Pranayama (in Savasana) 5min (14)

nerve energy control

(see Lesson Index, page 177)

Note: numbered arrows show sequence and location of the stages in inhalation and exhalation. Don't 'try' doing it correctly. Merely find an intuitive sense of the process and let nature take its course gradually. Simply said, once you intuitively know, you can't help but do it correctly. No effort needed. Avoid "*egging on the breathe*", as the Tao Te Ching puts it.

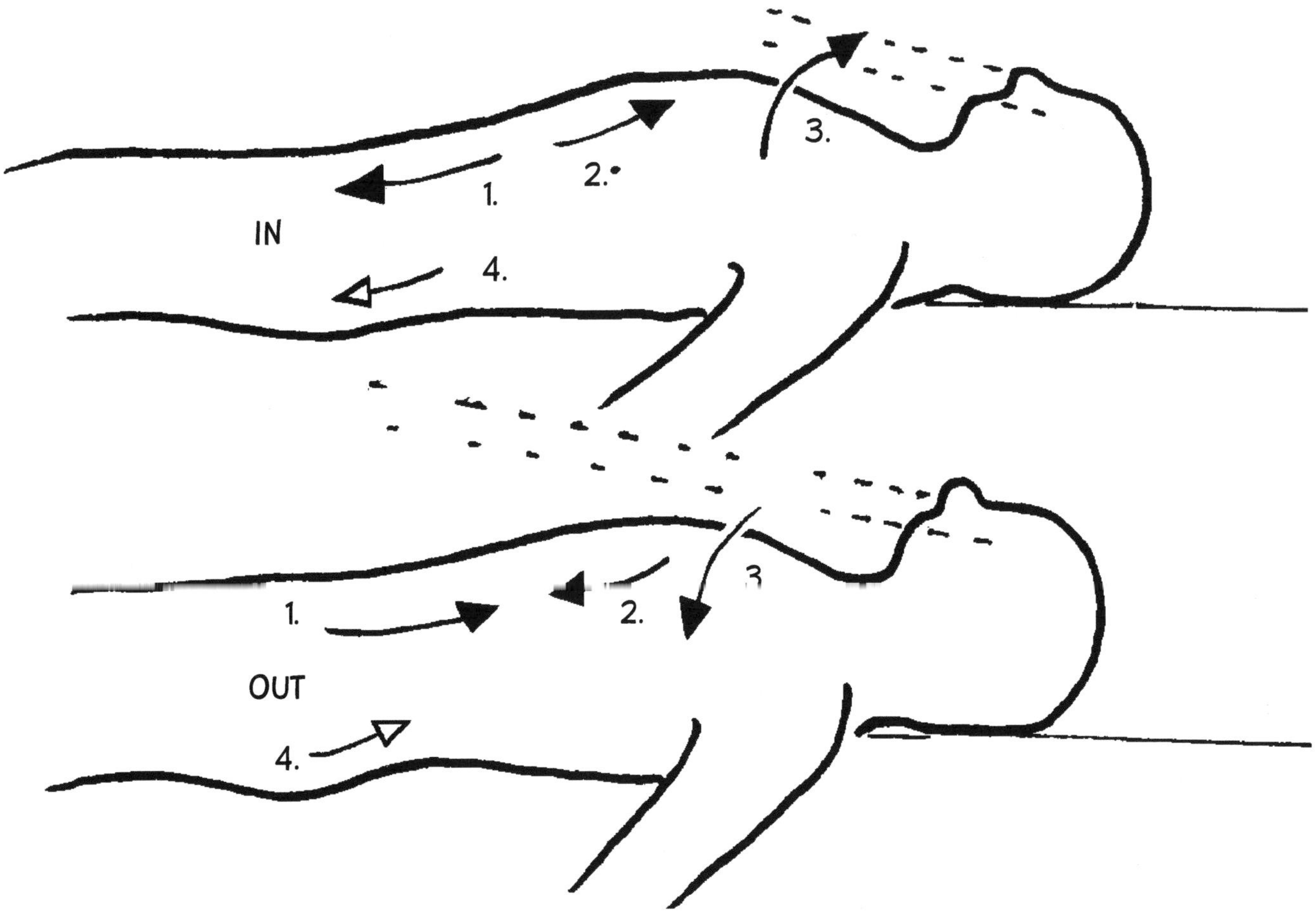
3.
2.
1.
IN
4.
3
1.
2.
OUT
4.

Note: in this or in upright Pranayama, never force exhalations, i.e., by depressing chest and/ or contracting air passage (or abdominal) areas. Instead, try to allow diaphragm to return to a completely relaxed and natural state.

Hold the eyes at nose level. This means the eyes gaze downward past the tip of the nose. The focus of the eyes is either at infinity or 3-5' in front of you (not crosseyed or focused on the tip of the nose). You can occasionally close the eye lids momentarily to help keep the muscles around the eyes relaxed totally.

Also Note: I prefer sui Zen (blowing Zen) for doing the pranayama side of yoga. This is done using a shakuhachi (end blown Japanese bamboo flute).
For more information, go to **centertao.org/essays/blowingzen**

Paripurna Navasana 30-60s (15)

complete boat

(see Lesson Index, page 177)

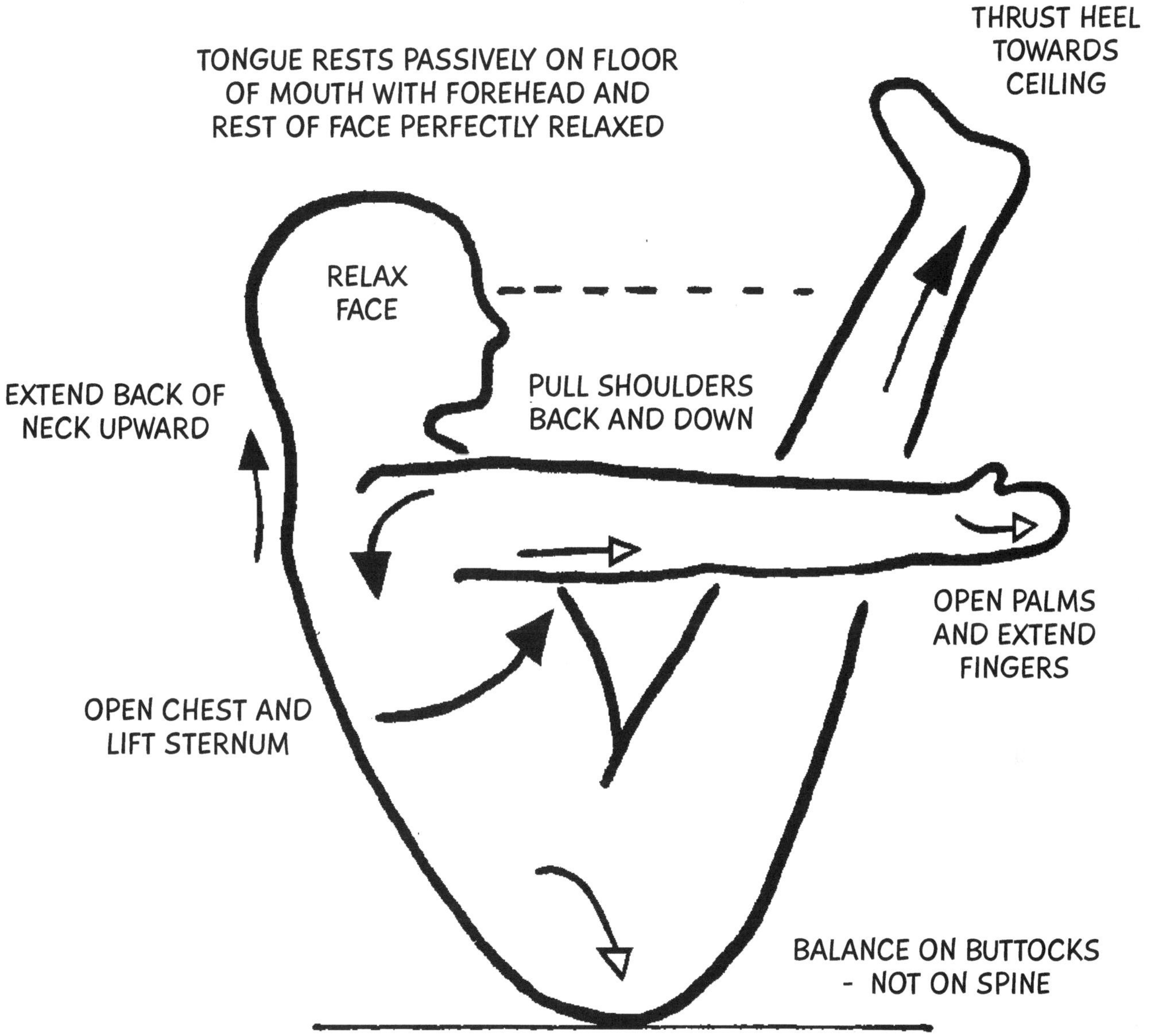

TONGUE RESTS PASSIVELY ON FLOOR OF MOUTH WITH FOREHEAD AND REST OF FACE PERFECTLY RELAXED
THRUST HEEL TOWARDS CEILING
RELAX FACE
EXTEND BACK OF NECK UPWARD
PULL SHOULDERS BACK AND DOWN
OPEN PALMS AND EXTEND FINGERS
OPEN CHEST AND LIFT STERNUM
BALANCE ON BUTTOCKS - NOT ON SPINE

Var: you can rest your legs on a chair and/or hold the legs up by the back of the knees with your hands. Concentrate on extending the chest and pulling the shoulders back and down.

Later on, raise you arm until the palms are level with the feet, as though doing a forward bend.

Ardha Navasana 30-60s

half boat

(see Lesson Index, page 177)

Var: you can extend the arms out straight and position the hands on the thighs. Keep the legs on the floor and slide the hands down the thighs as you lift the upper trunk off the floor a few inches.

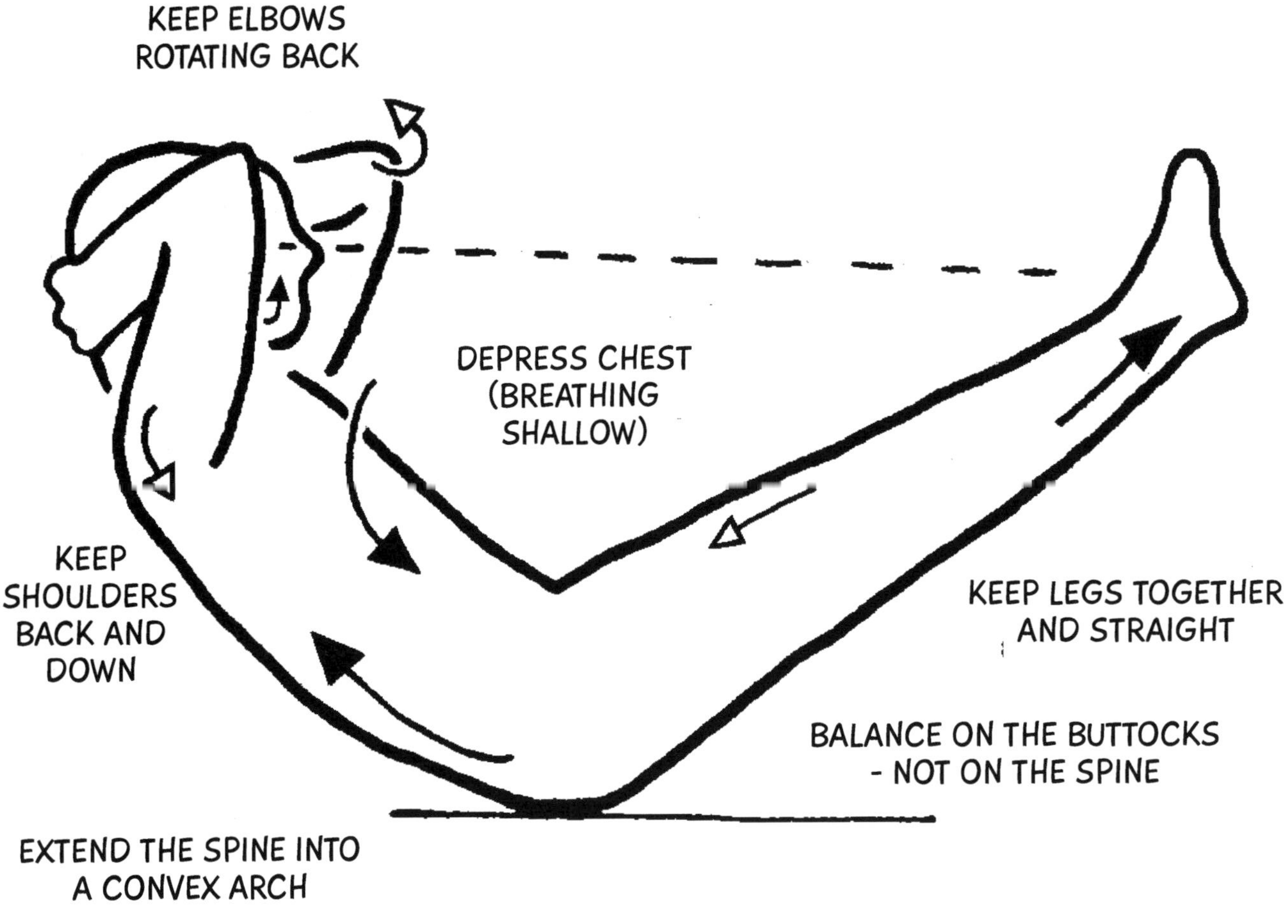

KEEP ELBOWS ROTATING BACK
DEPRESS CHEST (BREATHING SHALLOW)
KEEP SHOULDERS BACK AND DOWN
KEEP LEGS TOGETHER AND STRAIGHT
BALANCE ON THE BUTTOCKS - NOT ON THE SPINE
EXTEND THE SPINE INTO A CONVEX ARCH

Urdhva Prasarita Padasana 30-60s (17)

up stretched out foot

(see Lesson Index, page 177)

Var: first extend the legs perpendicular to the floor. Gradually lower the legs to increase the challenge, but never any further than you can keep the lower back pressed firmly to the floor.

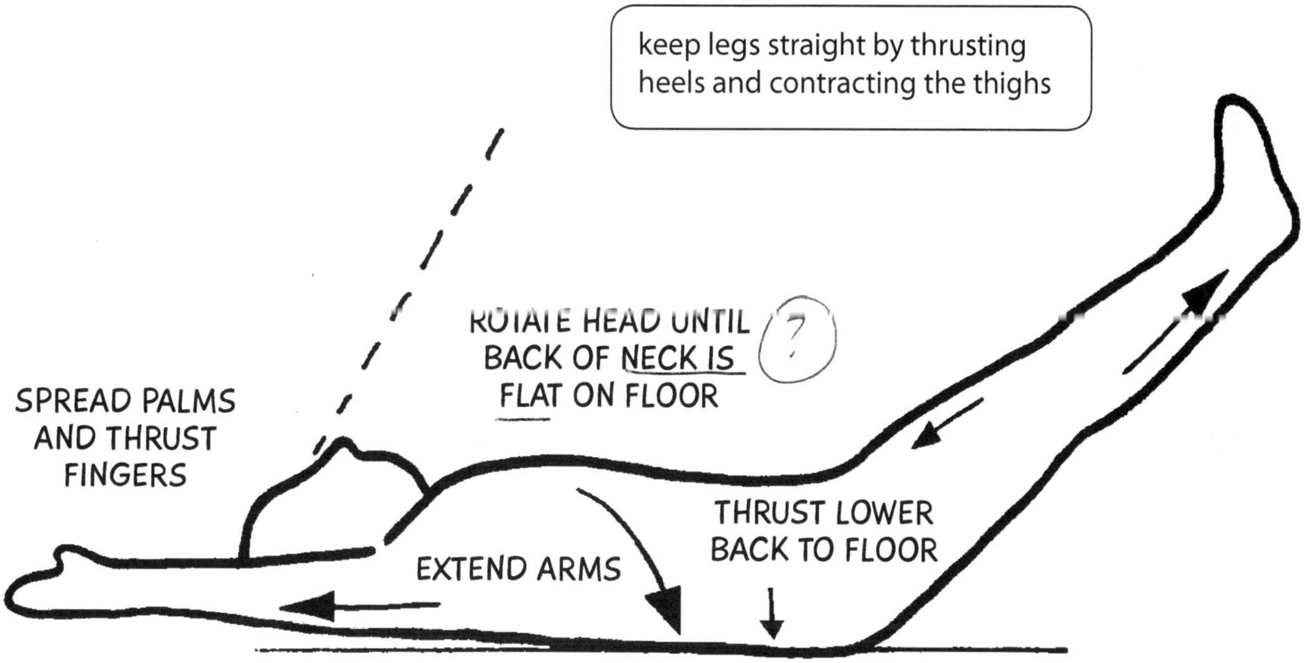

keep legs straight by thrusting heels and contracting the thighs
ROTATE HEAD UNTIL BACK OF NECK IS FLAT ON FLOOR
SPREAD PALMS AND THRUST FINGERS
EXTEND ARMS
THRUST LOWER BACK TO FLOOR

Note: in this and most other postures in this manual, the eyes are held at nose level. This means the eyes gaze downward past the tip of the nose. The focus of the eyes is either at infinity or 3-5' in front of you (not crosseyed or focused on the tip of the nose). You can occasionally close the eye lids momentarily to help keep the muscles around the eyes relaxed totally.

Adho Mukha Svanasana 60s (18)

downward face dog

(see Lesson Index, page 177)

Var: place hands next to a wall and thrust them into it to help stabilize the posture.

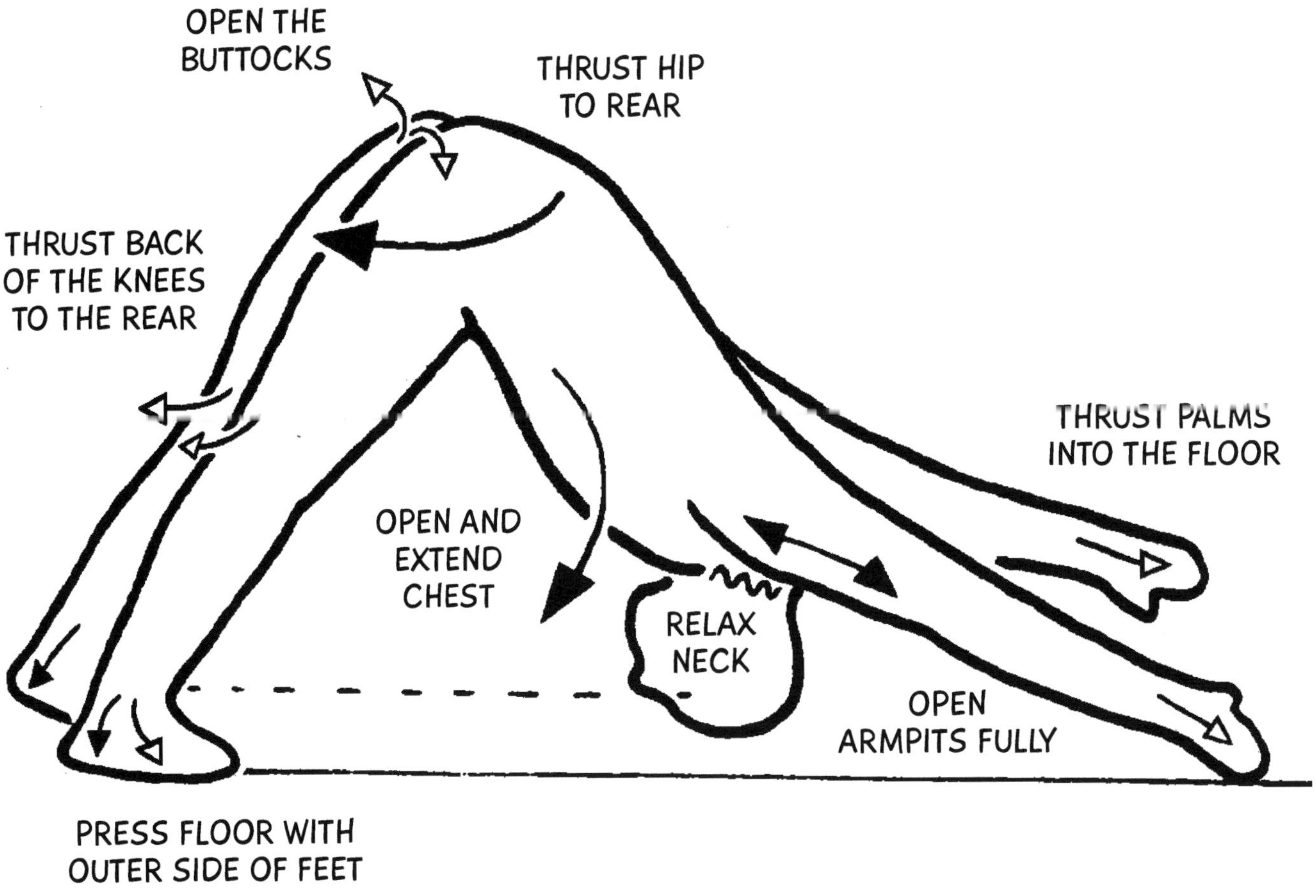
OPEN THE BUTTOCKS
THRUST HIP TO REAR
THRUST BACK OF THE KNEES TO THE REAR
THRUST PALMS INTO THE FLOOR
OPEN AND EXTEND CHEST
RELAX NECK
OPEN ARMPITS FULLY
PRESS FLOOR WITH OUTER SIDE OF FEET

Note: You should strive to keep the chest open and vigorously extended at all times, even during exhalations. Breathing is done with the diaphragm. This is true for all postures - but it may take some time before you can accomplish this.

Urdhva Mukha Svanasana 30-60s (19)

upward face dog

(see Lesson Index, page 177)

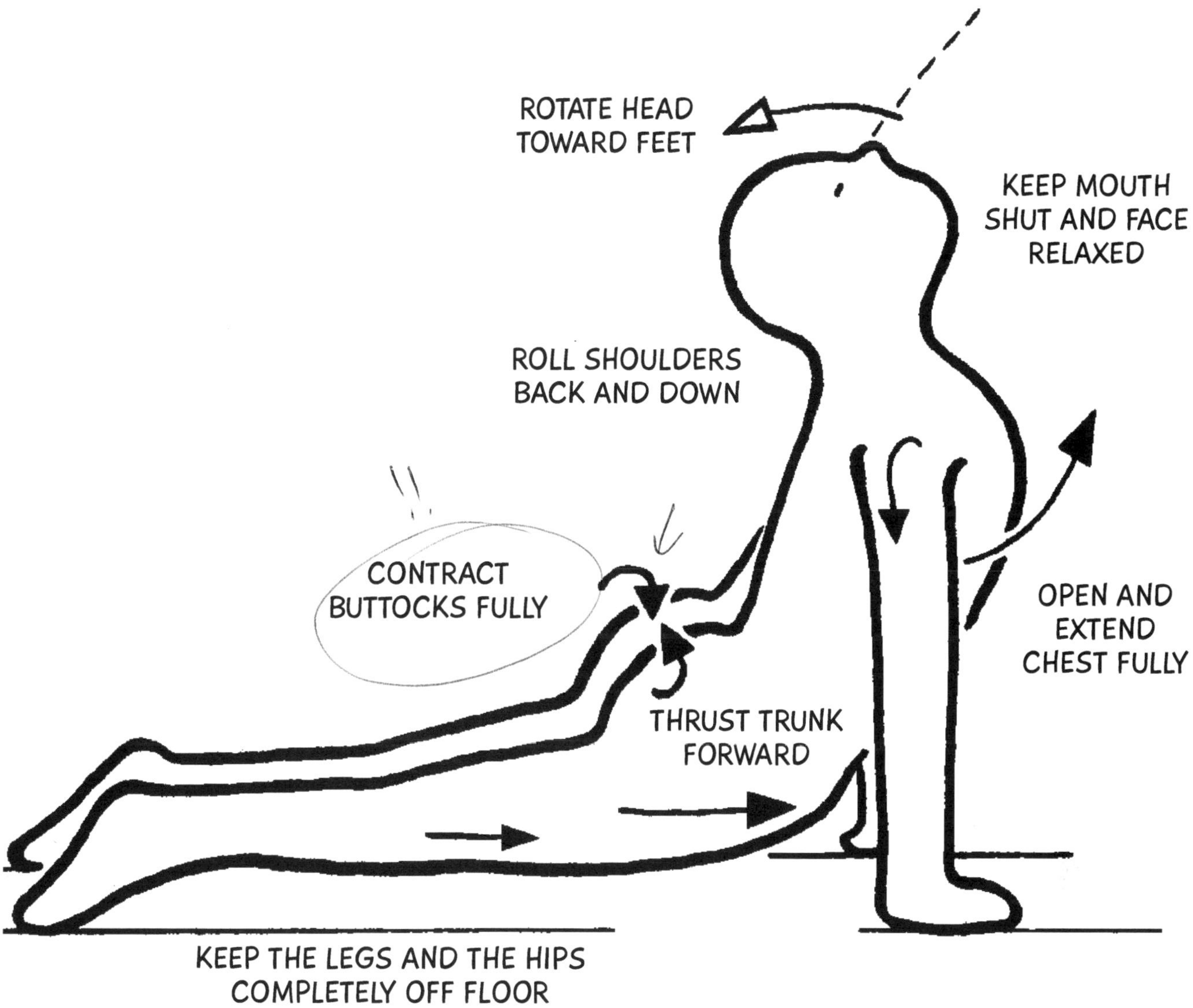
ROTATE HEAD
TOWARD FEET
KEEP MOUTH
SHUT AND FACE
RELAXED
ROLL SHOULDERS
BACK AND DOWN
CONTRACT
BUTTOCKS FULLY
OPEN AND
EXTEND
CHEST FULLY
THRUST TRUNK
FORWARD
KEEP THE LEGS AND THE HIPS
COMPLETELY OFF FLOOR

Note: support the legs on the upper side of the feet and toes - not on the tips or underside of the toes. Pull the hips toward the arms until the bend is greatest and you are at the edge of balance.

In this and other postures, never use strained exhalations. Instead, allow diaphragm to relax naturally - while still keeping chest fully extended.

Hold the eyes at nose level, gazing downward past the tip of the nose. The focus of the eyes is either at infinity or 3-5' in front of you. Occasionally close the eye lids momentarily to help keep the muscles around the eyes relaxed totally.

Chaturanga Dandasana 30-60s (20)

four limb staff

Rest your whole body on the floor, then raise it up evenly, keeping it parallel to the floor. Again, for help in learning how to move into or out of the Yoga postures, take a Hatha Yoga class from a competent teacher and/or refer to B.K.S, Iyengars' most excellent book - ***Light on Yoga.***

Var: you can rest the knees on the floor during the posture, and keep the rest of the body off the floor.

Note: for ***Nakrasana,*** support the legs on the underside of the toes. On the exhalation, jump forward a foot or so on all fours. Use a hopping motion but keep the body as straight and close to the floor as possible.

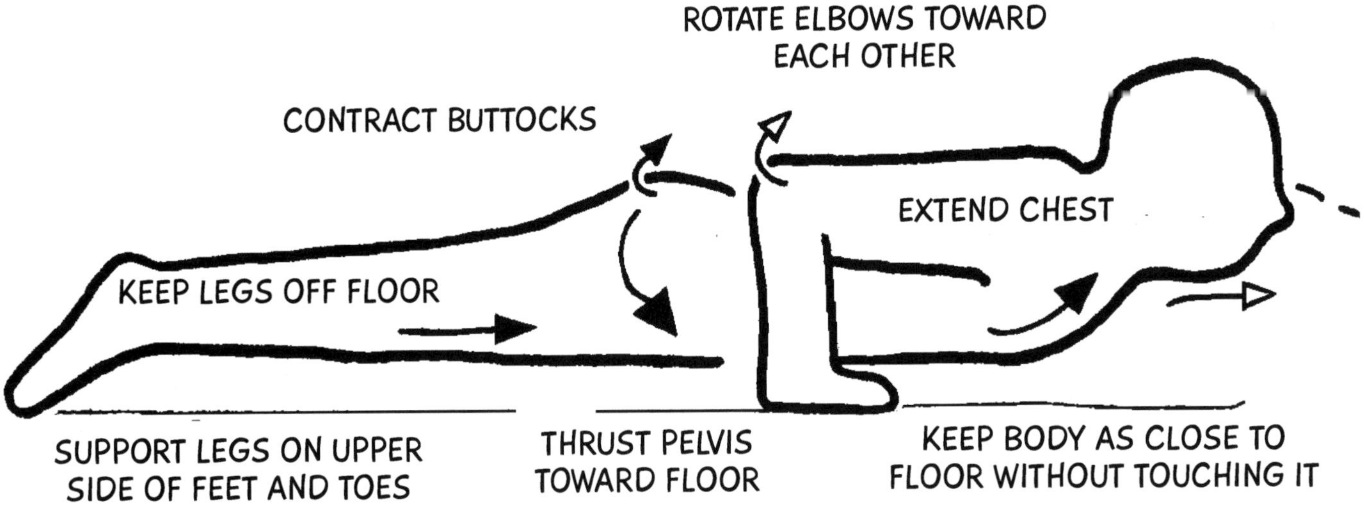

ROTATE ELBOWS TOWARD EACH OTHER
CONTRACT BUTTOCKS
EXTEND CHEST
KEEP LEGS OFF FLOOR
SUPPORT LEGS ON UPPER SIDE OF FEET AND TOES
THRUST PELVIS TOWARD FLOOR
KEEP BODY AS CLOSE TO FLOOR WITHOUT TOUCHING IT

Note: as in all postures, the tongue rest passively on the floor of the mouth, with the forehead and the rest of the face perfectly relaxed.

Salabhasana 60s (21)

locust

(see Lesson Index, page 177)

Var: lift only the legs or the trunk off the floor.

Note: first extend the chest and lift the trunk off the floor. On the next exhalation lift the legs off the floor.

Needless to say, you are unlikely to ever match the lift shown here. All these drawings show the 'ideal' you are striving towards. If and when you actually match the drawing, you'll have to figure out a way to make it still work. The goal is not to become strong and flexible; the goal of yoga is to balance work and rest. The more flexible and stronger you become, they more you need to find ways to make the posture work (challenging) enough to keep you as a 'beginner' on the frontier of your own personal limits.

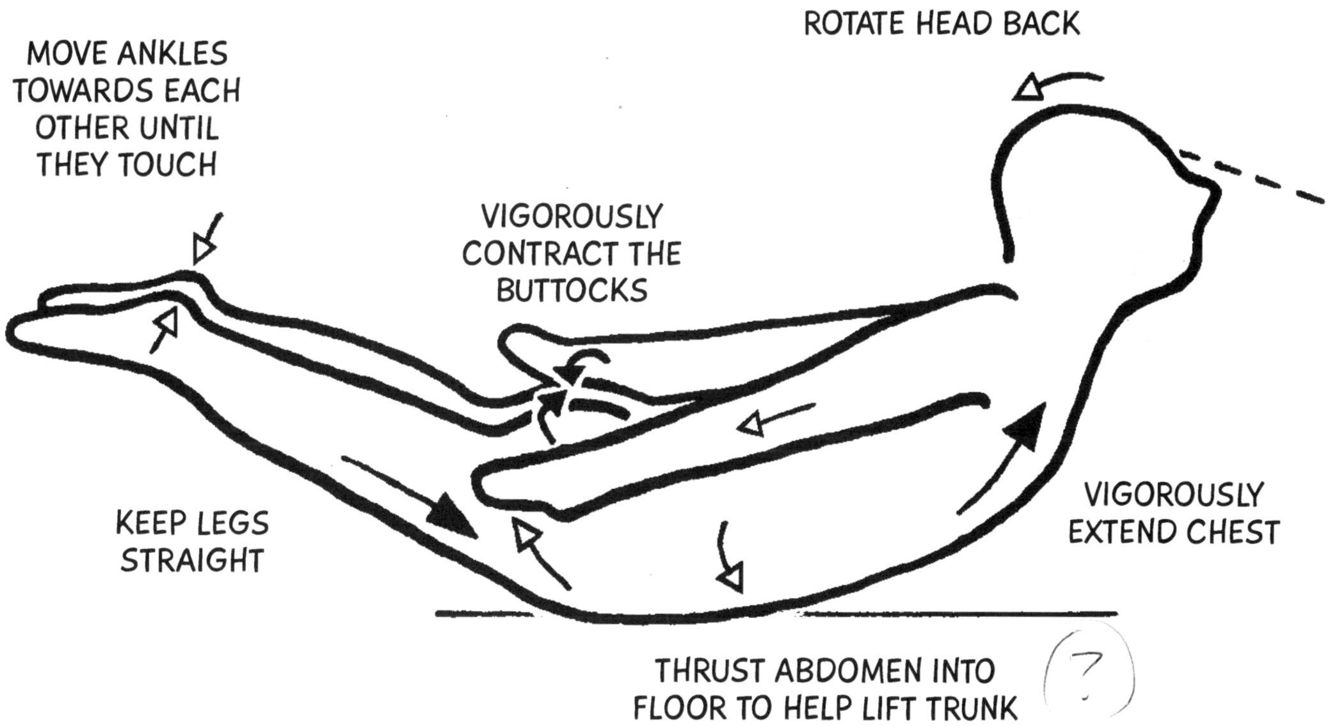
ROTATE HEAD BACK
MOVE ANKLES TOWARDS EACH OTHER UNTIL THEY TOUCH
VIGOROUSLY CONTRACT THE BUTTOCKS
KEEP LEGS STRAIGHT
VIGOROUSLY EXTEND CHEST
THRUST ABDOMEN INTO FLOOR TO HELP LIFT TRUNK
?

Ustrasana 30s (22)

camel

(see Lesson Index, page 177)

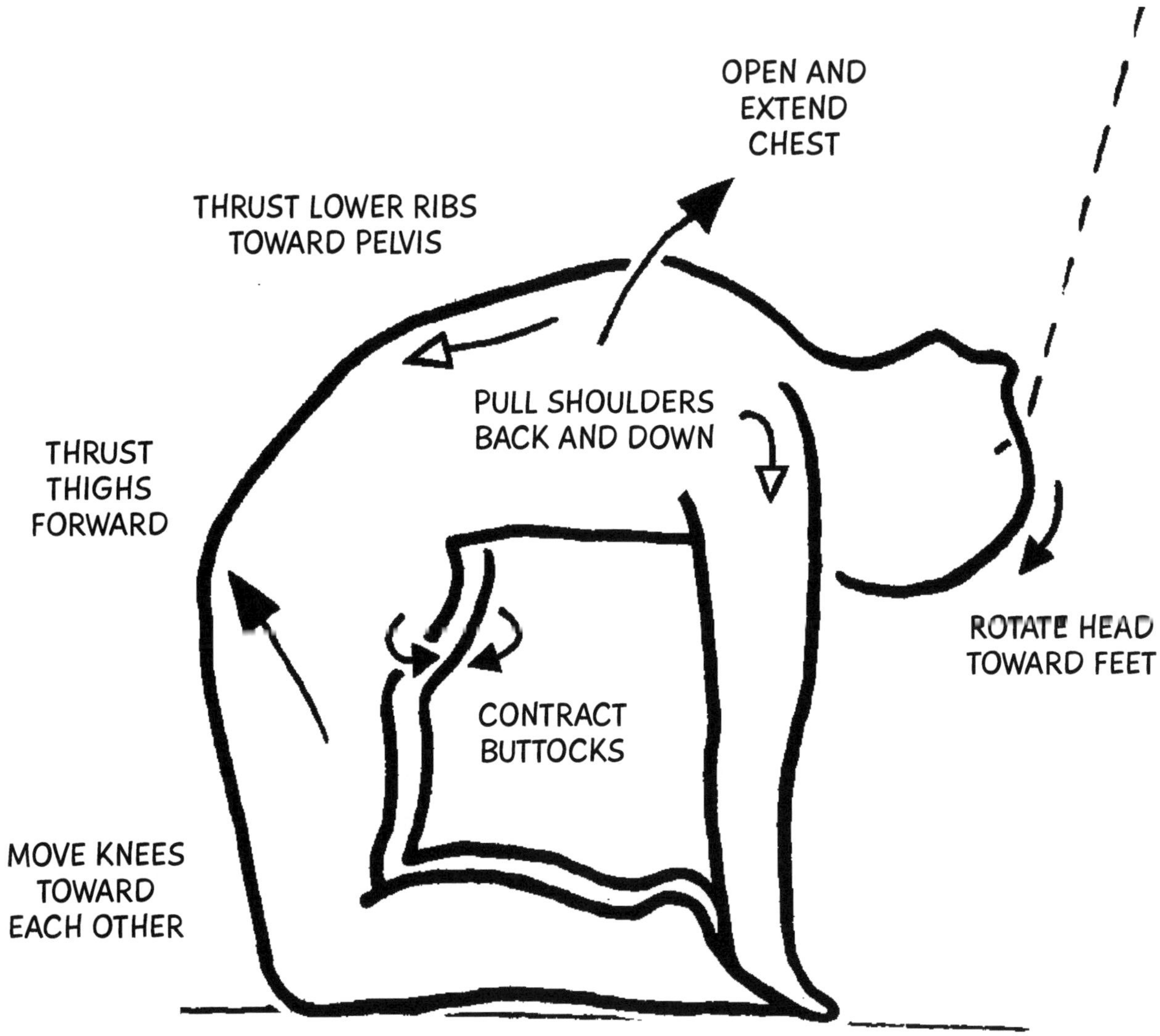
OPEN AND
EXTEND
CHEST
THRUST LOWER RIBS
TOWARD PELVIS
PULL SHOULDERS
BACK AND DOWN
THRUST
THIGHS
FORWARD
ROTATE HEAD
TOWARD FEET
CONTRACT
BUTTOCKS
MOVE KNEES
TOWARD
EACH OTHER

Var: you can first do this posture with the knees spread apart 12" or so. Then repeat it with the knees as close together as possible.

Note: in this and other back bend postures, keep the buttocks contracted as firmly as possible while moving into or out of the posture.

Virasana I and II 60s (23)

(hero)

(see Lesson Index, page 177)

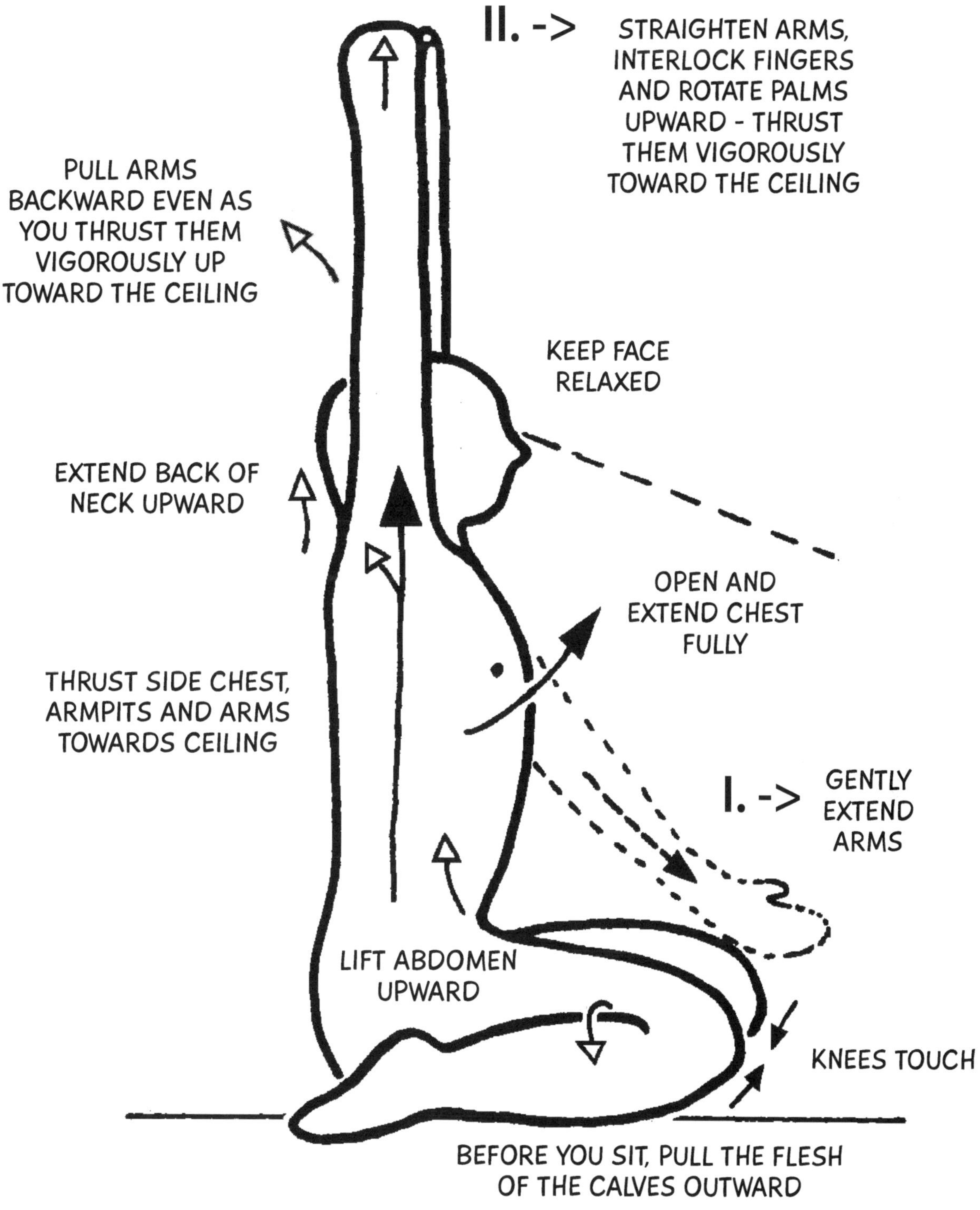

II. ->
STRAIGHTEN ARMS, INTERLOCK FINGERS AND ROTATE PALMS UPWARD - THRUST THEM VIGOROUSLY TOWARD THE CEILING
PULL ARMS BACKWARD EVEN AS YOU THRUST THEM VIGOROUSLY UP TOWARD THE CEILING
KEEP FACE RELAXED
EXTEND BACK OF NECK UPWARD
OPEN AND EXTEND CHEST FULLY
THRUST SIDE CHEST, ARMPITS AND ARMS TOWARDS CEILING
I. ->
GENTLY EXTEND ARMS
LIFT ABDOMEN UPWARD
KNEES TOUCH
BEFORE YOU SIT, PULL THE FLESH OF THE CALVES OUTWARD

Var: if the knees are very stiff, place a folded blanket under the buttocks.

Virasana III 60s (24)

hero

(see Lesson Index, page 177)

Note: in this and other postures, never use strained exhalations.

As this becomes easier, raise your arms so only your finger tips, knees, and lower legs touch the floor. You press yourself as close to the floor as possible, while making as minimal contact as possible.

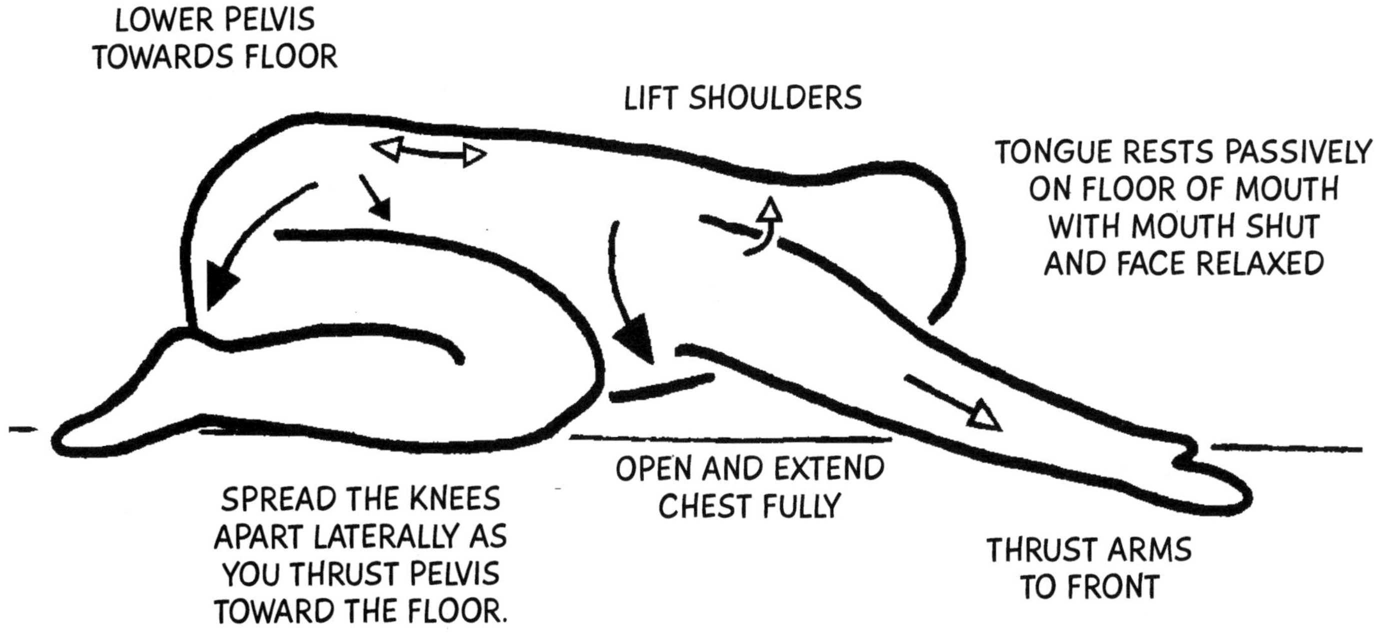
LOWER PELVIS TOWARDS FLOOR
LIFT SHOULDERS
TONGUE RESTS PASSIVELY ON FLOOR OF MOUTH WITH MOUTH SHUT AND FACE RELAXED
SPREAD THE KNEES APART LATERALLY AS YOU THRUST PELVIS TOWARD THE FLOOR.
OPEN AND EXTEND CHEST FULLY
THRUST ARMS TO FRONT

Janu Sirsasana   30-60s   (25)

knee head

(see Lesson Index, page 177)

Var: if you can't grasp the toes, you can grasp the knees and strive to slide the hand down the shin toward the foot. Concentrate on keeping the chest extended and the leg straight.

Note: in this and other forward bends, gently rotate the head upward slightly and with the gaze at nose level, look out beyond the feet throughout the posture. Later, when you can lay the trunk on the legs, rest the forehead on the shins. Rather than grasping your wrist, you can simply thrust your arms forward as far as they can go. You are effectively reaching to touch the wall beyond your reach!

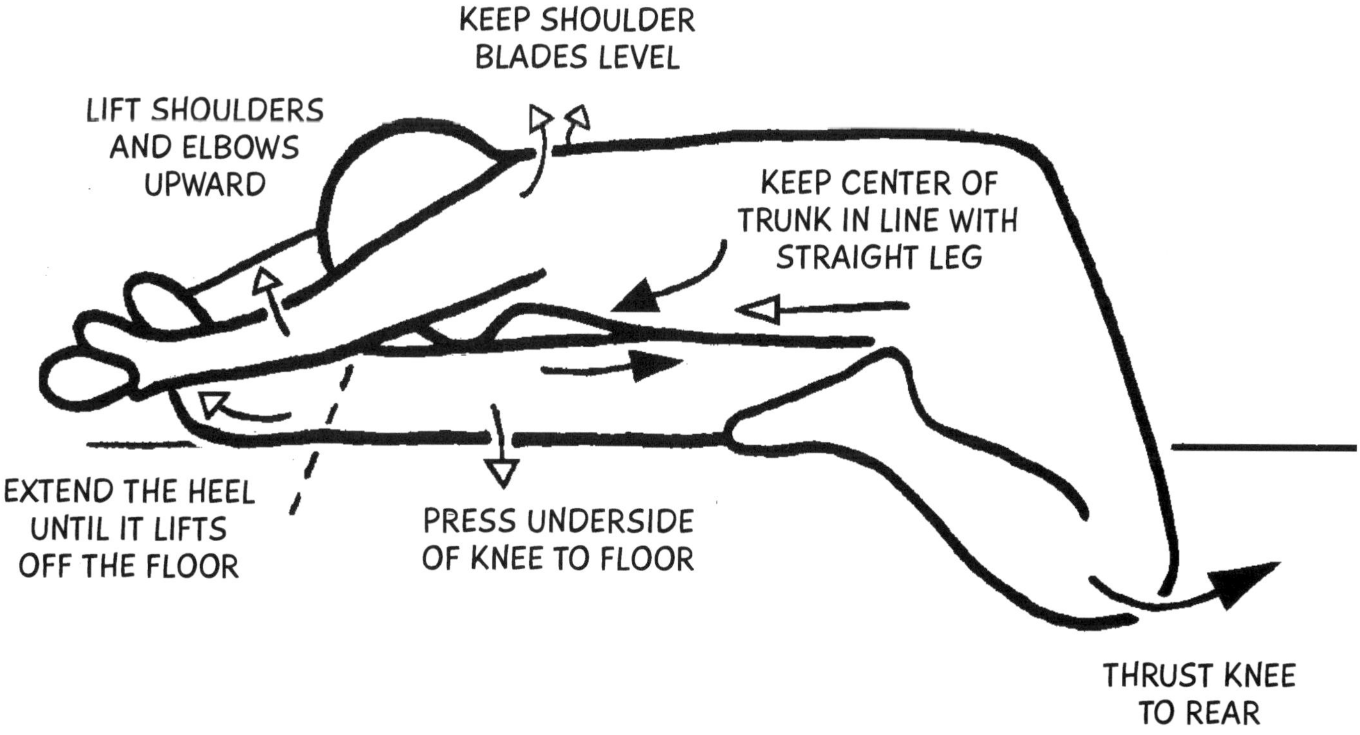
KEEP SHOULDER BLADES LEVEL
LIFT SHOULDERS AND ELBOWS UPWARD
KEEP CENTER OF TRUNK IN LINE WITH STRAIGHT LEG
EXTEND THE HEEL UNTIL IT LIFTS OFF THE FLOOR
PRESS UNDERSIDE OF KNEE TO FLOOR
THRUST KNEE TO REAR

Bharadvajasana I 30s (26)

father of Drona

(see Lesson Index, page 177)

Var: place bent arm a few inches behind buttock and straighten it, thrust its palm into the floor. Use this arm to pivot the trunk around.

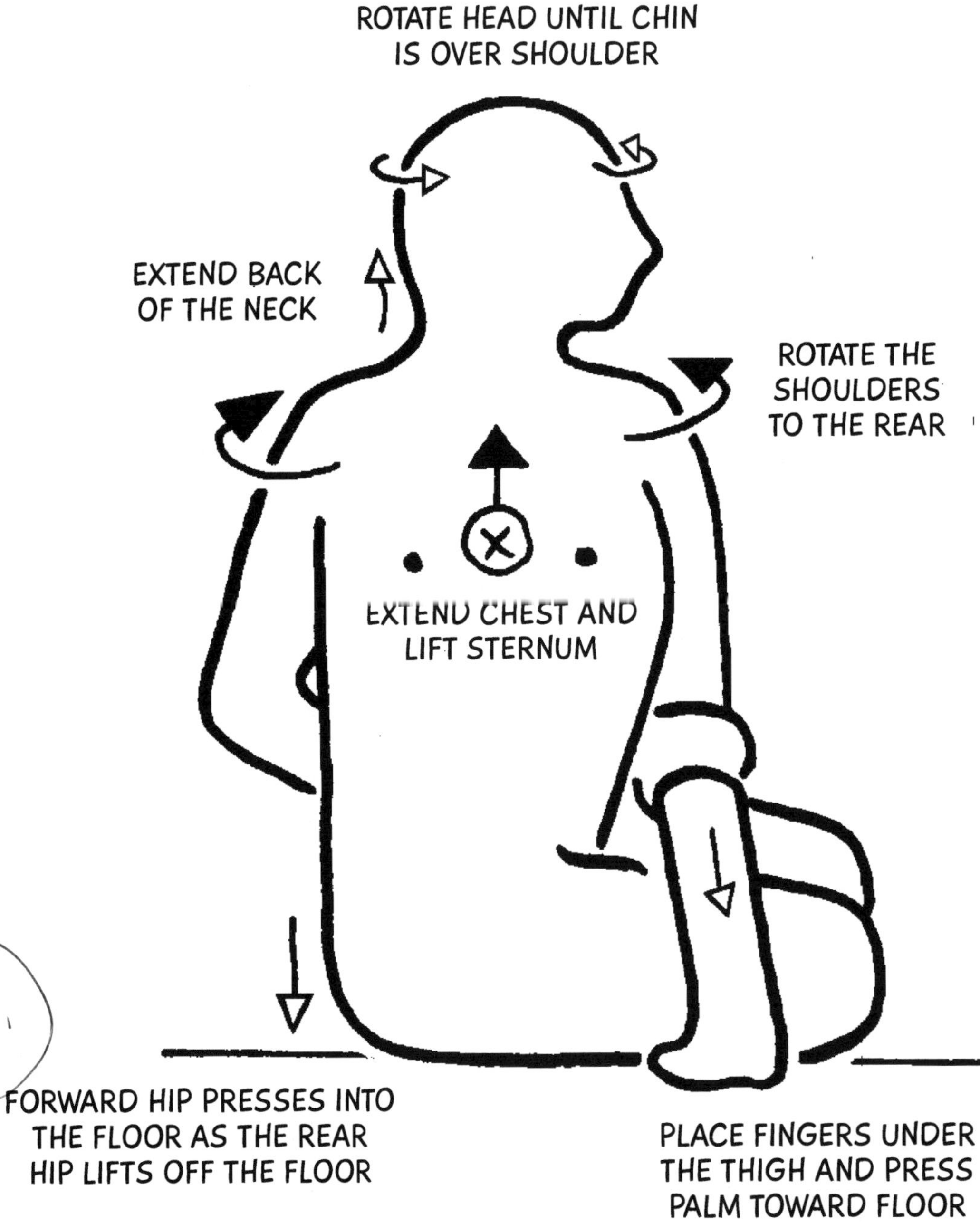
ROTATE HEAD UNTIL CHIN IS OVER SHOULDER
EXTEND BACK OF THE NECK
ROTATE THE SHOULDERS TO THE REAR
EXTEND CHEST AND LIFT STERNUM
FORWARD HIP PRESSES INTO THE FLOOR AS THE REAR HIP LIFTS OFF THE FLOOR
PLACE FINGERS UNDER THE THIGH AND PRESS PALM TOWARD FLOOR

Note: In this and other twist postures, avoid looking out of the side of your eyes when rotating your head side ways. Instead look straight ahead. Review Note for posture #17.

Program 3: First Day

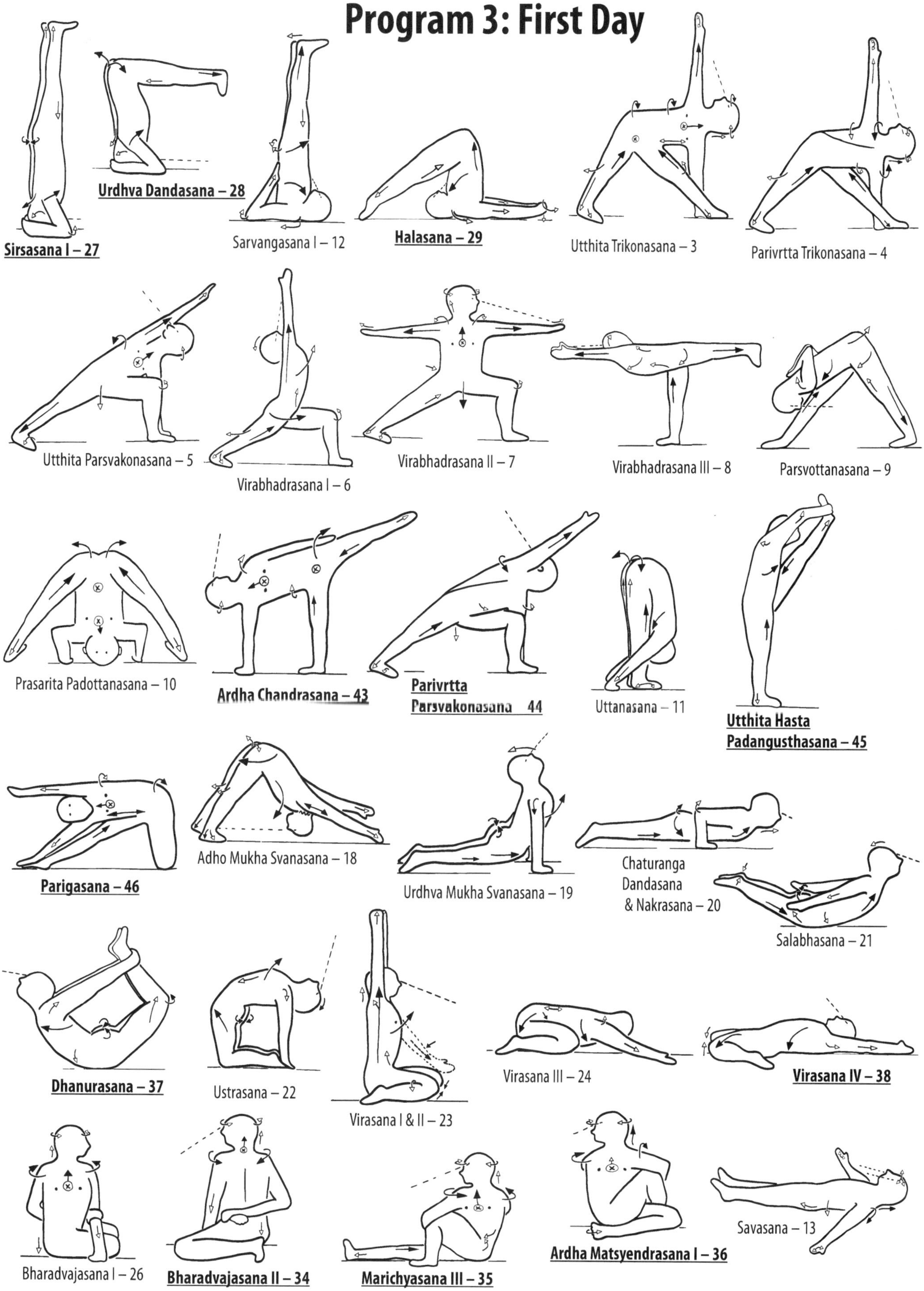

Sirsasana I – 27
Urdhva Dandasana – 28
Sarvangasana I – 12
Halasana – 29
Utthita Trikonasana – 3
Parivrtta Trikonasana – 4
Utthita Parsvakonasana – 5
Virabhadrasana I – 6
Virabhadrasana II – 7
Virabhadrasana III – 8
Parsvottanasana – 9
Prasarita Padottanasana – 10
Ardha Chandrasana – 43
Parivrtta Parsvakonasana 44
Uttanasana – 11
Utthita Hasta Padangusthasana – 45
Parigasana – 46
Adho Mukha Svanasana – 18
Urdhva Mukha Svanasana – 19
Chaturanga Dandasana & Nakrasana – 20
Salabhasana – 21
Dhanurasana – 37
Ustrasana – 22
Virasana I & II – 23
Virasana III – 24
Virasana IV – 38
Bharadvajasana I – 26
Bharadvajasana II – 34
Marichyasana III – 35
Ardha Matsyendrasana I – 36
Savasana – 13

Program 3: Second Day

TIP: For a more intense daily routine, do the **First Day Program** up to posture #11 (Uttanasana). Then do the entire sequence below, beginning with posture #15 Navasana, Paripoorna.

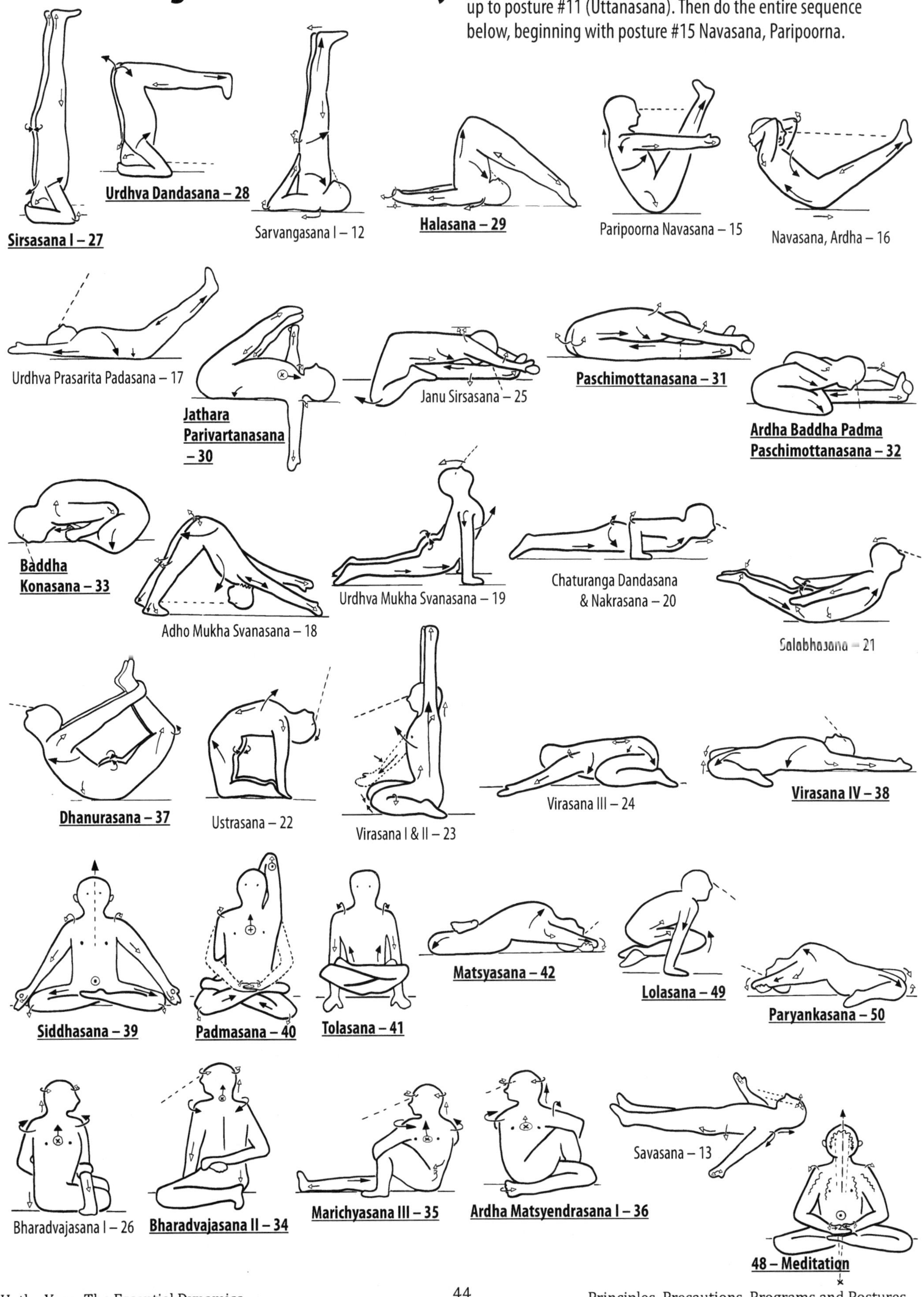
Sirsasana I – 27
Urdhva Dandasana – 28
Sarvangasana I – 12
Halasana – 29
Paripoorna Navasana – 15
Navasana, Ardha – 16
Urdhva Prasarita Padasana – 17
Jathara Parivartanasana – 30
Janu Sirsasana – 25
Paschimottanasana – 31
Ardha Baddha Padma Paschimottanasana – 32
Baddha Konasana – 33
Adho Mukha Svanasana – 18
Urdhva Mukha Svanasana – 19
Chaturanga Dandasana & Nakrasana – 20
Salabhasana – 21
Dhanurasana – 37
Ustrasana – 22
Virasana I & II – 23
Virasana III – 24
Virasana IV – 38
Siddhasana – 39
Padmasana – 40
Tolasana – 41
Matsyasana – 42
Lolasana – 49
Paryankasana – 50
Bharadvajasana I – 26
Bharadvajasana II – 34
Marichyasana III – 35
Ardha Matsyendrasana I – 36
Savasana – 13
48 – Meditation

Sirsasana I 1-5min (27)

head

(see Lesson Index, page 177)

Note: SIRSASANA is like an upside down TADASANA. Body is kept as straight as possible without back arch and with base of neck extending backward.

Var: Place head and interlocked hands next to wall. Straighten legs and walk them up toward the head, pressing as much of spine flat on wall as possible. Now practice lifting the shoulders and extending the neck.

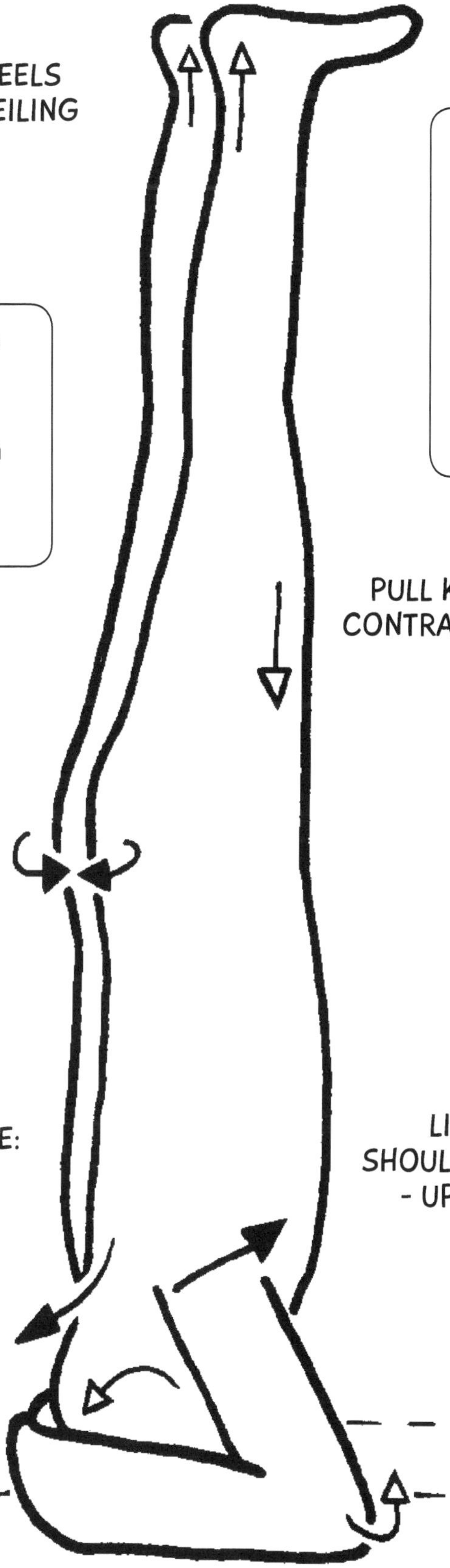
THRUST HEELS TOWARD CEILING
PULL KNEE CAPS UP BY CONTRACTING THE THIGHS
CONTRACT BUTTOCKS
EXTEND BACK OF THE NECK (SEE NOTE: FOR POSTURE #1)
LIFT AND THRUST THE SHOULDERS IN THIS DIRECTION - UPWARD AND OUTWARD
DISTANCE BETWEEN ELBOWS IS EQUAL TO SHOULDER WIDTH.
(SEE NOTE: FOR POSTURE 52 & 79).
ROTATE HEAD SLIGHTLY UNTIL BALANCE POINT IS ON THE CROWN OF THE HEAD

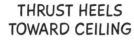

Urdhva Dandasana   1-5 min   (28)

up staff

Var: Initially just lower the legs a little bit at a time, keeping them perfectly straight at all times. Also, keep lifting the shoulders and extending the neck during the entire range of movement.

Note: Eventually you want to go up to or down from SIRSASANA with the legs perfectly straight. You do this by walking the feet in toward the head. This moves the trunk backwards until the body weight is carried by the head. Then it is easy to lift the straightened legs off the floor. (see Var: for posture 51). Another variation: Spread the legs fully, as in Supta Konasana [56], and lower (or raise if going up) the feet fully spread apart to the ground.

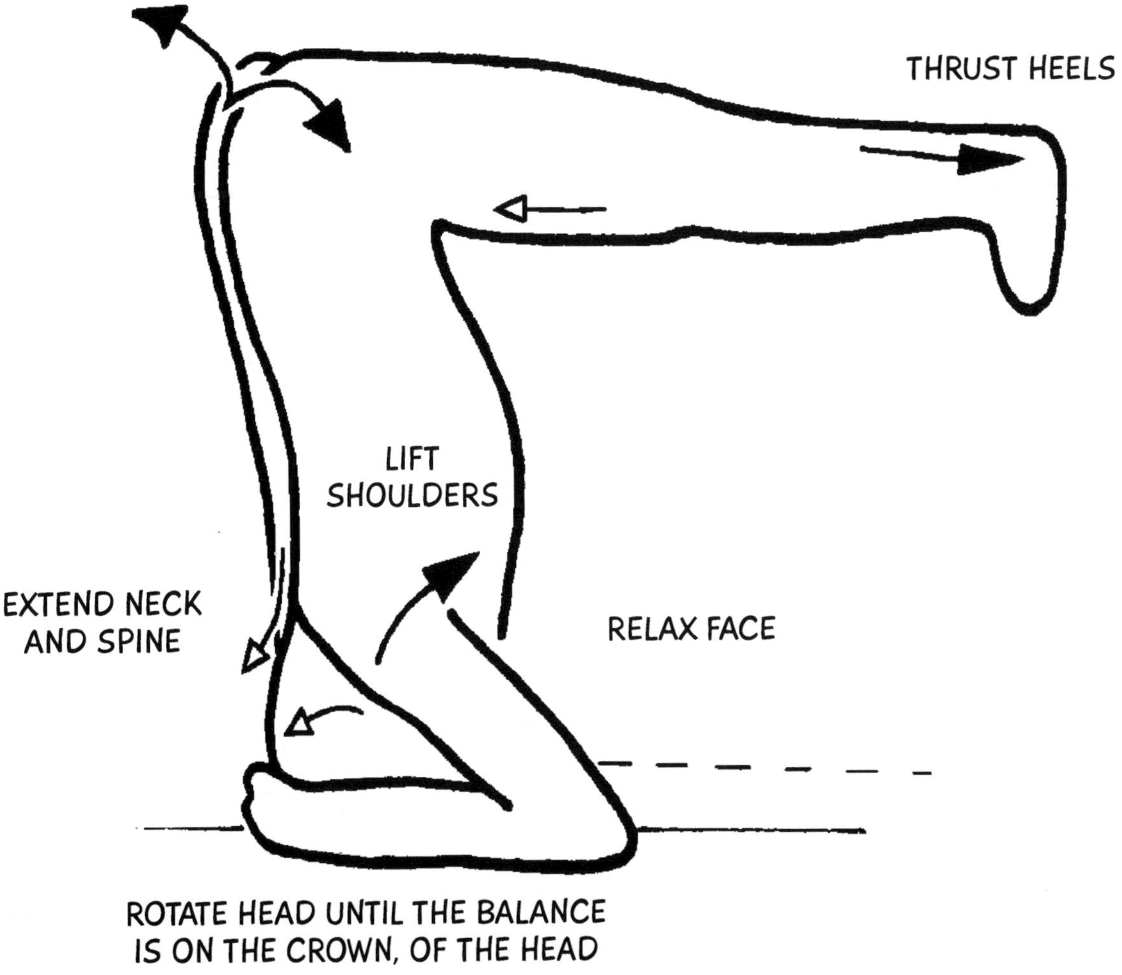

OPEN BUTTOCKS
THRUST HEELS
LIFT SHOULDERS
EXTEND NECK AND SPINE
RELAX FACE
ROTATE HEAD UNTIL THE BALANCE IS ON THE CROWN, OF THE HEAD

Halasana 1-5min (29)

plow

(see Lesson Index, page 177)

Var: For the first year, bend the arms and support the trunk with the palms thrusting into the lower ribs (as in SARVANGASANA). Also curl the toes in towards the feet and thrust the heels. If it is very difficult to do properly with your toes on the floor, you may place a chair behind, and rest the legs on this - be sure to contract the thighs vigorously, pulling the knee caps up.

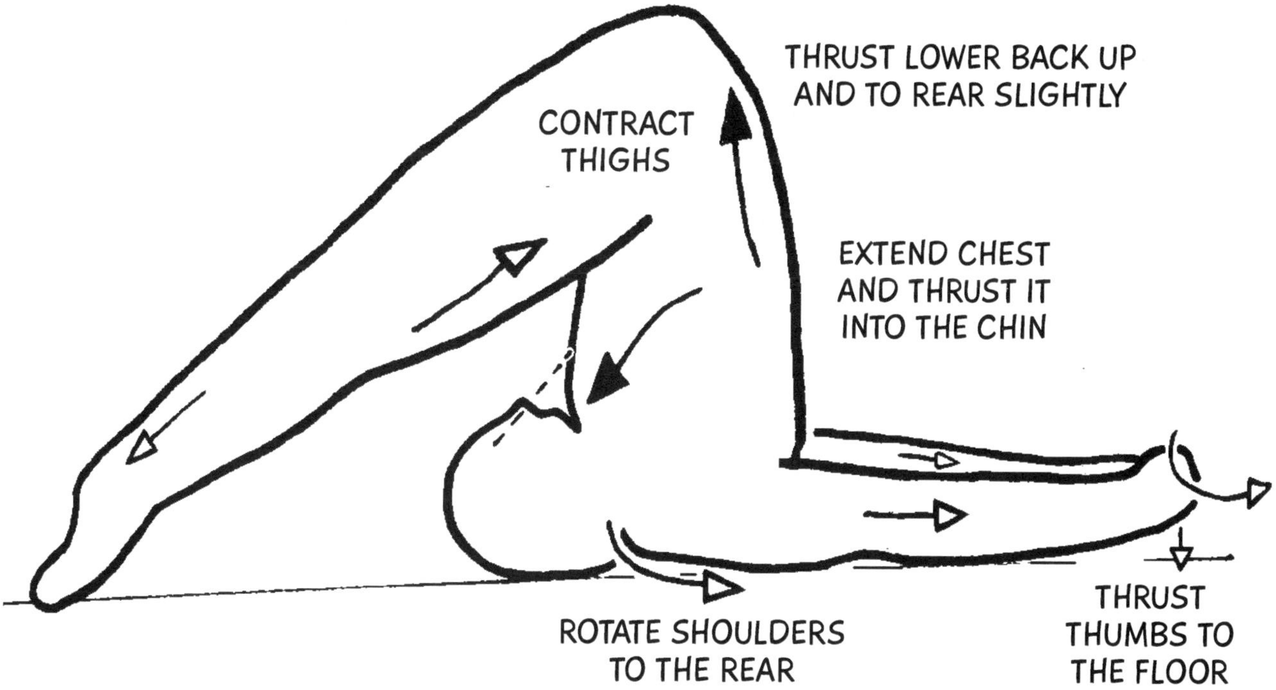
THRUST LOWER BACK UP AND TO REAR SLIGHTLY
CONTRACT THIGHS
EXTEND CHEST AND THRUST IT INTO THE CHIN
ROTATE SHOULDERS TO THE REAR
THRUST THUMBS TO THE FLOOR

Note: When returning to the floor from Halasana, extend the arms straight back on the floor, and lower the body very slowly. Keep the back of the neck thrust toward the floor throughout this transition, i.e. don't allow the chin to rise, Eventually you'll be 'rolling' down to the floor vertebrae by vertebrae.

Jathara Parivartanasana 20s (30)

stomach turn around

Var: In the beginning, lower the legs only part way from perpendicular - and never lower them so far that they bend or that the shoulders leave the floor.

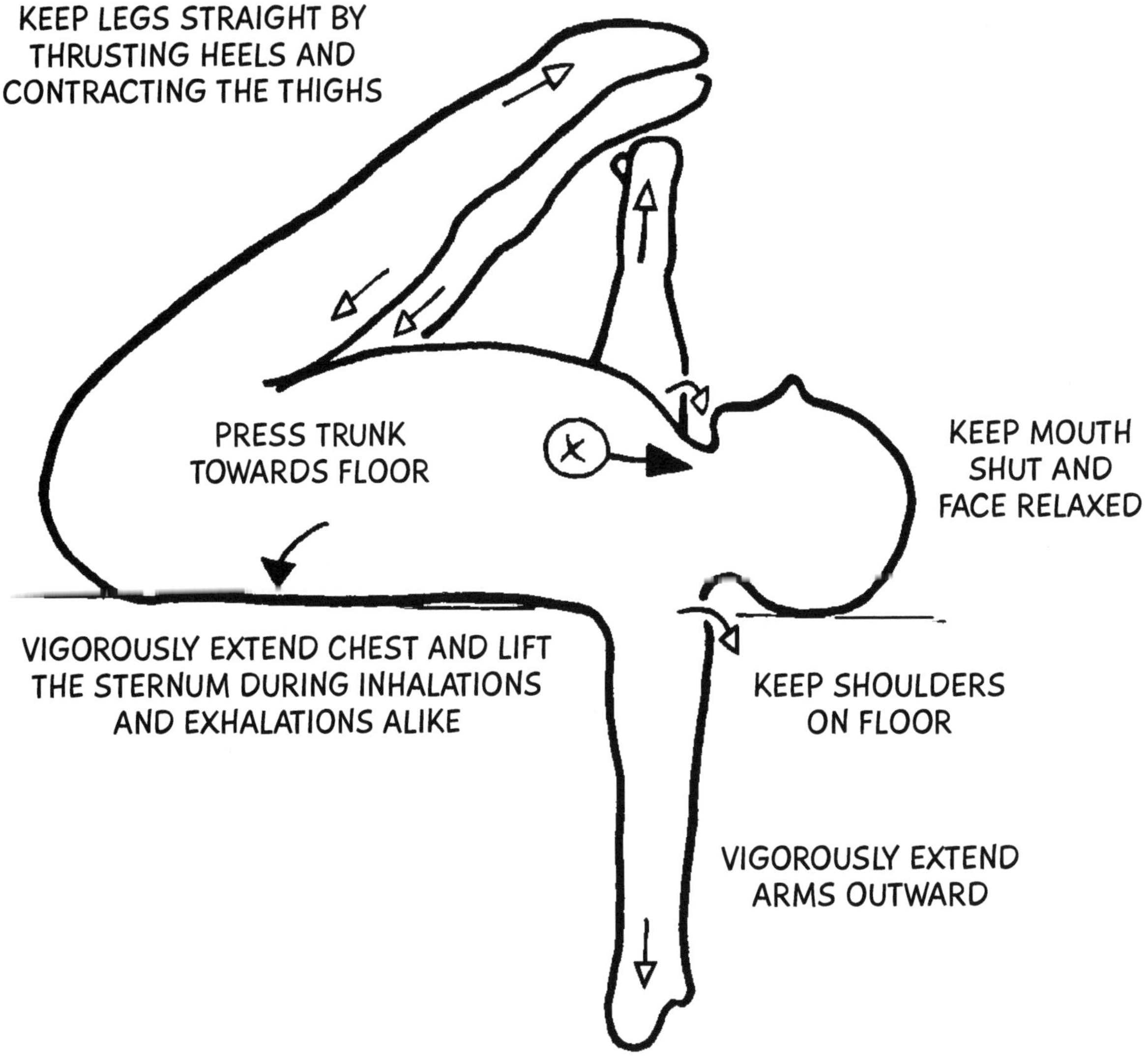

KEEP LEGS STRAIGHT BY THRUSTING HEELS AND CONTRACTING THE THIGHS
PRESS TRUNK TOWARDS FLOOR
KEEP MOUTH SHUT AND FACE RELAXED
VIGOROUSLY EXTEND CHEST AND LIFT THE STERNUM DURING INHALATIONS AND EXHALATIONS ALIKE
KEEP SHOULDERS ON FLOOR
VIGOROUSLY EXTEND ARMS OUTWARD

Note: Use the abdominal muscle to pull the feet toward the hand. Don't turn the head; hold the gaze downward at nose level and focused at infinity or 3-5' in front of you.

Again, for help in learning how to move into or out of the Yoga postures, take a Hatha Yoga class from a competent teacher and/or refer to **B.K.S, Iyengar's** most excellent book - *Light on Yoga*.

Paschimottanasana 1-5min (31)

west stretch

(see Lesson Index, page 177)

Var: If you can't grasp the toes, place the hand as far down on the leg as possible. You can also grasp a short rope, looped around the feet, and pull the trunk forward. In any case, concentrate on extending the chest and keeping the legs straight.

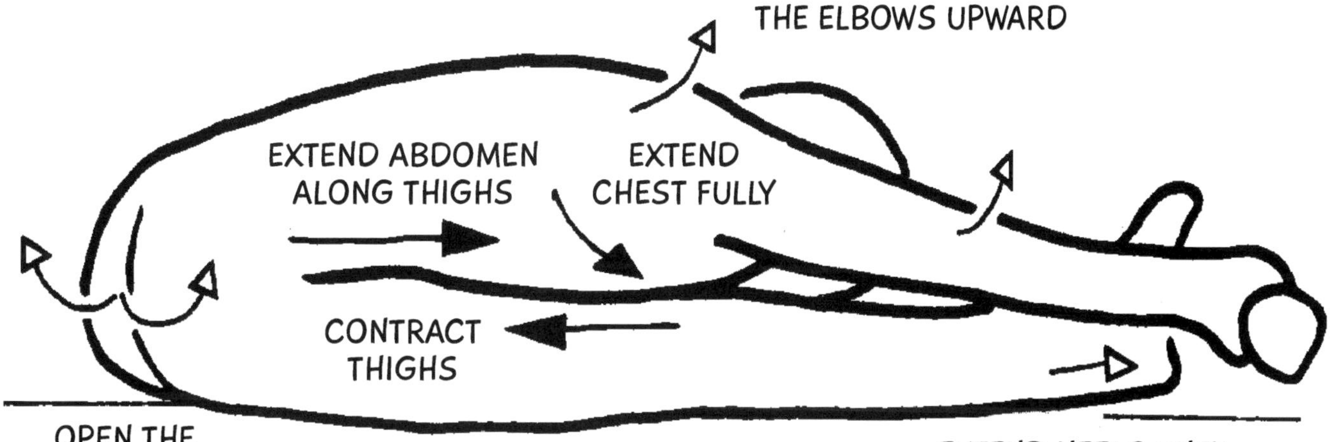
LIFT THE SHOULDERS AND THE ELBOWS UPWARD
EXTEND ABDOMEN ALONG THIGHS
EXTEND CHEST FULLY
CONTRACT THIGHS
OPEN THE BUTTOCKS
EXTEND HEELS UNTIL THEY RISE SLIGHTLY OFF THE FLOOR

Note: Begin by pulling the fleshy part of the buttocks outward from under the pelvis. This allows you to bring more of the lower front of the pelvic bone in firm contact with the floor.

In this and other forward bends, vigorously lift the sternum and thrust the chest forward on the inhalations. On the exhalations strive to bend forward a little more each time. Bend as little as possible from the upper spine. Instead bend from the lowest part of the spine (lumbar vertebrae).

Gently rotate the head upward slightly and with the gaze at nose level, look out beyond the feet throughout the posture. Later, when you can lay the trunk on the legs, rest the forehead on the shins.

To encourage bending from the lower spine, extend the arms straight out, level with the toes, instead of grasping your hands or wrist. Simply thrust your arms forward as far as they can go. You are effectively reaching to touch the wall beyond your reach!

Ardha Baddha Padma Paschimottanasana 30-60s (32)

half bound lotus west stretch

(see Lesson Index, page 177)

Var.: Instead of grasping the toe of the bent leg, extend this arm along the straight leg (next to the other arm).

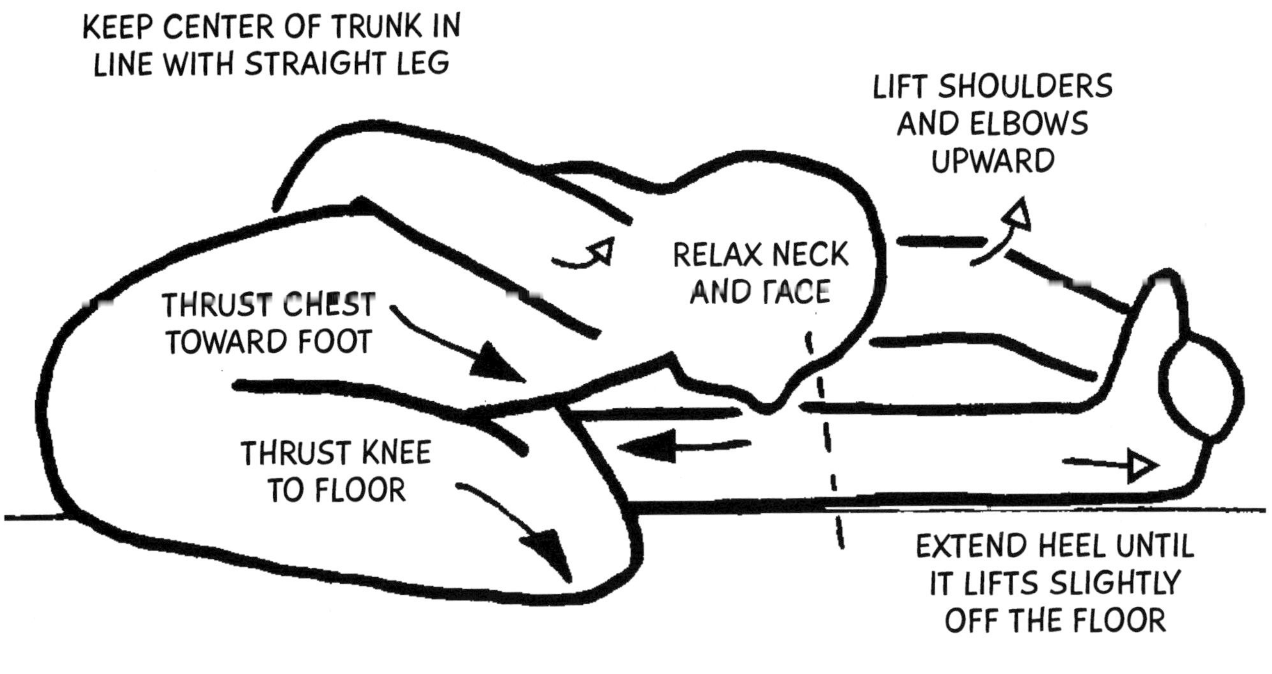
KEEP CENTER OF TRUNK IN LINE WITH STRAIGHT LEG
LIFT SHOULDERS AND ELBOWS UPWARD
RELAX NECK AND FACE
THRUST CHEST TOWARD FOOT
THRUST KNEE TO FLOOR
EXTEND HEEL UNTIL IT LIFTS SLIGHTLY OFF THE FLOOR

Note: Don't bob up and down as in calisthenics to get a deeper bend. Instead extend the trunk forward continuously, going a little further with each exhalation.

Baddha Konasana 30-60s (33)

bound angle

(see Lesson Index, page 177)

Var: Before you begin bending the trunk forward, practice extending the chest and trunk upward and keep arms straight. Then gradually 'surrender' yourself into the bend.

Note: In this or in any other variation you do, try to eliminate the variation as soon as possible and do the posture as near to what is shown as possible.

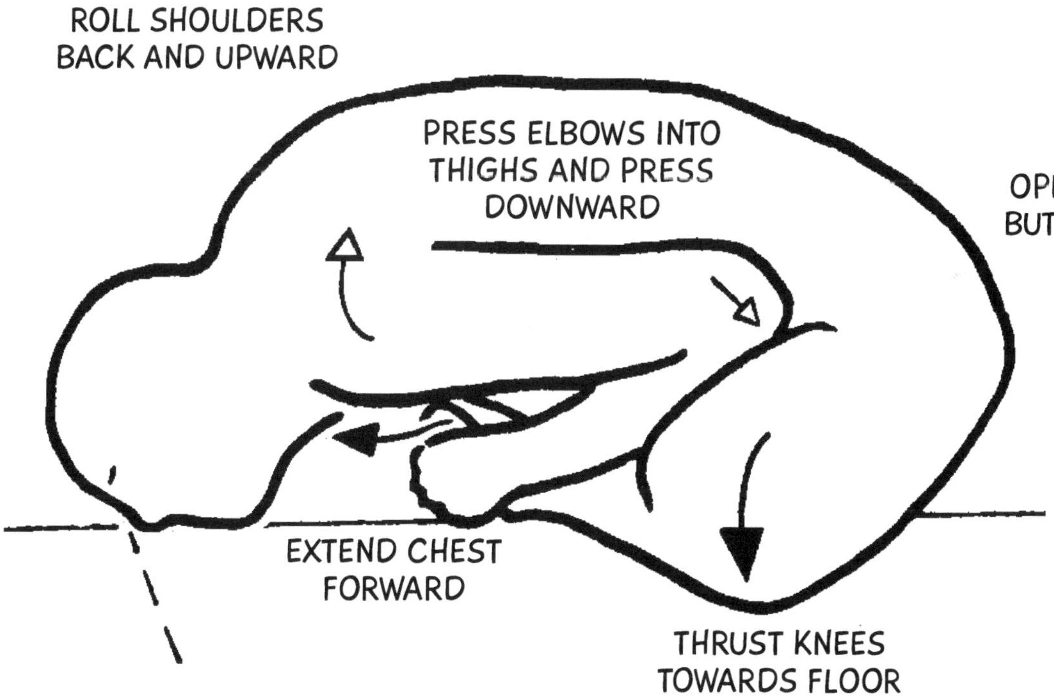
ROLL SHOULDERS BACK AND UPWARD
PRESS ELBOWS INTO THIGHS AND PRESS DOWNWARD
OPEN THE BUTTOCKS
EXTEND CHEST FORWARD
THRUST KNEES TOWARDS FLOOR

Bharadvajasana II 30-60s (34)

father of Drona

(see Lesson Index, page 177)

Var: Loop a rope around foot of bent leg and grasp it with bent arm and pull.

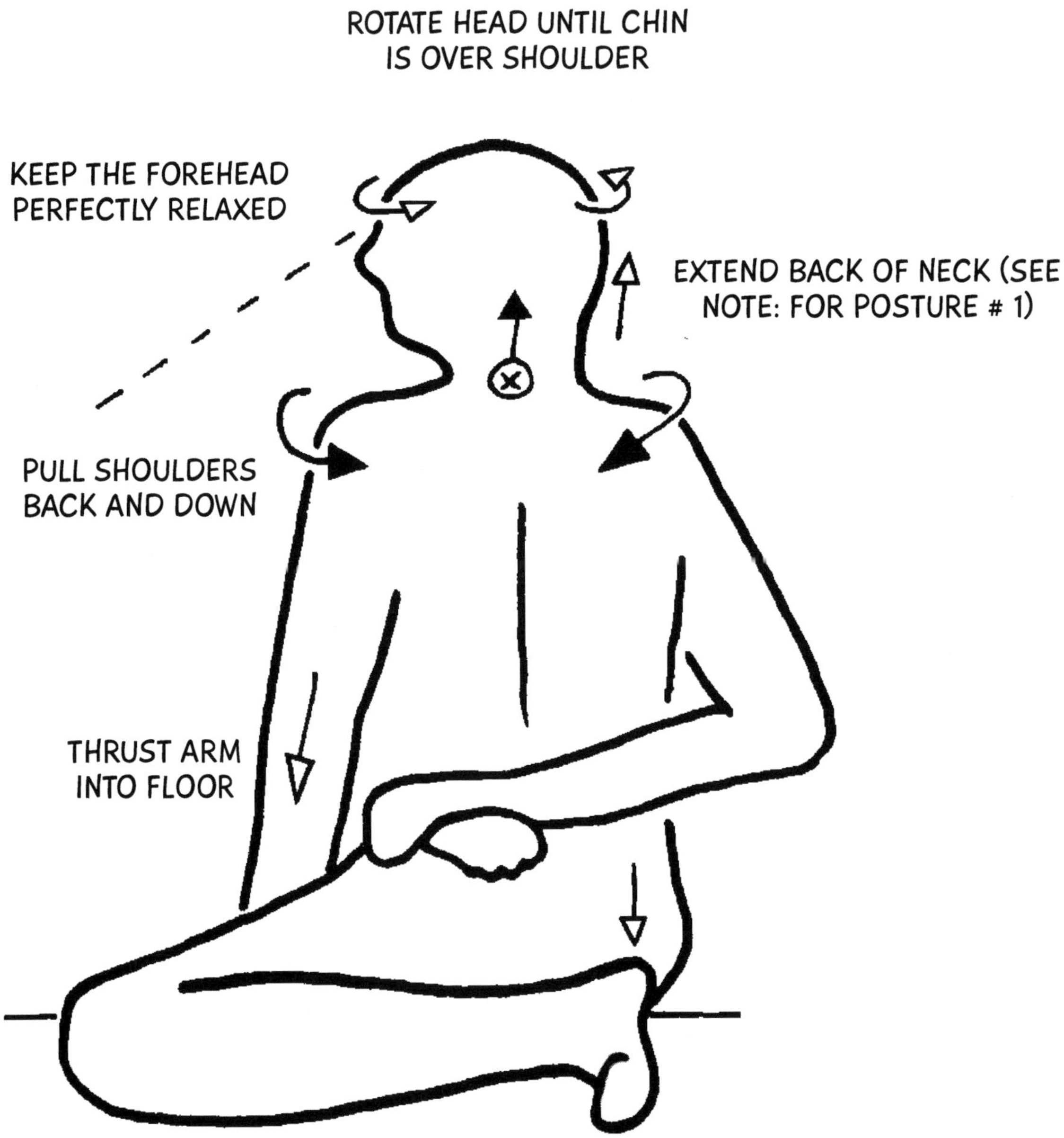
ROTATE HEAD UNTIL CHIN IS OVER SHOULDER
KEEP THE FOREHEAD PERFECTLY RELAXED
EXTEND BACK OF NECK (SEE NOTE: FOR POSTURE # 1)
PULL SHOULDERS BACK AND DOWN
THRUST ARM INTO FLOOR

Note: In this and other twist postures, avoid looking out of the side of your eyes when rotating your head side ways. Instead look straight ahead.

Marichyasana III 30-60s (35)

son of Brahma

(see Lesson Index, page 177)

Var: Instead of bending arm around bent leg, extend it past the bent knee and grasp the shin. Place the rear arm to the rear a few inches from the hip.

In twist postures you can place a folded blanket under the buttocks to help thrust the trunk forward.

Any variations or props you use for a postures should be eliminated as soon as possible.

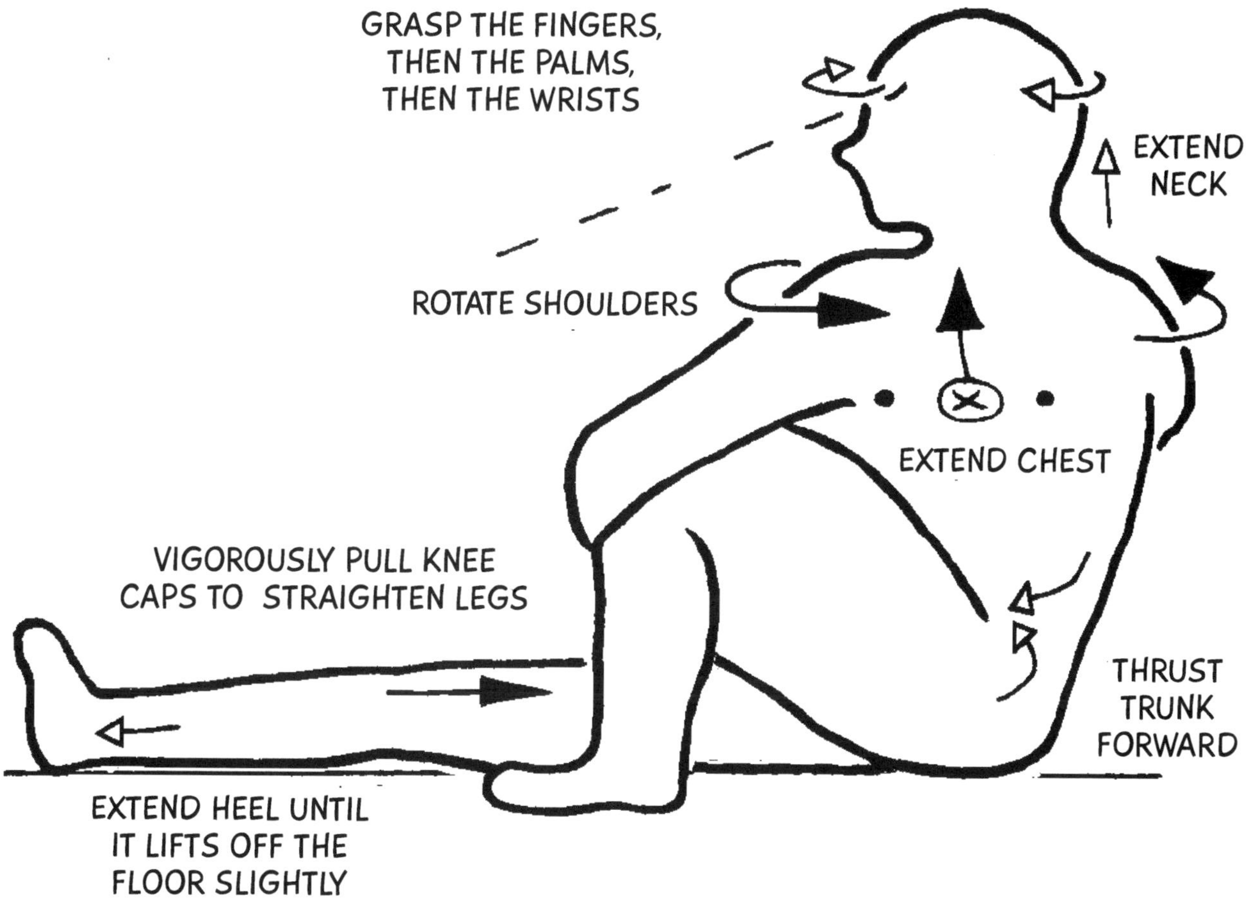
GRASP THE FINGERS, THEN THE PALMS, THEN THE WRISTS
EXTEND NECK
ROTATE SHOULDERS
EXTEND CHEST
VIGOROUSLY PULL KNEE CAPS TO STRAIGHTEN LEGS
THRUST TRUNK FORWARD
EXTEND HEEL UNTIL IT LIFTS OFF THE FLOOR SLIGHTLY

Note: In this and other twist postures where the arm is passed around a bent leg, press the back of the arm-pit as firmly into the lower thigh as possible.

In twisting postures, you always bring as much of the trunk (chest and abdomen) to one side of the leg (or body) as possible.

Ardha Matsyendrasana I 30-60s (36)

a founder of Yoga

(see Lesson Index, page 177)

Var: Instead of sitting on the ankle, move this ankle outward and sit on the floor. Also, similar to Marichyasana III [35], you can take the bent arm and instead, extend it straight and grasp the forward ankle (or knee).

It helps to lift your truck slightly off the floor and vigorously thrust it forward, then reaching around the leg, grasp as much of the other hand (if any) as possible.

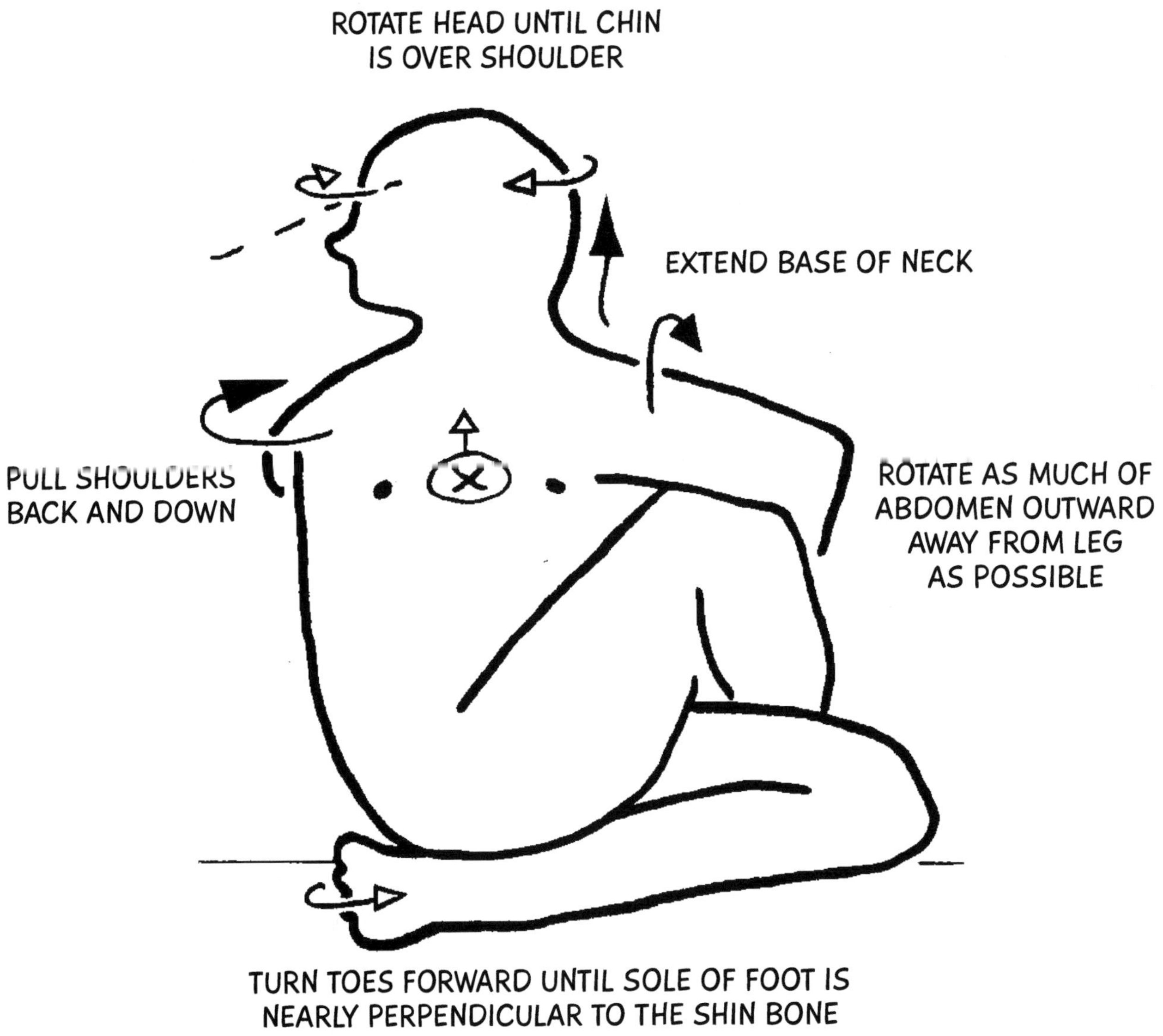
ROTATE HEAD UNTIL CHIN IS OVER SHOULDER
EXTEND BASE OF NECK
PULL SHOULDERS BACK AND DOWN
ROTATE AS MUCH OF ABDOMEN OUTWARD AWAY FROM LEG AS POSSIBLE
TURN TOES FORWARD UNTIL SOLE OF FOOT IS NEARLY PERPENDICULAR TO THE SHIN BONE

Note: Press the back of the arm-pit as firmly into the thigh as possible. Avoid looking out of the side of your eyes when rotating your head side ways. Instead look straight ahead with gaze held at nose level and focused towards infinity.

Dhanurasana 20-60s (37)

bow

(see Lesson Index, page 177)

Note: First lift the chest, and then on the next exhalation lift the legs with the knees apart 18" or so. When you reach your maximum bend, pull the knees in toward each other while maintaining as much bend as possible.

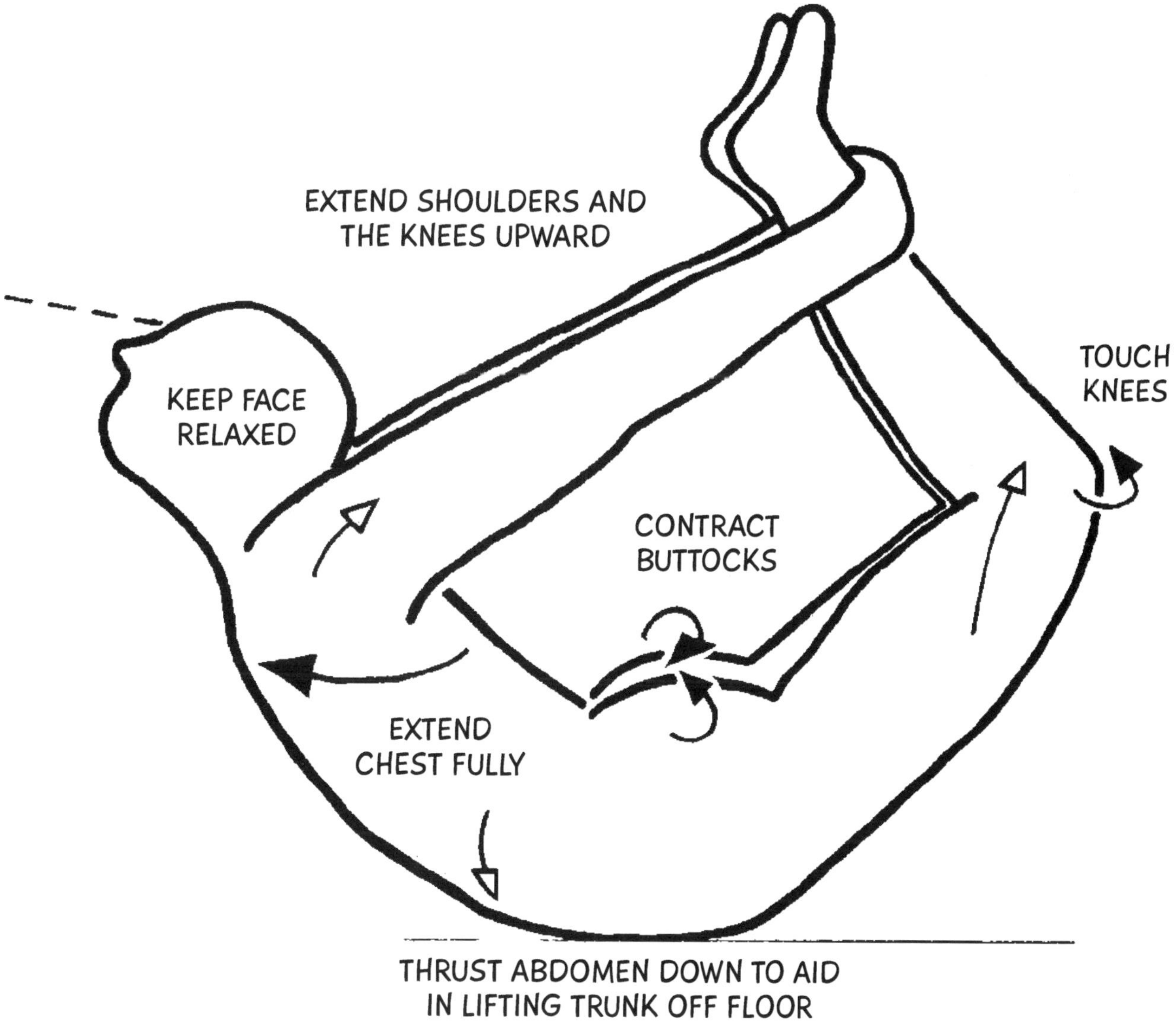

EXTEND SHOULDERS AND THE KNEES UPWARD
KEEP FACE RELAXED
TOUCH KNEES
CONTRACT BUTTOCKS
EXTEND CHEST FULLY
THRUST ABDOMEN DOWN TO AID IN LIFTING TRUNK OFF FLOOR

Virasana IV 1-5min (38)

hero

(see Lesson Index, page 177)

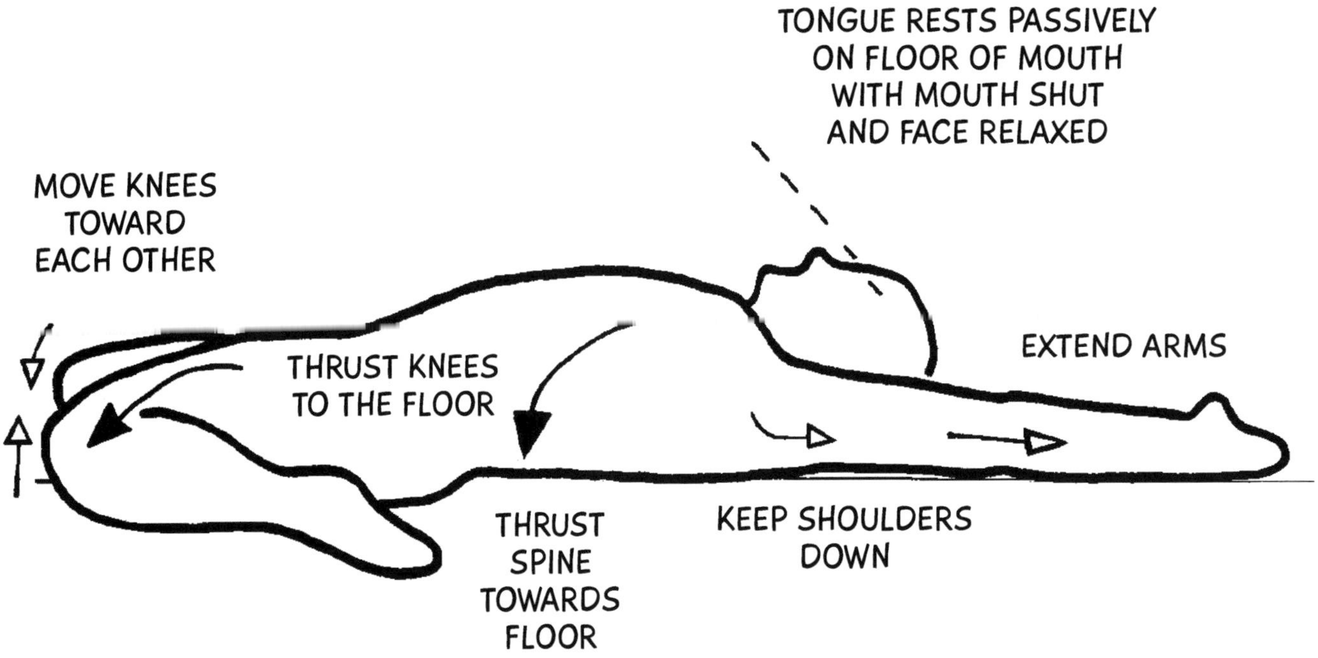
TONGUE RESTS PASSIVELY ON FLOOR OF MOUTH WITH MOUTH SHUT AND FACE RELAXED
MOVE KNEES TOWARD EACH OTHER
THRUST KNEES TO THE FLOOR
EXTEND ARMS
THRUST SPINE TOWARDS FLOOR
KEEP SHOULDERS DOWN

Note: In this and most other postures in this manual, the eyes are held at nose level. This means the eyes gaze downward past the tip of the nose. The focus of the eyes is either at infinity or 3-5' in front of you (not cross-eyed or focus on the tip of the nose). You can occasionally close the eye lids momentarily to help keep the muscles around the eyes relaxed totally.

Siddhasana 30-60s+ (39)

semi divine

(see Lesson Index, page 177)

Var: Instead of putting right foot on left calf, you can place this foot on the floor in front of the calf. Practice this posture or Padmasana as much as possible in your daily life, i.e. while eating, reading, watching T.V., etc.

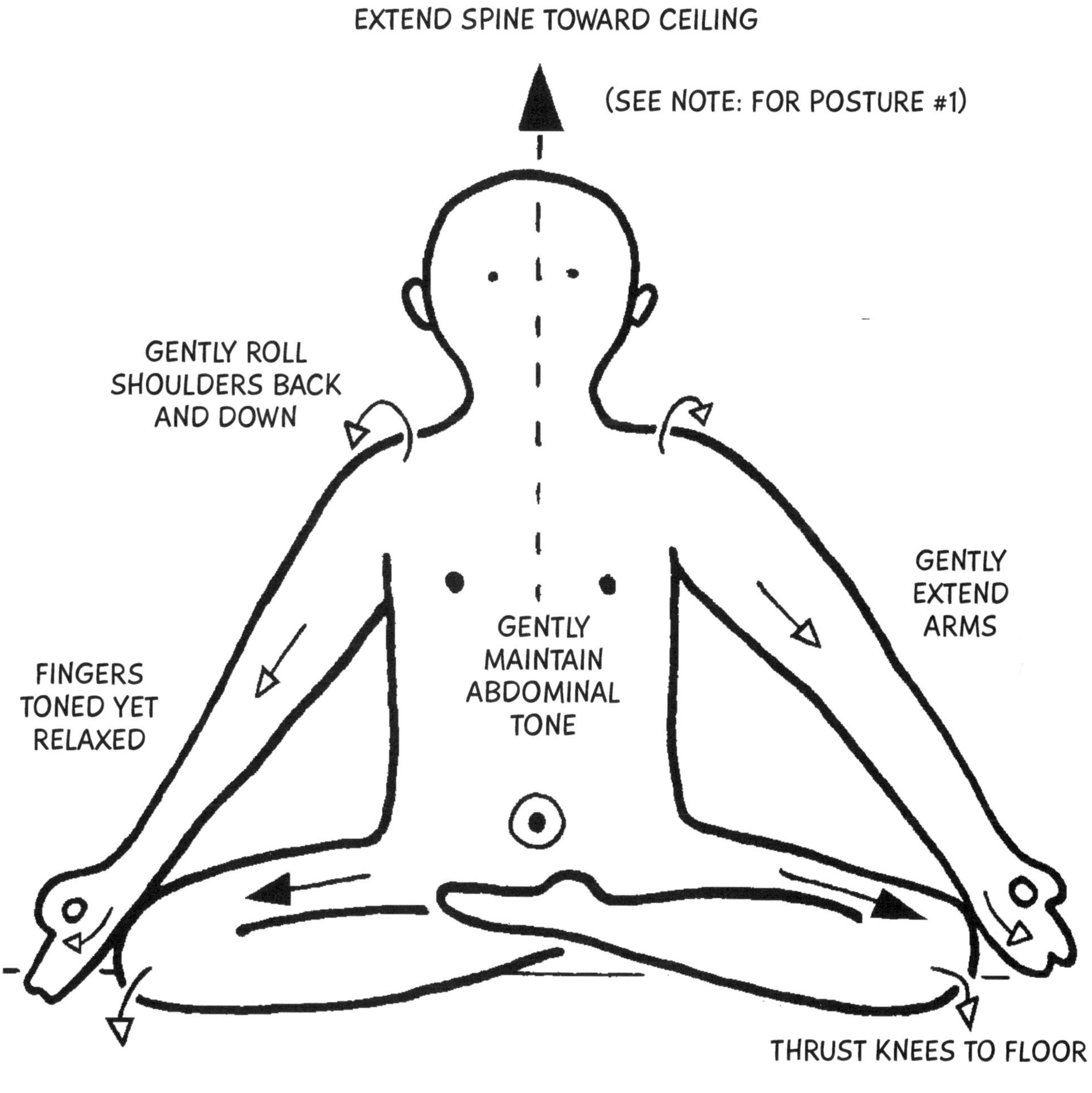

EXTEND SPINE TOWARD CEILING
(SEE NOTE: FOR POSTURE #1)
GENTLY ROLL SHOULDERS BACK AND DOWN
GENTLY EXTEND ARMS
GENTLY MAINTAIN ABDOMINAL TONE
FINGERS TONED YET RELAXED
THRUST KNEES TO FLOOR

Thumb and forefinger are held less than a hairs' width apart - on the edge of sensation. Deviation from this during meditation indicates a drifting, non-presence of mind.

Padmasana I, II 30-60s (40)

lotus

(see Lesson Index, page 177)

Var: Instead of interlocking the legs, place the left foot on the floor and then place the right foot on the left thigh. (then visa versa)

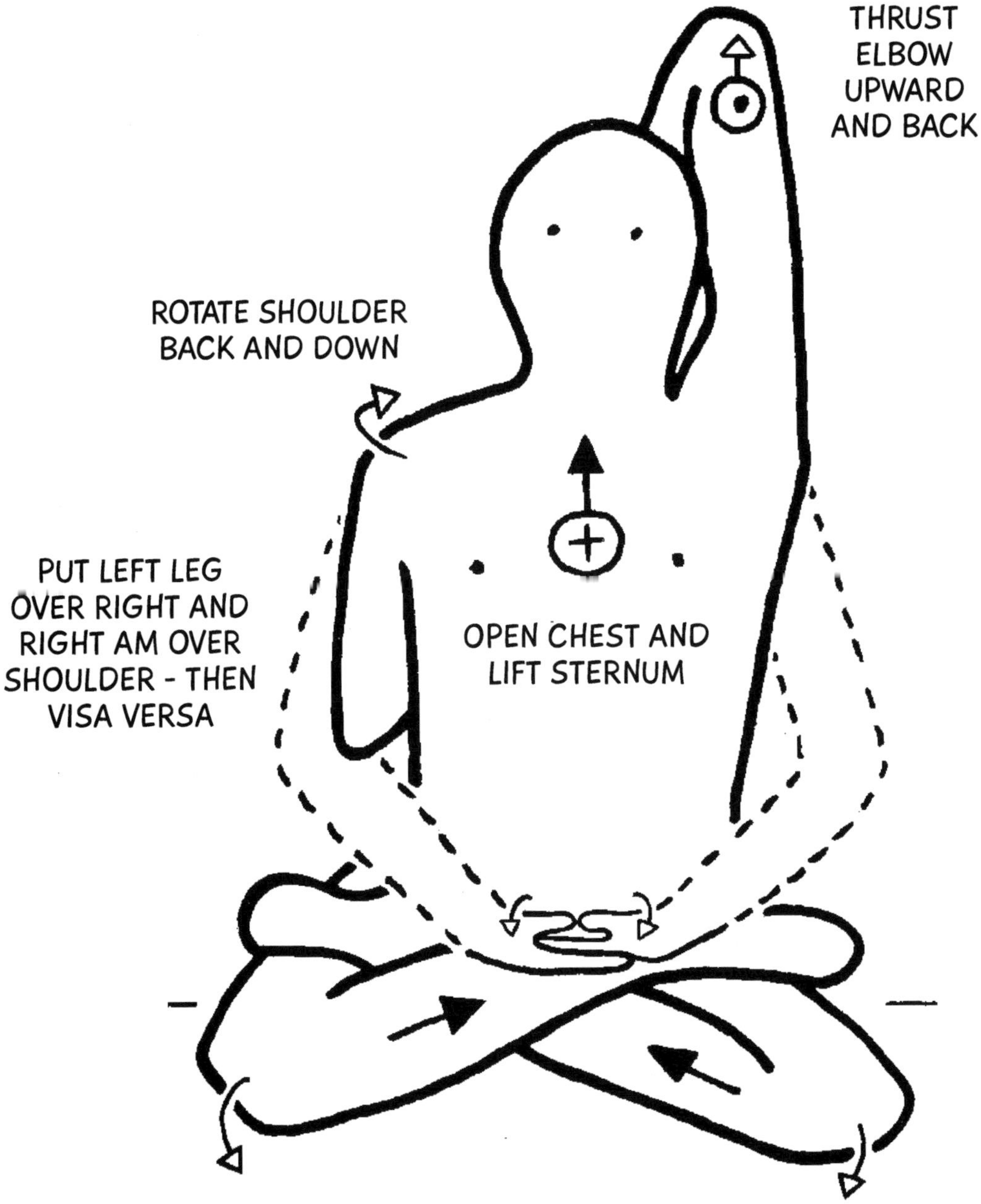
THRUST
ELBOW
UPWARD
AND BACK
ROTATE SHOULDER
BACK AND DOWN
PUT LEFT LEG
OVER RIGHT AND
RIGHT AM OVER
SHOULDER - THEN
VISA VERSA
OPEN CHEST AND
LIFT STERNUM

Note: Once this becomes fairly comfortable, strive to bring the feet up onto the thigh as high as possible, until the ankles rest on the upper part of the thighs. This produces a very firm interlocking of the legs. Obviously, don't force this on your legs and knees before they are ready!

Tolasana 60s (41)

scales

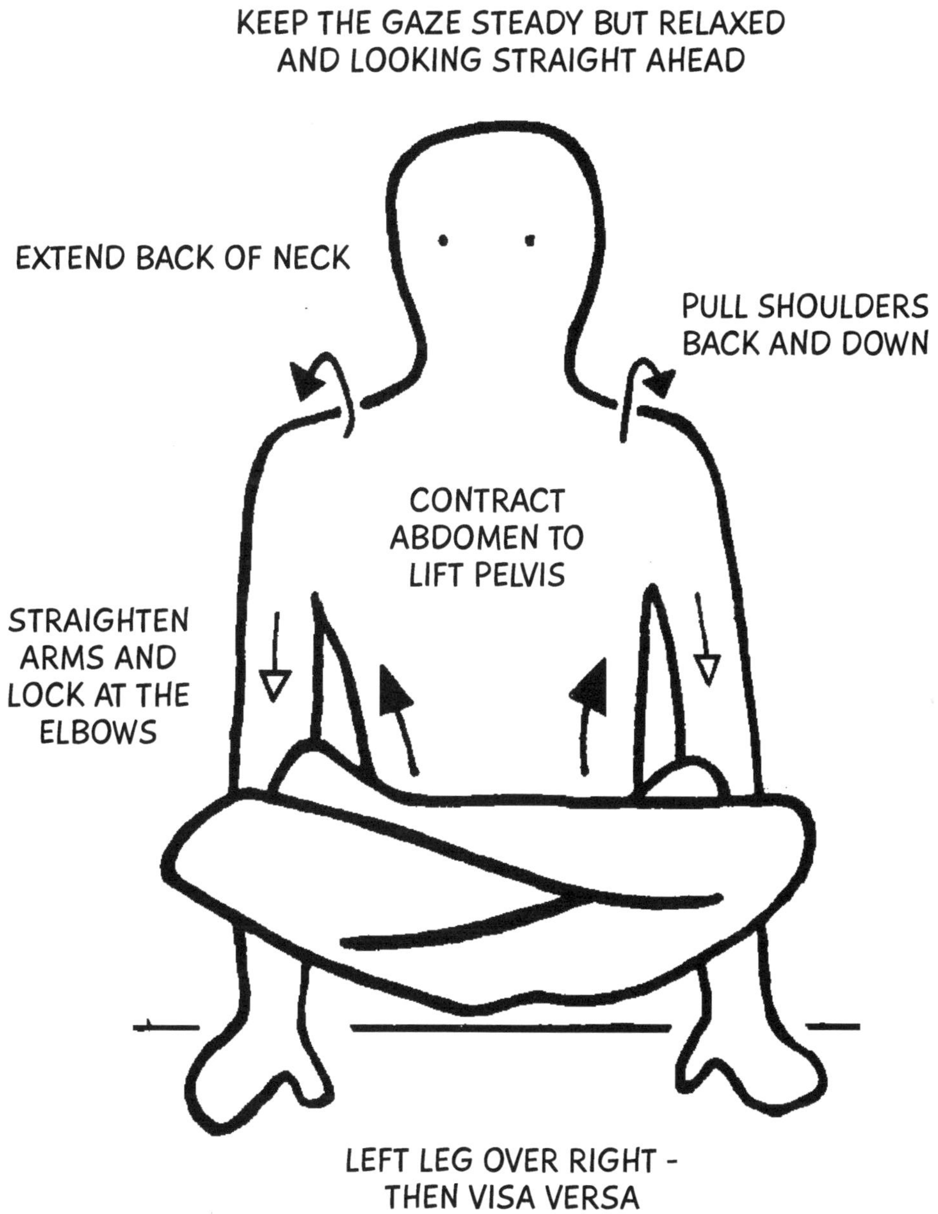
KEEP THE GAZE STEADY BUT RELAXED AND LOOKING STRAIGHT AHEAD
EXTEND BACK OF NECK
PULL SHOULDERS BACK AND DOWN
CONTRACT ABDOMEN TO LIFT PELVIS
STRAIGHTEN ARMS AND LOCK AT THE ELBOWS
LEFT LEG OVER RIGHT - THEN VISA VERSA

Matsyasana 30-60s (42)

fish

(see Lesson Index, page 177)

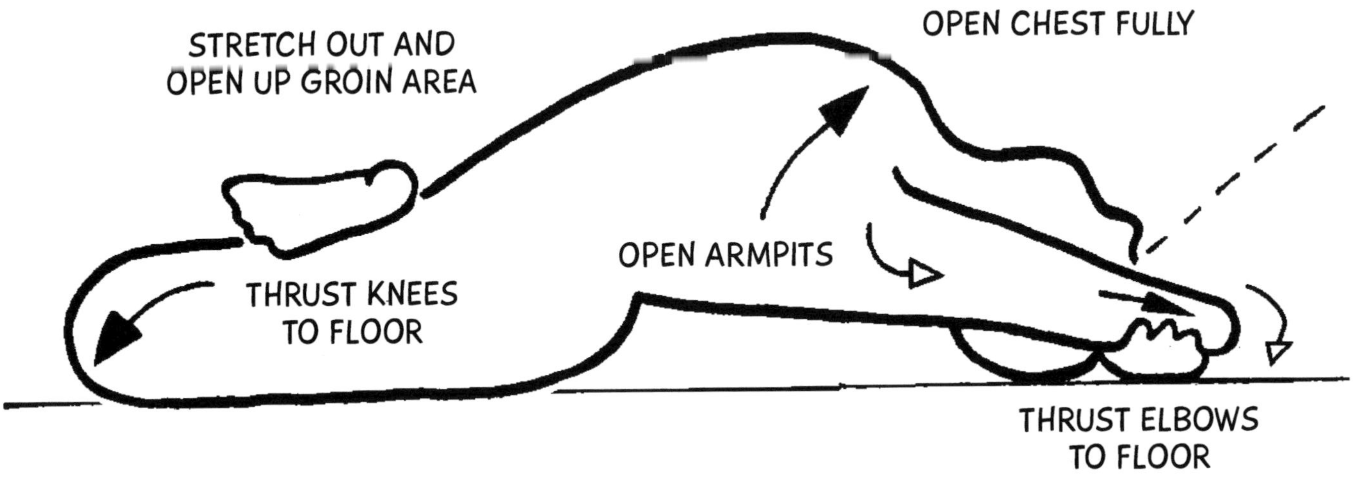

STRETCH OUT AND OPEN UP GROIN AREA
OPEN CHEST FULLY
OPEN ARMPITS
THRUST KNEES TO FLOOR
THRUST ELBOWS TO FLOOR

AS IN ALL POSTURES, THE TONGUE RESTS PASSIVELY ON THE FLOOR OF THE MOUTH - WITH THE FOREHEAD AND THE REST OF THE FACE PERFECTLY RELAXED.

Ardha Chandrasana 20-30s **43)**

half moon

(see Lesson Index, page 177)

Var: Do this posture with the back to a wall. Rotate the upper trunk backward and press the upper hip and shoulder into the wall.

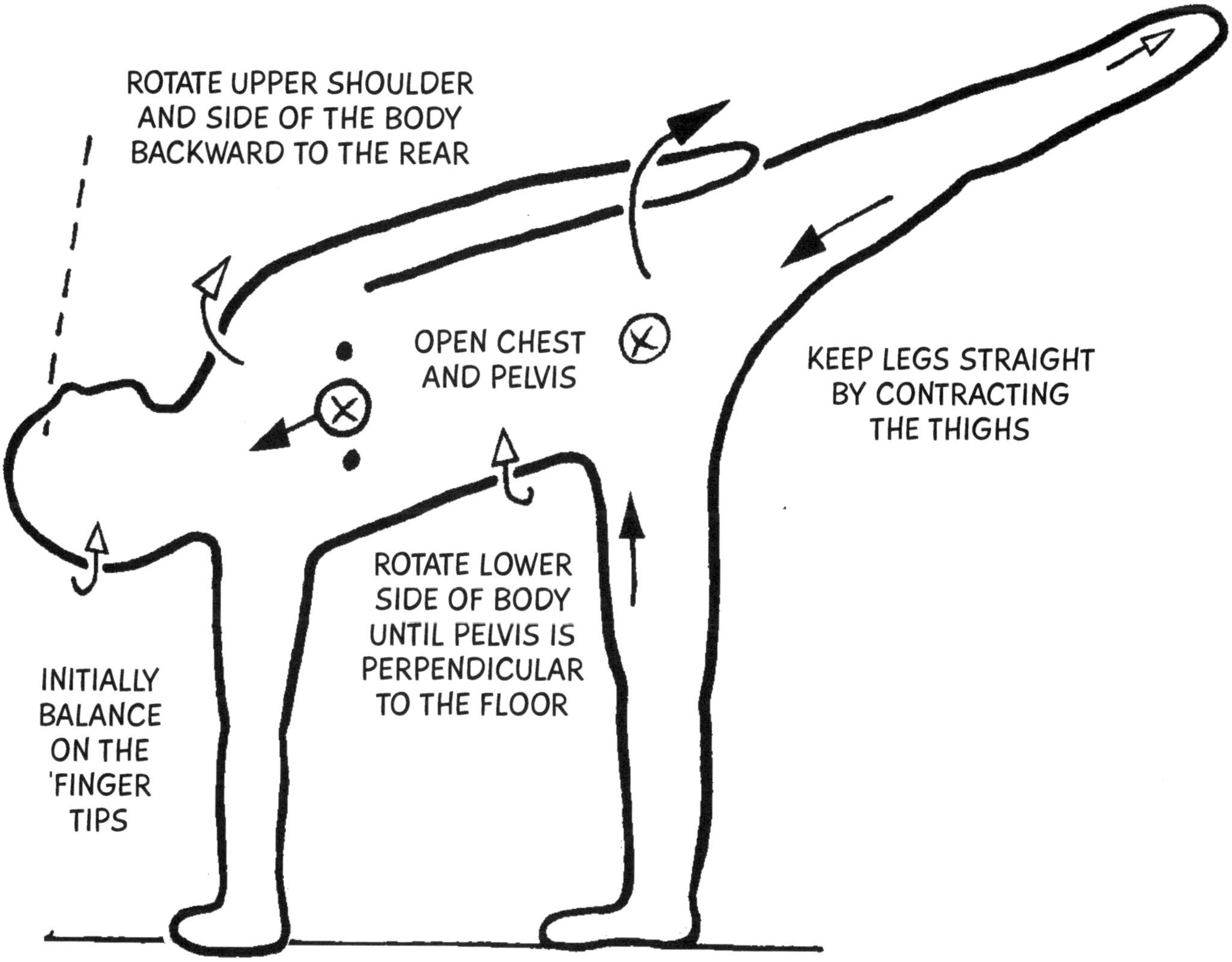

ROTATE UPPER SHOULDER AND SIDE OF THE BODY BACKWARD TO THE REAR
OPEN CHEST AND PELVIS
KEEP LEGS STRAIGHT BY CONTRACTING THE THIGHS
ROTATE LOWER SIDE OF BODY UNTIL PELVIS IS PERPENDICULAR TO THE FLOOR
INITIALLY BALANCE ON THE 'FINGER TIPS

Note: First do TRIKONASANA UTTHITA. Bend knee and place hand 18" in front of front foot and then lift rear leg. Keep the upper side of the body rotating backward at all times. Concentrate on pulling the knee caps on the lower leg upward vigorously. Keep the ankle firm and imagine that your foot is a root extending down into the floor.

For an added challenge after hold this, rotate the body parallel to the floor and extend the arms straight out like you're an airplane. Then continue the rotation, twisting around, until the other hand rests on the floor.

Parivrtta Parsvakonasana 20-60s (44)

revolved side angle

(see Lesson Index, page 177)

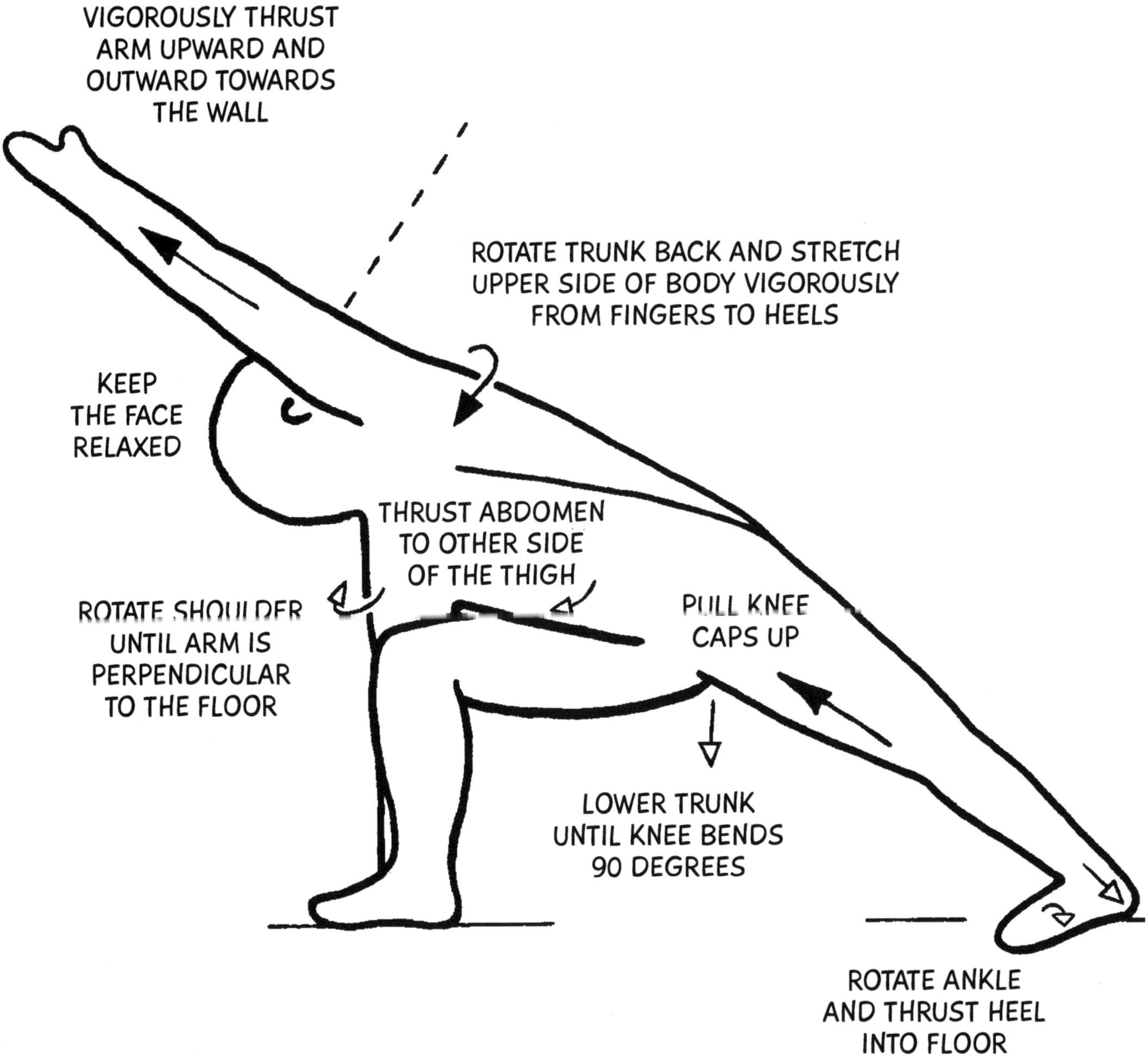

VIGOROUSLY THRUST ARM UPWARD AND OUTWARD TOWARDS THE WALL
ROTATE TRUNK BACK AND STRETCH UPPER SIDE OF BODY VIGOROUSLY FROM FINGERS TO HEELS
KEEP THE FACE RELAXED
THRUST ABDOMEN TO OTHER SIDE OF THE THIGH
ROTATE SHOULDER UNTIL ARM IS PERPENDICULAR TO THE FLOOR
PULL KNEE CAPS UP
LOWER TRUNK UNTIL KNEE BENDS 90 DEGREES
ROTATE ANKLE AND THRUST HEEL INTO FLOOR

Var: You may let the rear heel lift off the floor. This is an intense twisting standing posture combination which demands all the rotation and extention you can muster. Recall the two giants pulling you apart earlier on.

Utthita Hasta Padangusthasana 30s (45)

extended hand leg-toe

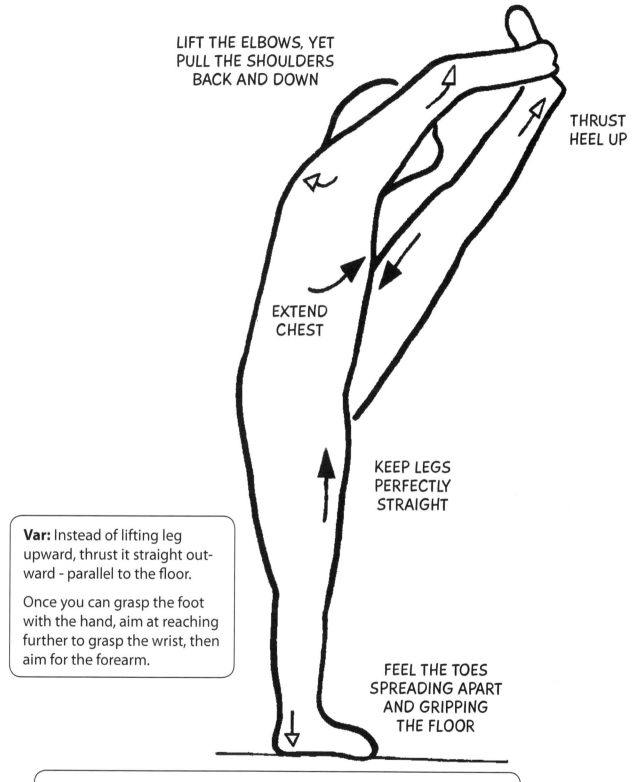

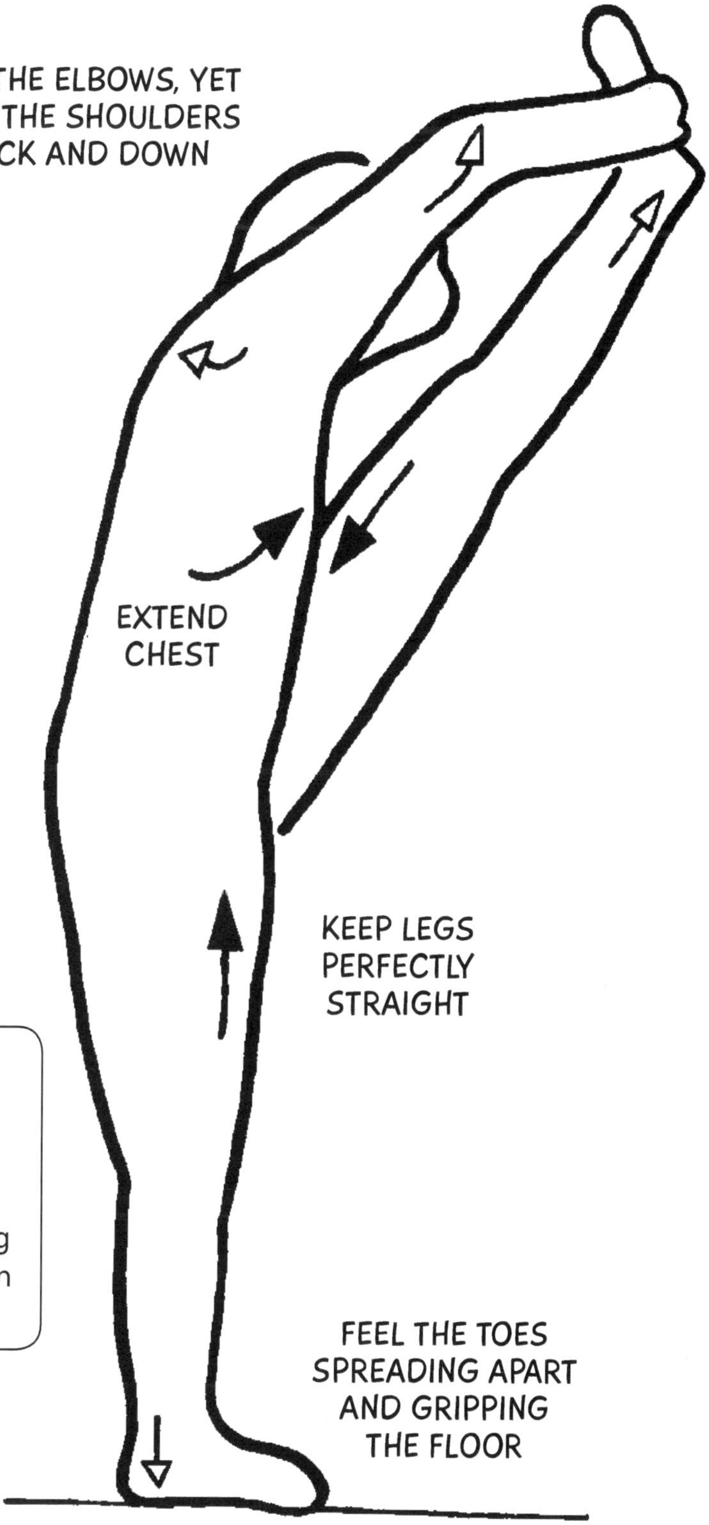
LIFT THE ELBOWS, YET PULL THE SHOULDERS BACK AND DOWN
THRUST HEEL UP
EXTEND CHEST
KEEP LEGS PERFECTLY STRAIGHT
FEEL THE TOES SPREADING APART AND GRIPPING THE FLOOR

Var: Instead of lifting leg upward, thrust it straight outward - parallel to the floor.

Once you can grasp the foot with the hand, aim at reaching further to grasp the wrist, then aim for the forearm.

Note: In this and all postures where you balance on one leg, concentrate primarily on keeping this lower leg perfectly straight by pulling the knee caps upward vigorously. Also keeping the ankle firm and feeling it rooted to the floor will increase stability and balance greatly.

Parigasana 20-60s (46)

gate cross beam

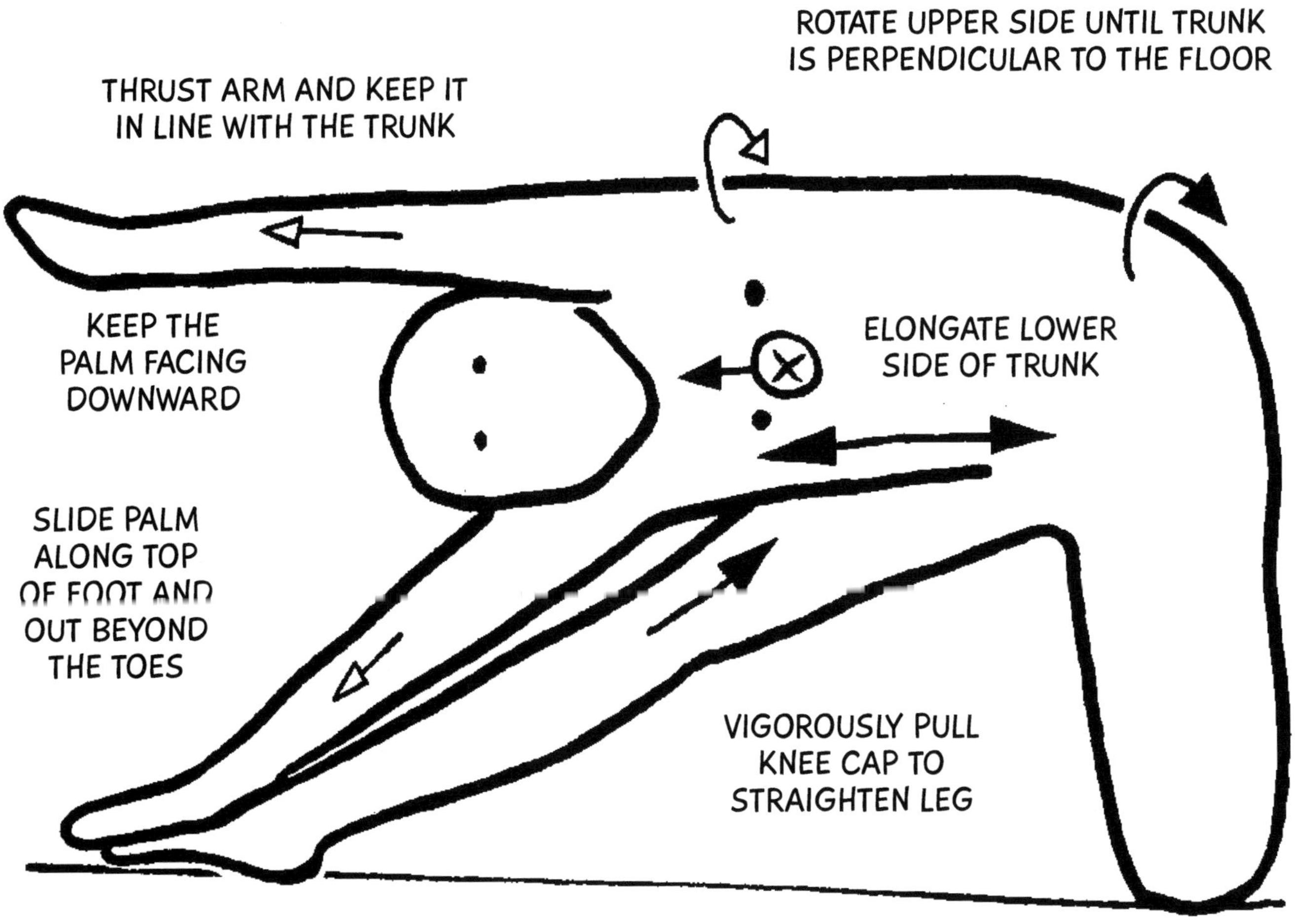
ROTATE UPPER SIDE UNTIL TRUNK
IS PERPENDICULAR TO THE FLOOR
THRUST ARM AND KEEP IT
IN LINE WITH THE TRUNK
KEEP THE
PALM FACING
DOWNWARD
ELONGATE LOWER
SIDE OF TRUNK
SLIDE PALM
ALONG TOP
OF FOOT AND
OUT BEYOND
THE TOES
VIGOROUSLY PULL
KNEE CAP TO
STRAIGHTEN LEG

Note: On each' inhalation vigorously extend the chest and elongate the lower side of the trunk. Then on the exhalation, hold this elongation and strive to bend sideways a little further. Eventually you will extend your lower hand out beyond your foot bringing your trunk nearly flat on you outstretched leg.

Although as a beginner you began Hatha Yoga doing standing postures, they are among the most difficult of all the postures to perfect. You can only perfect these basic postures by going on to the more advanced postures. Well, that's not exactly right. More to the point, as strength and flexibility increase you 'advance' in order to remain a beginner. As you do so, you naturally bring more integrity to these 'beginner' postures. In a way, you are striving to always remain a beginner pushing against your limit. The advanced postures are merely a means of accomplishing this.

Pranayama (upright) 3-5min

nerve energy control

Var: Place a folded blanket under the buttocks to help keep the spine straight and the knees on the floor.

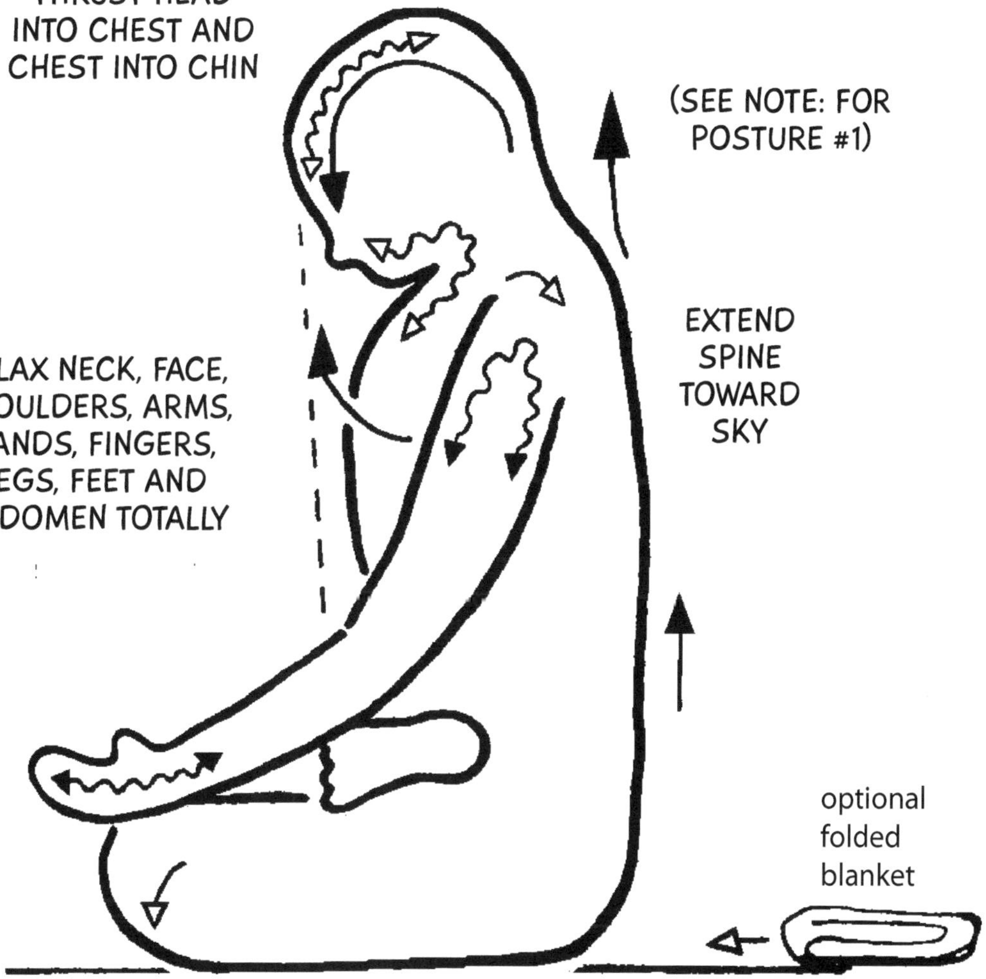
THRUST HEAD INTO CHEST AND CHEST INTO CHIN
(SEE NOTE: FOR POSTURE #1)
RELAX NECK, FACE, SHOULDERS, ARMS, HANDS, FINGERS, LEGS, FEET AND ABDOMEN TOTALLY
EXTEND SPINE TOWARD SKY
optional folded blanket

Note: In this formal Pranayama the chest (rib cage) in fully extended and the sternum is lifted upward during inhalations and exhalations alike. Breathing is accomplished with the diaphragm only. Except for the chin thrusting downward, this is the same thing which is done in most of the Hatha Yoga postures - however it takes years to perfect this.

Naturally, never force exhalations, i.e., by depressing chest and/or contracting air passage (or abdominal) areas. Instead, try to allow diaphragm to return to a completely relaxed and natural state.

Meditation 5 minutes minimum (48)

(see Lesson Index, page 177)

First mentally scan entire body to insure that it is symmetrical and relaxed (especially face and shoulders). Then watch the natural ebb and flow of the breath with the mantra 'SA-HA'. Mentally hear the sound 'SA' during your inhalations, and then the sound 'HA' during exhalations. Breath gently and evenly. Later you can try 'OM' and after that just silence the mind and watch.

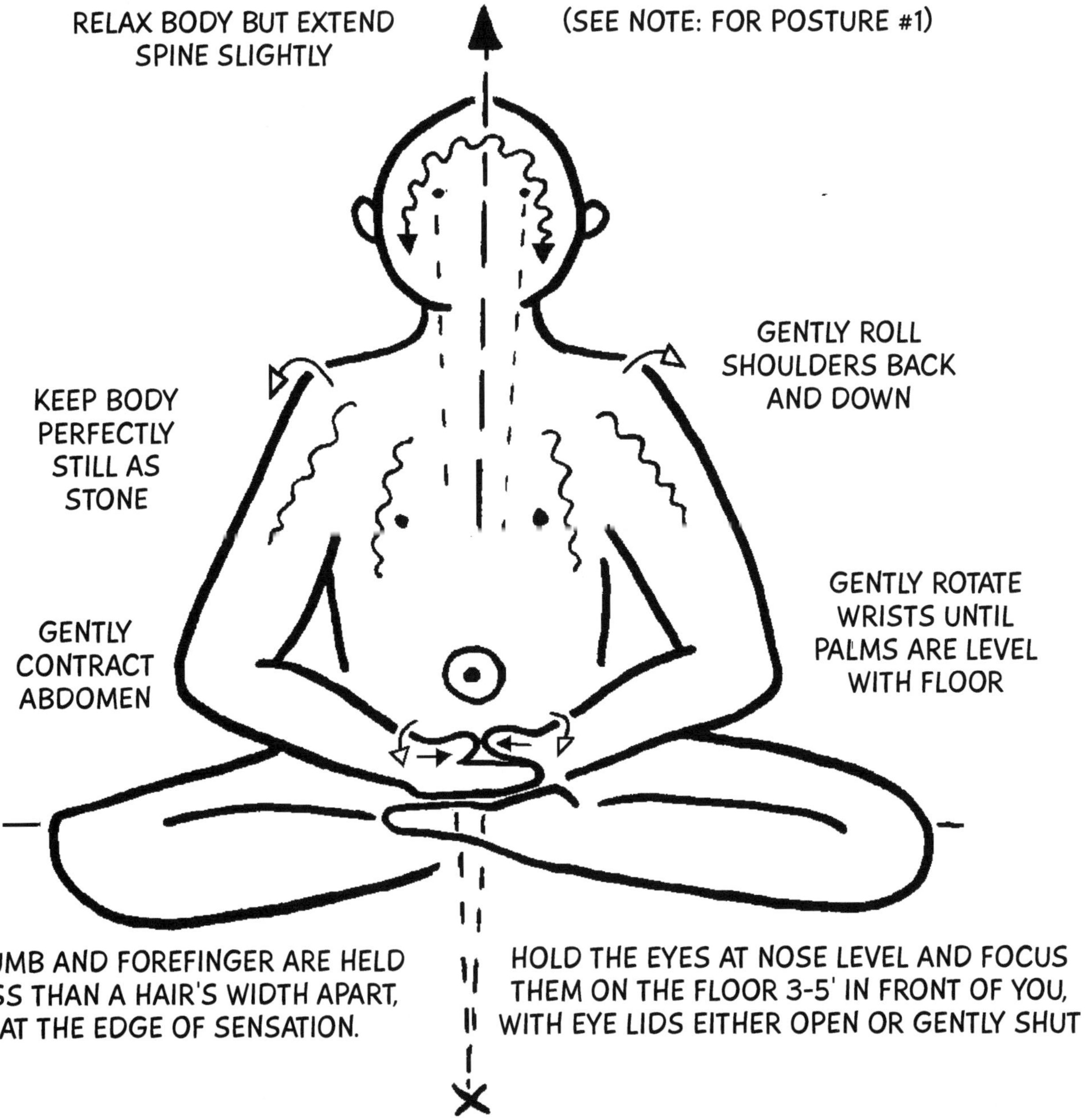

RELAX BODY BUT EXTEND SPINE SLIGHTLY
(SEE NOTE: FOR POSTURE #1)
KEEP BODY PERFECTLY STILL AS STONE
GENTLY ROLL SHOULDERS BACK AND DOWN
GENTLY CONTRACT ABDOMEN
GENTLY ROTATE WRISTS UNTIL PALMS ARE LEVEL WITH FLOOR
THUMB AND FOREFINGER ARE HELD LESS THAN A HAIR'S WIDTH APART, AT THE EDGE OF SENSATION.
HOLD THE EYES AT NOSE LEVEL AND FOCUS THEM ON THE FLOOR 3-5' IN FRONT OF YOU, WITH EYE LIDS EITHER OPEN OR GENTLY SHUT

Note: Breathing is accomplished with the diaphragm only. Naturally, never force breathing. Feel the diaphragm 'wax and wane' deep in the lower abdomen, relaxed and natural.

Lolasana 20-30s

dangling

Var: You can just lift the knees off the floor.

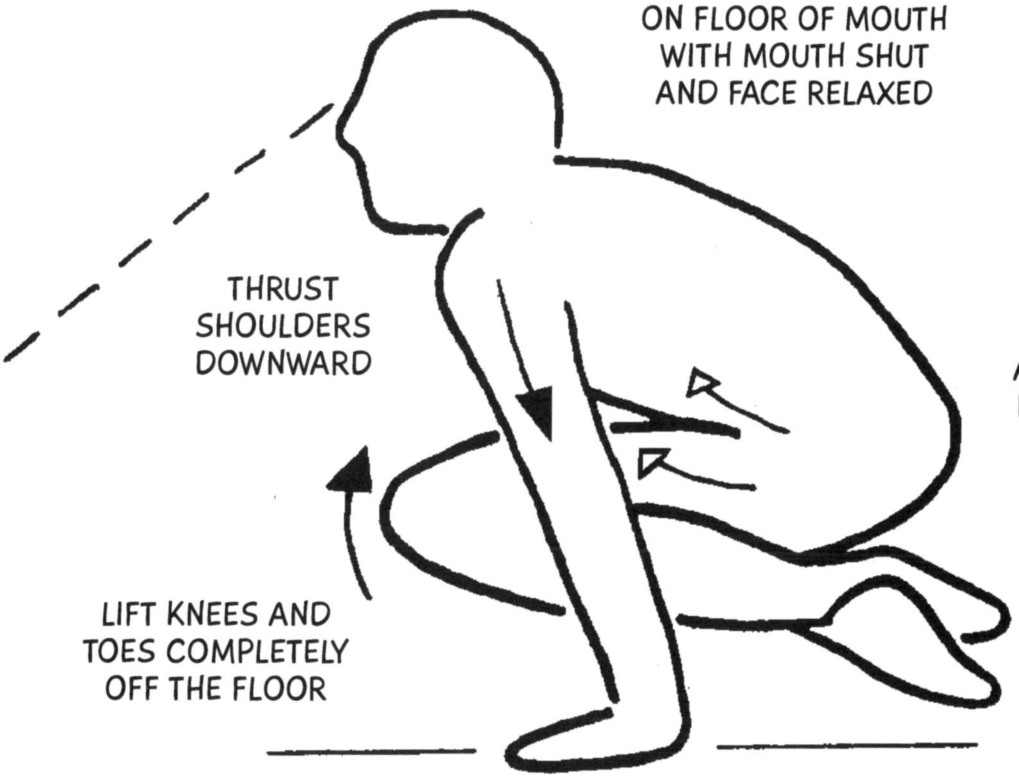
TONGUE RESTS PASSIVELY
ON FLOOR OF MOUTH
WITH MOUTH SHUT
AND FACE RELAXED
THRUST
SHOULDERS
DOWNWARD
CONTRACT
ABDOMEN TO
PROVIDE THE
LIFT NEEDED
LIFT KNEES AND
TOES COMPLETELY
OFF THE FLOOR

Note: In this or in any other variation you do, try to eliminate the variation as soon as possible and do the posture as near to what is shown as possible.

Paryankasana 60s (50)

couch

Note: In this and other postures, never use strained exhalations. Instead, allow diaphragm to relax naturally - while still keeping chest (rib cage) in fully extended and the sternum is lifted upward during inhalations and exhalations alike.

You can occasionally close the eye lids momentarily to help keep the muscles around the eyes relaxed totally.

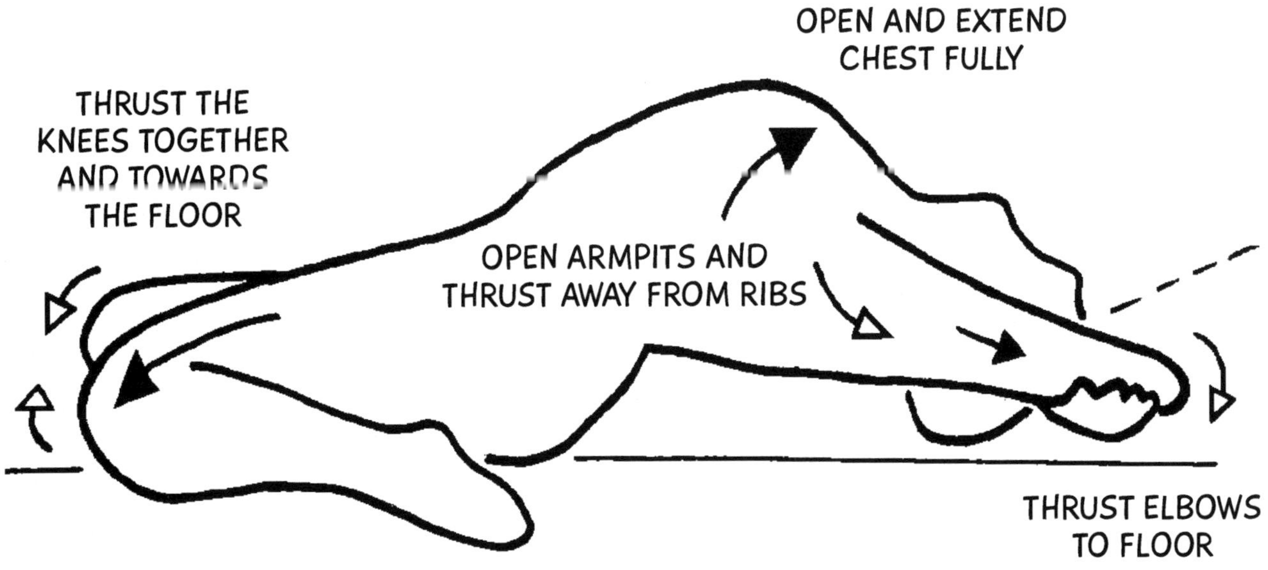
OPEN AND EXTEND CHEST FULLY
THRUST THE KNEES TOGETHER AND TOWARDS THE FLOOR
OPEN ARMPITS AND THRUST AWAY FROM RIBS
THRUST ELBOWS TO FLOOR

Program 4: First Day

NOTE: After doing Virasana IV – 38 (below) do the entire Padmasana (Lotus) Cycle (page 72). Afterwards, continue on with Urdhva Dhanurasana – 73. The Programs from here on take about 60 minutes daily.

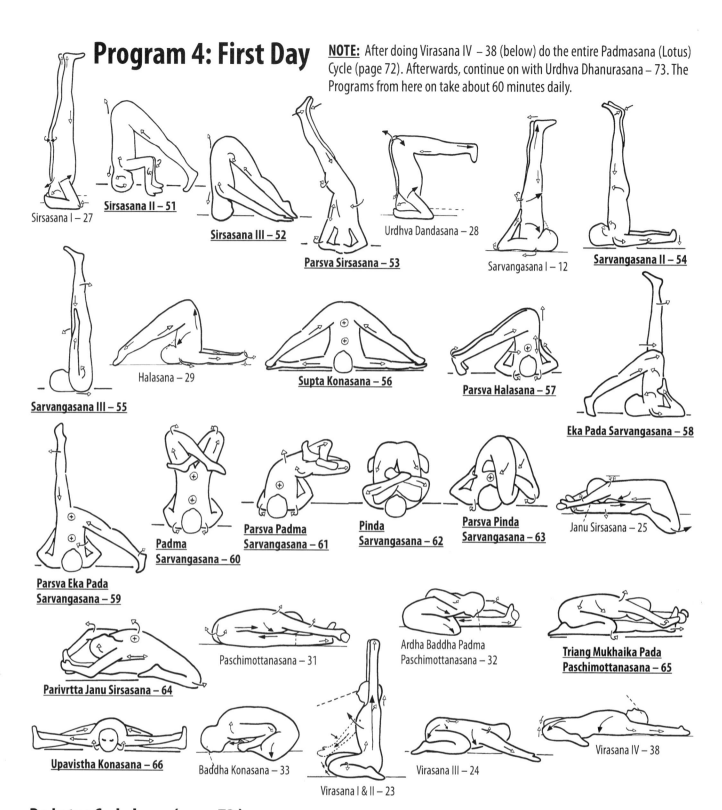

Sirsasana I – 27
Sirsasana II – 51
Sirsasana III – 52
Parsva Sirsasana – 53
Urdhva Dandasana – 28
Sarvangasana I – 12
Sarvangasana II – 54
Sarvangasana III – 55
Halasana – 29
Supta Konasana – 56
Parsva Halasana – 57
Eka Pada Sarvangasana – 58
Parsva Eka Pada Sarvangasana – 59
Padma Sarvangasana – 60
Parsva Padma Sarvangasana – 61
Pinda Sarvangasana – 62
Parsva Pinda Sarvangasana – 63
Janu Sirsasana – 25
Parivrtta Janu Sirsasana – 64
Paschimottanasana – 31
Ardha Baddha Padma Paschimottanasana – 32
Triang Mukhaika Pada Paschimottanasana – 65
Upavistha Konasana – 66
Baddha Konasana – 33
Virasana I & II – 23
Virasana III – 24
Virasana IV – 38

Do Lotus Cycle here: (page 72) The postures are arranged in the probable order of difficulty. You may find this order doesn't match your body, so rearrange the order to suit.

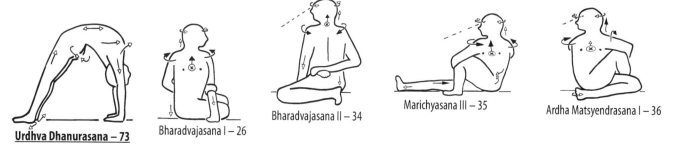

Urdhva Dhanurasana – 73
Bharadvajasana I – 26
Bharadvajasana II – 34
Marichyasana III – 35
Ardha Matsyendrasana I – 36

Program 4: Second Day

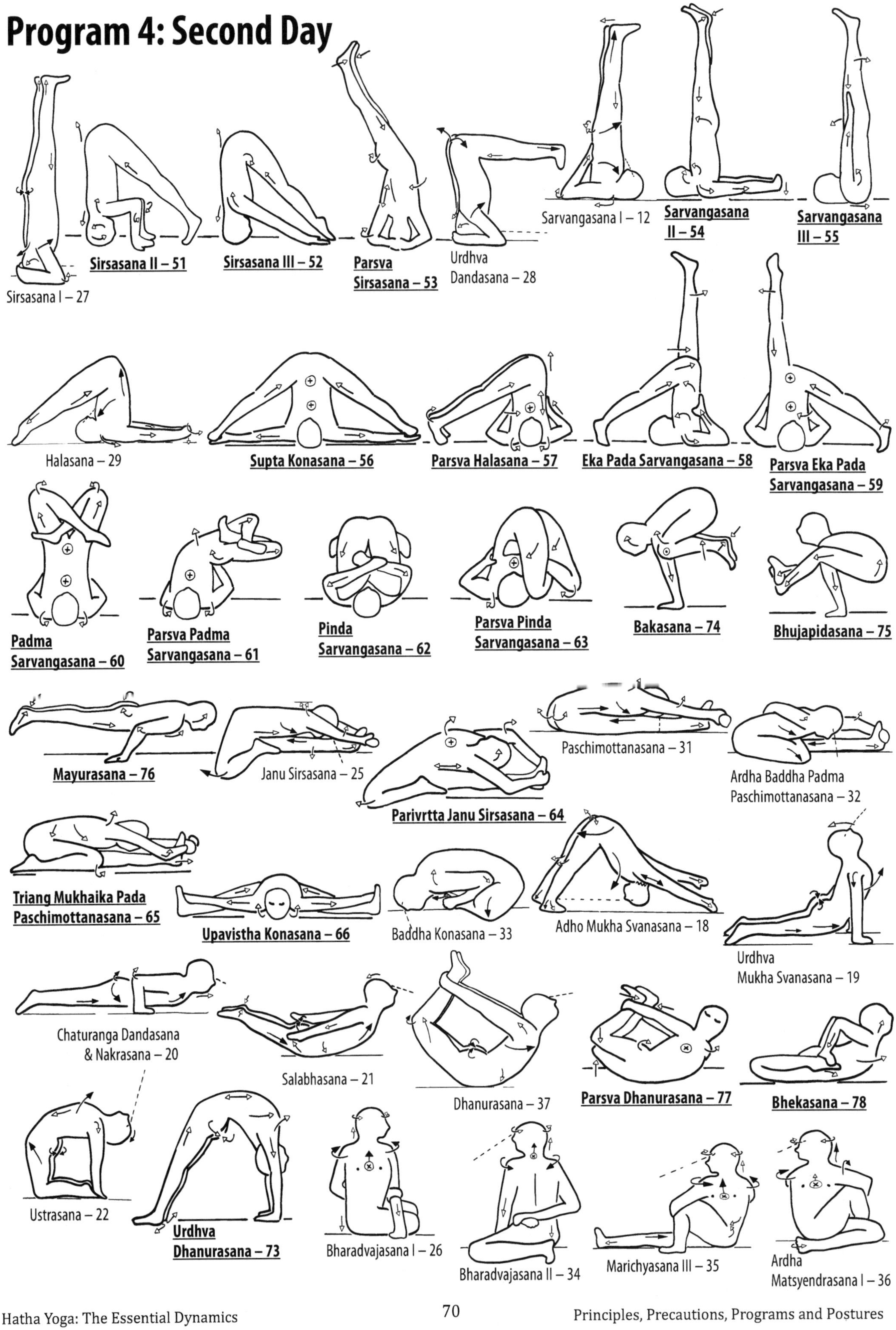
Sirsasana I – 27
Sirsasana II – 51
Sirsasana III – 52
Parsva Sirsasana – 53
Urdhva Dandasana – 28
Sarvangasana I – 12
Sarvangasana II – 54
Sarvangasana III – 55
Halasana – 29
Supta Konasana – 56
Parsva Halasana – 57
Eka Pada Sarvangasana – 58
Parsva Eka Pada Sarvangasana – 59
Padma Sarvangasana – 60
Parsva Padma Sarvangasana – 61
Pinda Sarvangasana – 62
Parsva Pinda Sarvangasana – 63
Bakasana – 74
Bhujapidasana – 75
Mayurasana – 76
Janu Sirsasana – 25
Parivrtta Janu Sirsasana – 64
Paschimottanasana – 31
Ardha Baddha Padma Paschimottanasana – 32
Triang Mukhaika Pada Paschimottanasana – 65
Upavistha Konasana – 66
Baddha Konasana – 33
Adho Mukha Svanasana – 18
Urdhva Mukha Svanasana – 19
Chaturanga Dandasana & Nakrasana – 20
Salabhasana – 21
Dhanurasana – 37
Parsva Dhanurasana – 77
Bhekasana – 78
Ustrasana – 22
Urdhva Dhanurasana – 73
Bharadvajasana I – 26
Bharadvajasana II – 34
Marichyasana III – 35
Ardha Matsyendrasana I – 36

Program 4: Review or Third Day

Do these few inverted postures below first. Stay longer in Sirsasana and Sarvangasana than usual, perhaps 10 minutes or so. Next do the Cycles below. Which you do first doesn't matter; just see what works best for you.

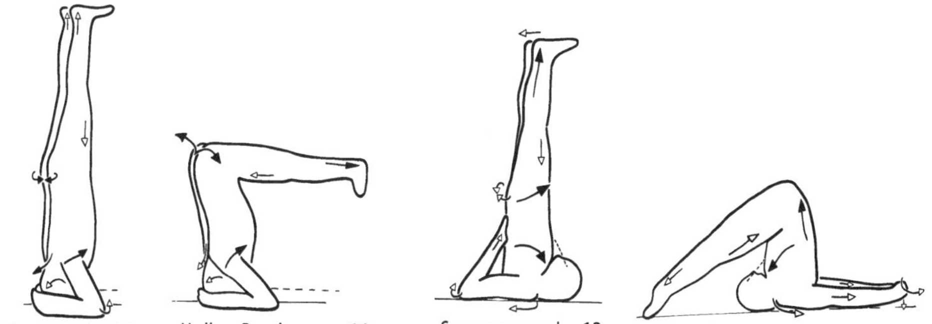

Sirsasana I – 27 Urdhva Dandasana – 28 Sarvangasana I – 12 Halasana – 29

<u>Basic Cycle here</u>: (page 73) The postures in each cycle are arranged in the common order of difficulty. Many folks will find that the order doesn't match their body to some degree. Simply rearrange the order of the program to suit your ability.

<u>Standing Cycle here</u>: (page 72) The standing cycle's posture order should not be a problem for most folk. If it is, just rearrange to suit your body's needs.

<u>About The 12 Cycles</u>: Again, it is very important to skip any postures that push your body beyond its limit (sharp pain or other acute symptoms are good indicators that you need to back off). By all means, take a few years to grow the necessary strength and flexibility.

Can I rearrange the order of the postures in the cycles? Each cycle's postures are arranged in an order that works very well for me. Feel free to rearrange them in any way that suits your body's needs best. Needless to say, do so thoughtfully and patiently.

How long should I do each cycle? Each cycle includes an rough guide to "about how many minutes" the cycle will take to complete. Don't let this frivolous bit of information get in the way. In the end, your own self-honest intuition will be your best guide for every facet of yoga.

<u>Now Relax</u>: Doing Savasana – 13, for 10 minutes after completing any Program can be wonderfully relaxing. Also, try out Pranayama – 14, first in Savasana, and later, the more formal, Pranayama – 47. Meditation (in Padmasana – 48, or in Siddhasana – 48) is also worth trying out. All these techniques take time to feel at home in. Doing them for awhile, then not for awhile, then returning to them can be helpful.

This *'not doing'* something can be a remarkably effective step in your journey. Sometimes totally letting go of whatever it is that you are struggling with helps you get over yourself and enter the activity from another angle, another level. Failure is often (if not always) the secret of success. At some point totally letting go of what ever success goal you harbor allows you to transcend. This is another aspect of what I've found to be a universal principle. As ironic and paradoxical as it sounds: *you can only have that of which you let go.*

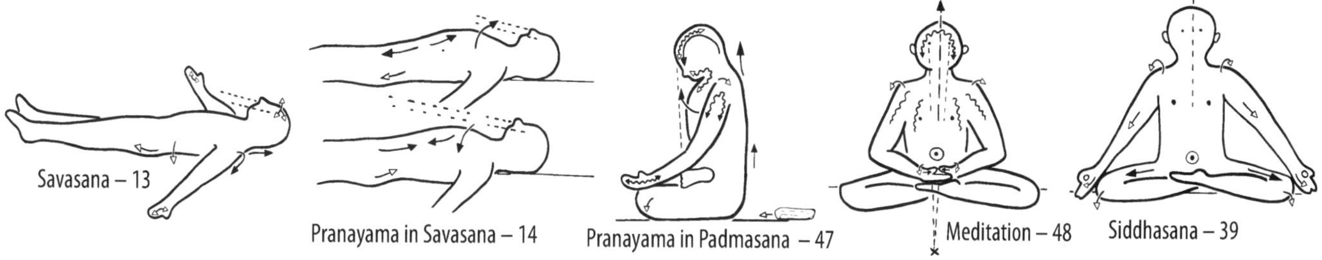

Savasana – 13 Pranayama in Savasana – 14 Pranayama in Padmasana – 47 Meditation – 48 Siddhasana – 39

Standing Cycle (About 15 minutes)

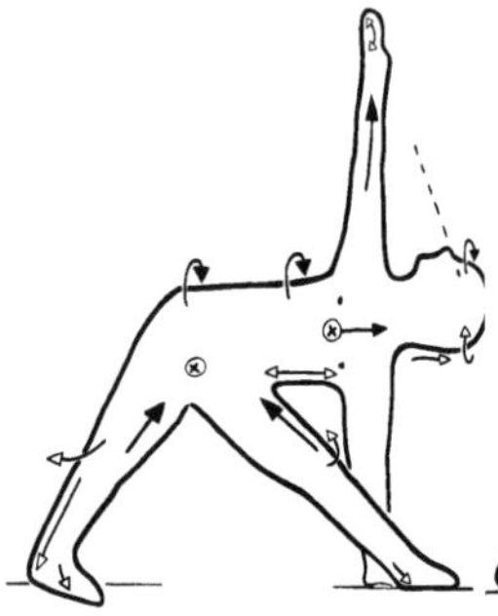
Utthita Trikonasana – 3

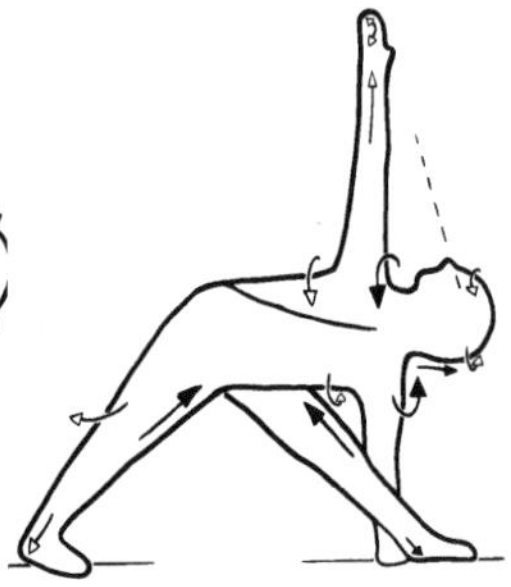
Parivrtta Trikonasana – 4

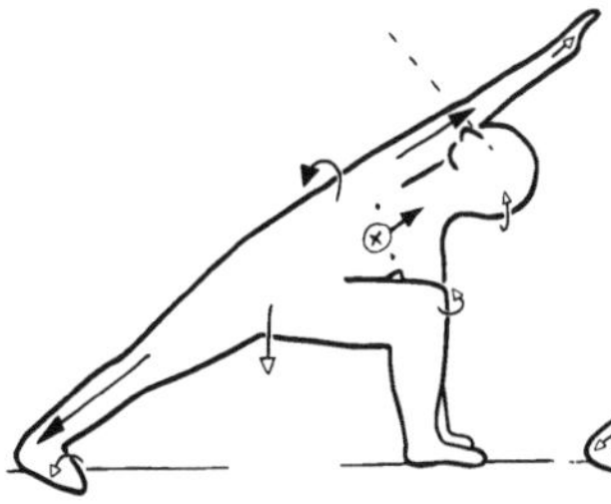
Utthita Parsvakonasana – 5

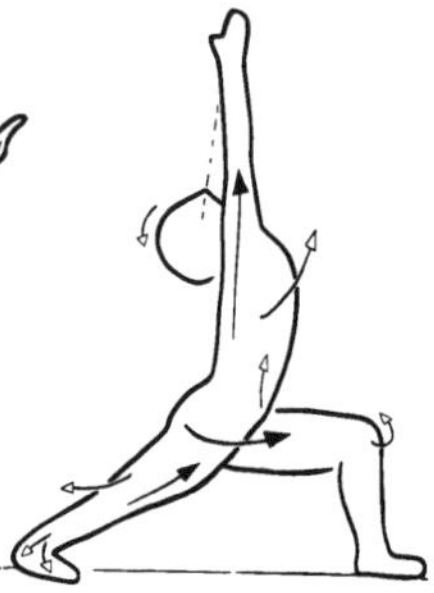
Virabhadrasana I – 6

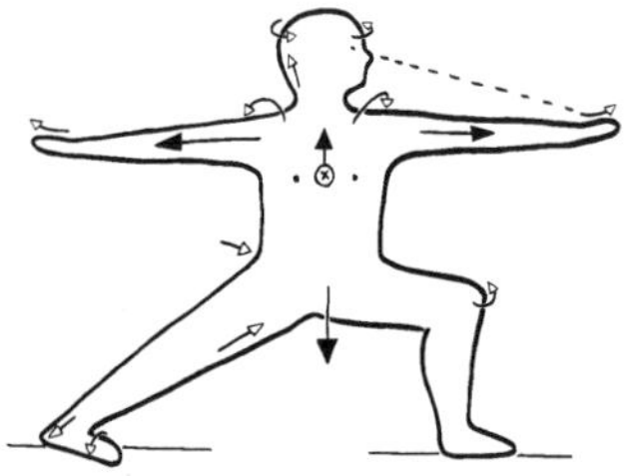
Virabhadrasana II – 7

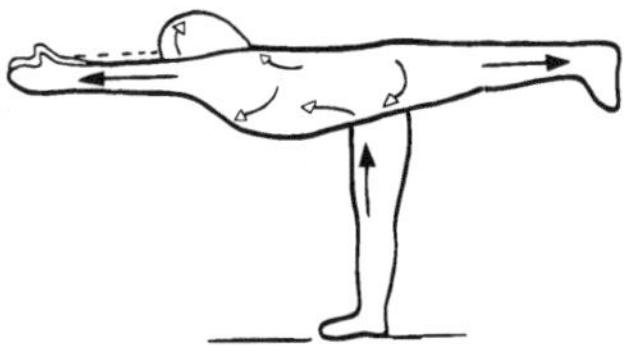
Virabhadrasana III – 8

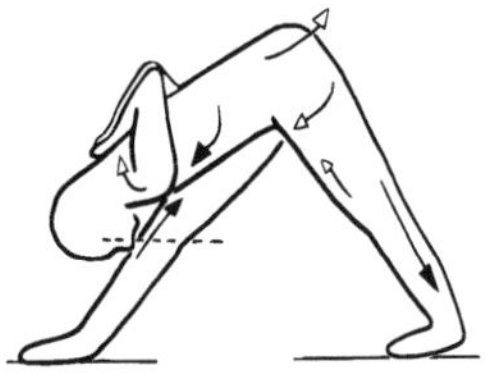
Parsvottanasana – 9

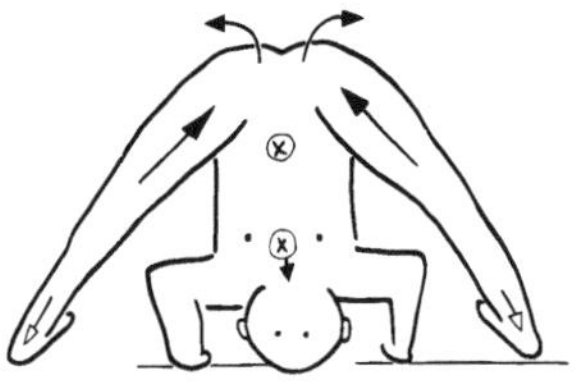
Prasarita Padottanasana – 10

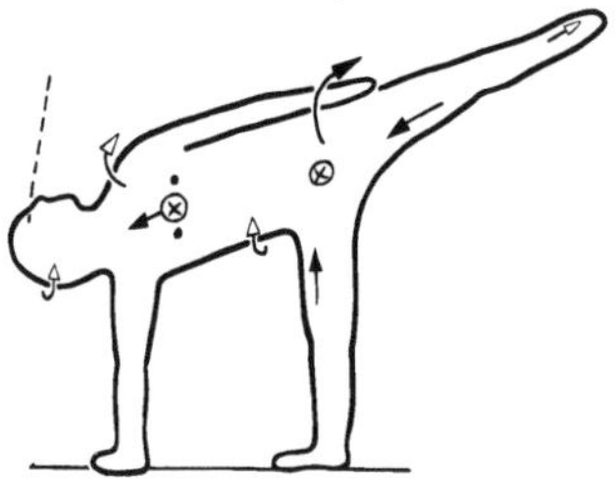
Ardha Chandrasana – 43

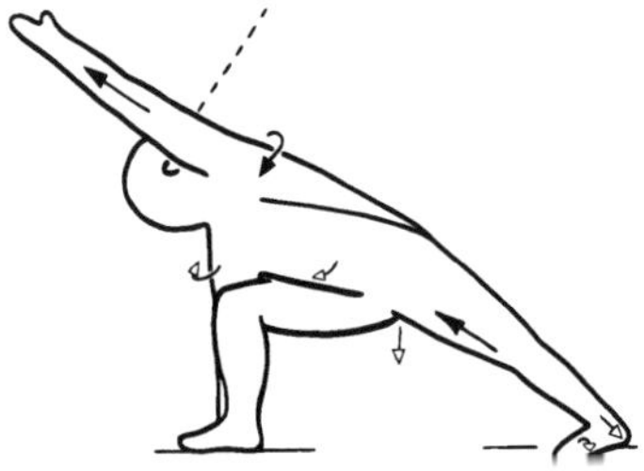
Parivrtta Parsvakonasana – 44

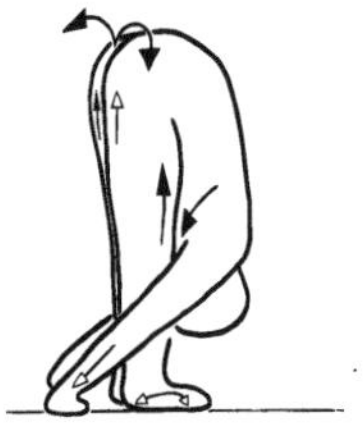
Uttanasana – 11

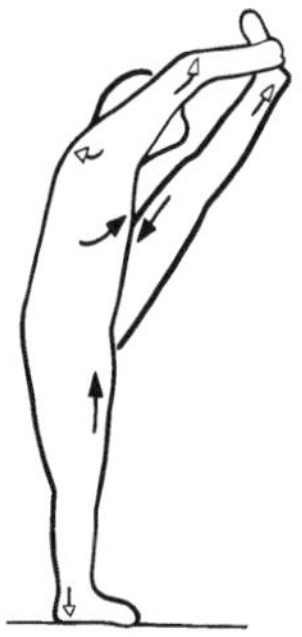
Utthita Hasta Padangusthasana – 45

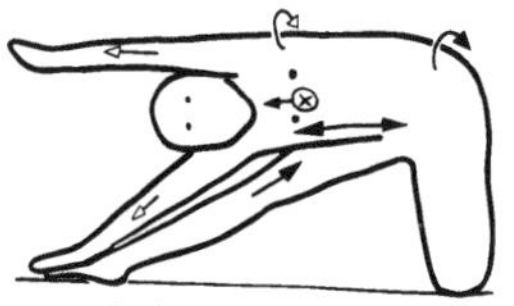
Parigasana – 46

Lotus Cycle (About 14minutes)

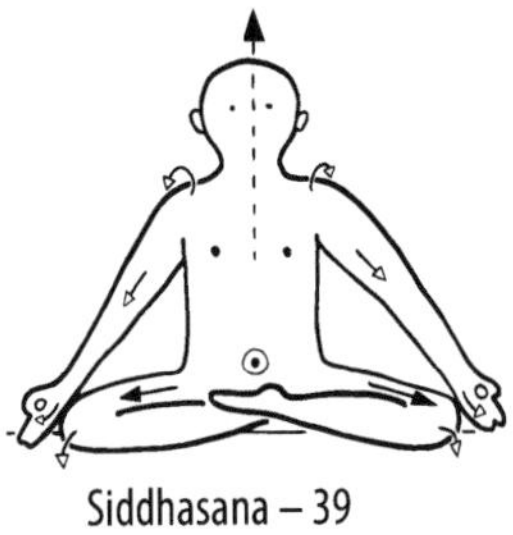
Siddhasana – 39

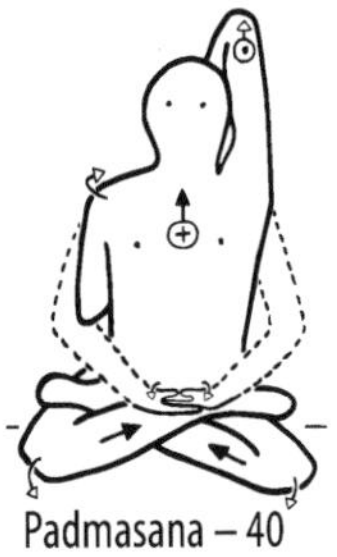
Padmasana – 40

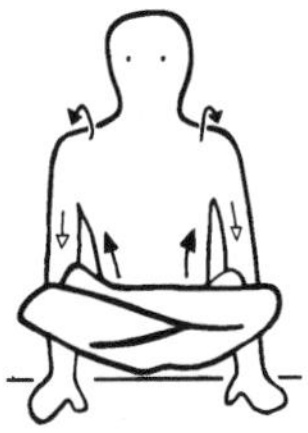
Tolasana – 41

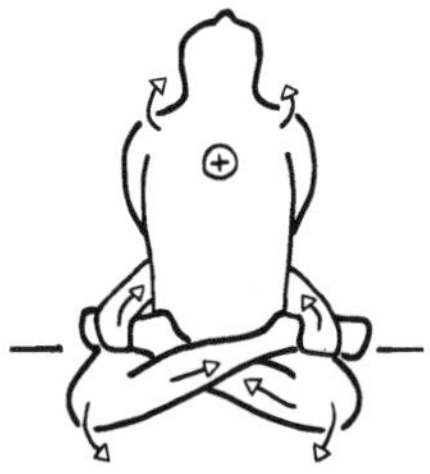
Baddha Padmasana – 67

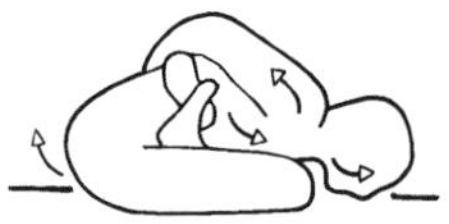
Yoga Mudrasana – 68

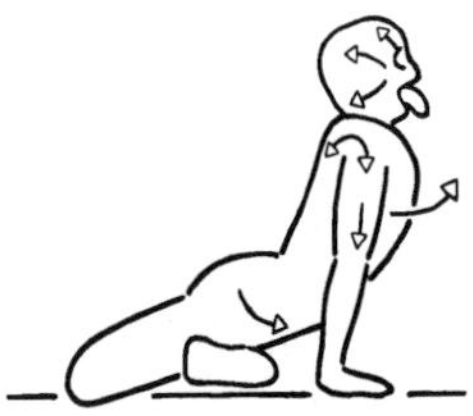
Simhasana – 69

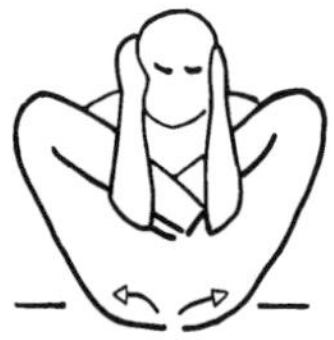
Garbha Pindasana – 70

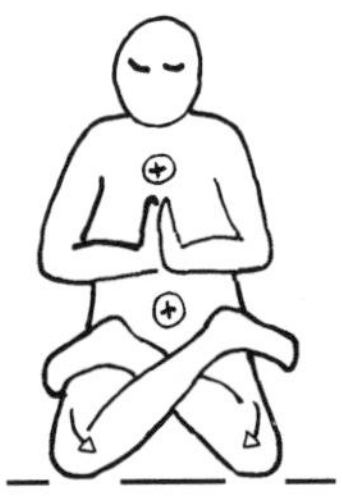
Goraksasana – 71

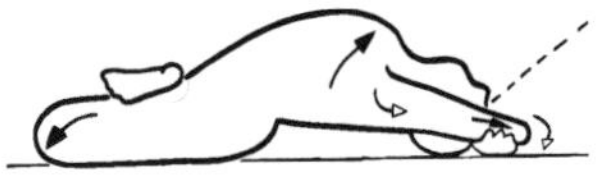
Matsyasana – 42

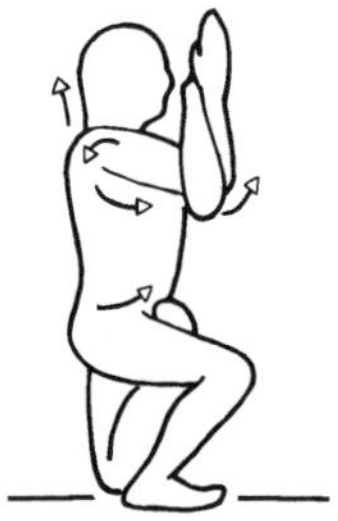
Vatayanasana – 72

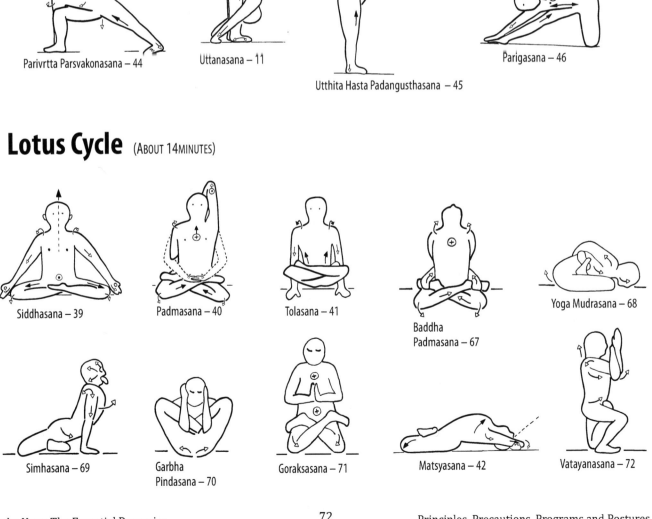

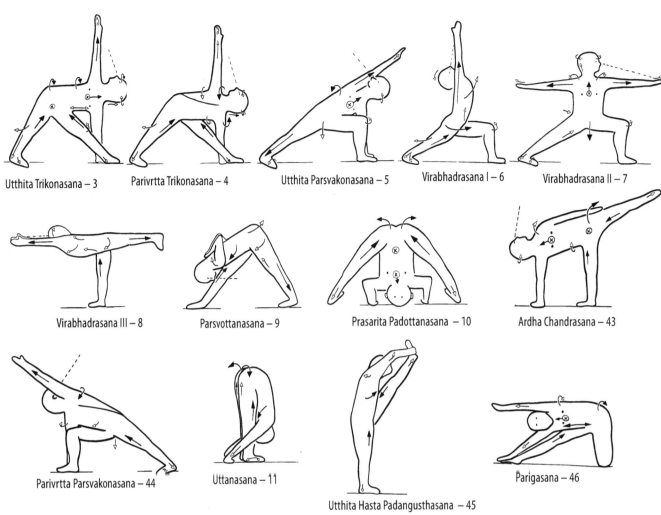

Basic Cycle (About 13 minutes)

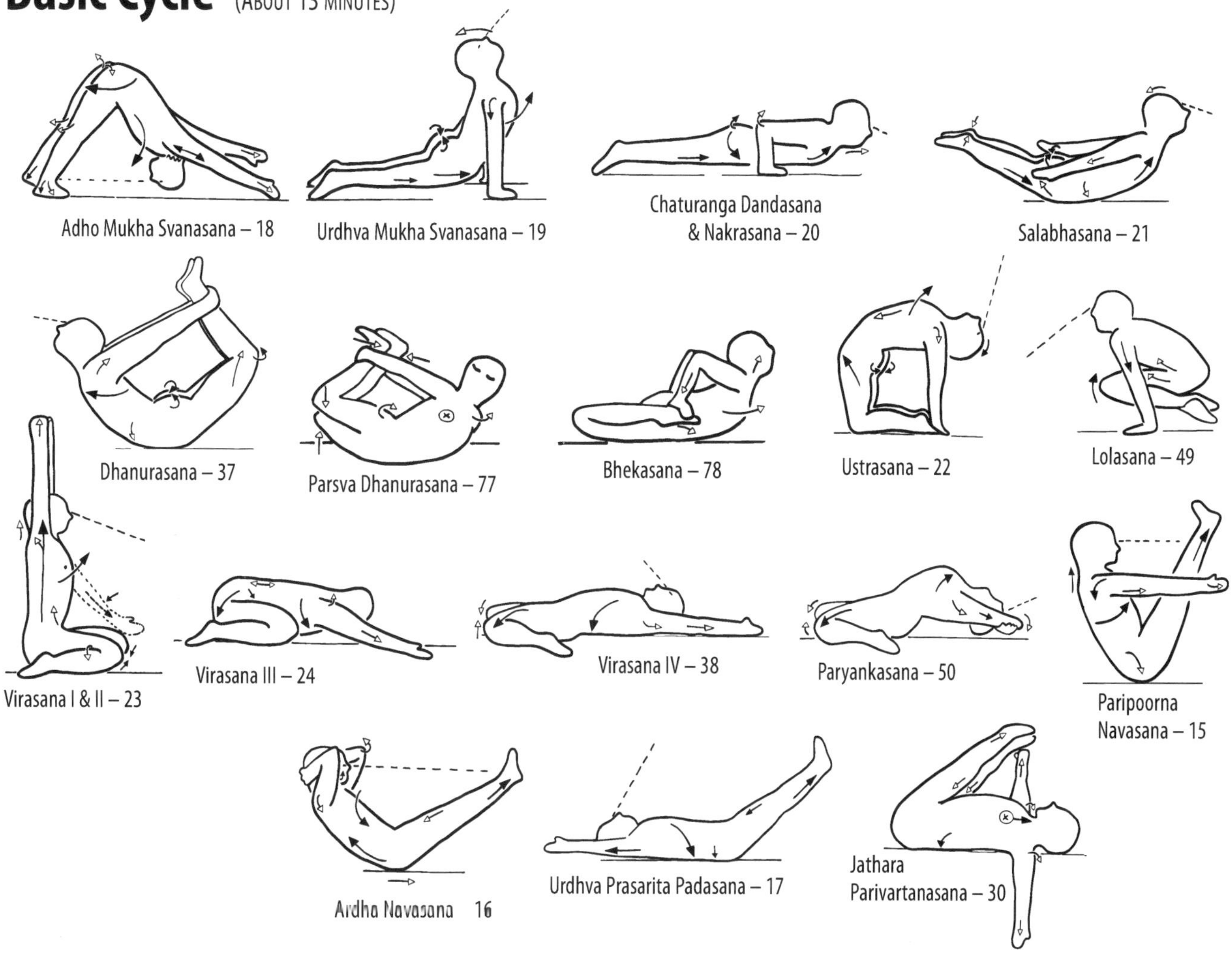

Adho Mukha Svanasana – 18

Urdhva Mukha Svanasana – 19

Chaturanga Dandasana & Nakrasana – 20

Salabhasana – 21

Dhanurasana – 37

Parsva Dhanurasana – 77

Bhekasana – 78

Ustrasana – 22

Lolasana – 49

Virasana I & II – 23

Virasana III – 24

Virasana IV – 38

Paryankasana – 50

Paripoorna Navasana – 15

Ardha Navasana 16

Urdhva Prasarita Padasana – 17

Jathara Parivartanasana – 30

Forward Cycle (About 20 minutes)

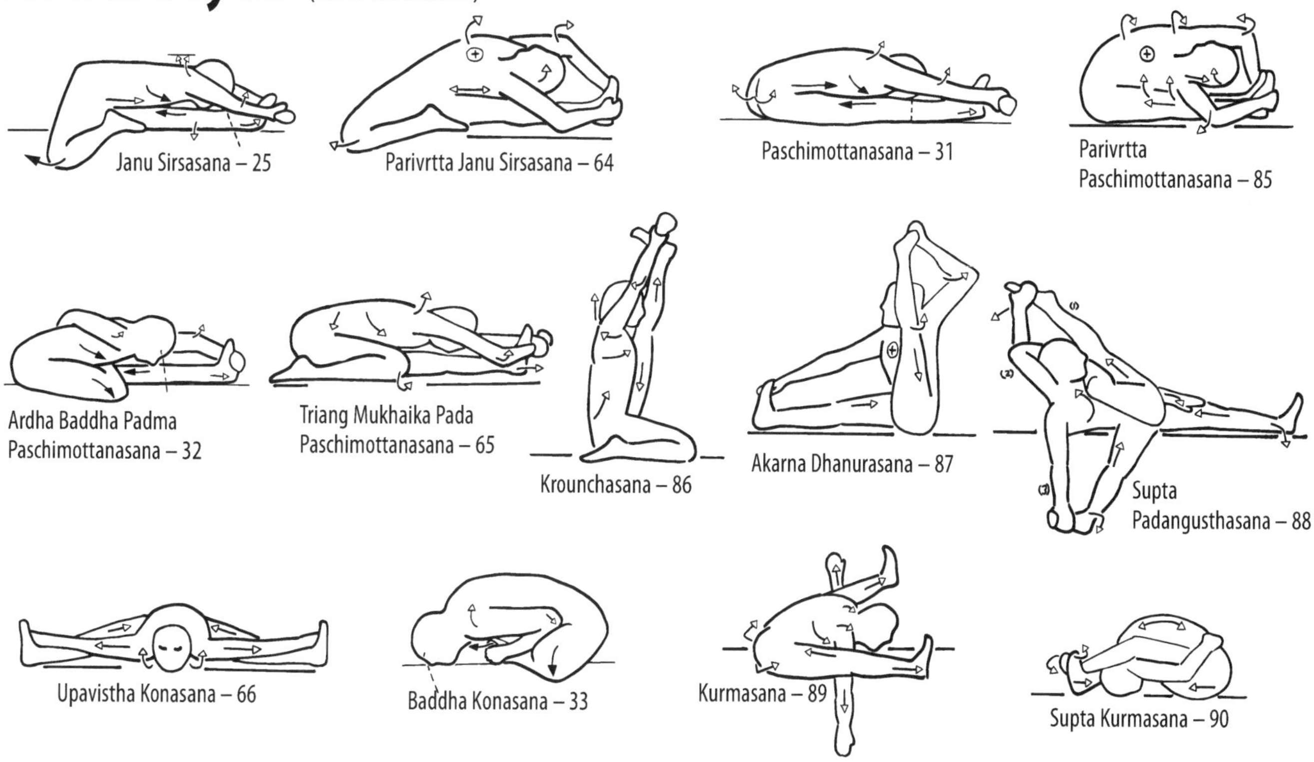

Janu Sirsasana – 25

Parivrtta Janu Sirsasana – 64

Paschimottanasana – 31

Parivrtta Paschimottanasana – 85

Ardha Baddha Padma Paschimottanasana – 32

Triang Mukhaika Pada Paschimottanasana – 65

Krounchasana – 86

Akarna Dhanurasana – 87

Supta Padangusthasana – 88

Upavistha Konasana – 66

Baddha Konasana – 33

Kurmasana – 89

Supta Kurmasana – 90

Sirsasana II 60s (51)

head

Var: Instead of moving into this posture from Sirsasana, begin it with the feet on the floor. Gradually shift the body weight backward until the feet leave the floor. You may also separate the hands and elbows 12-18".

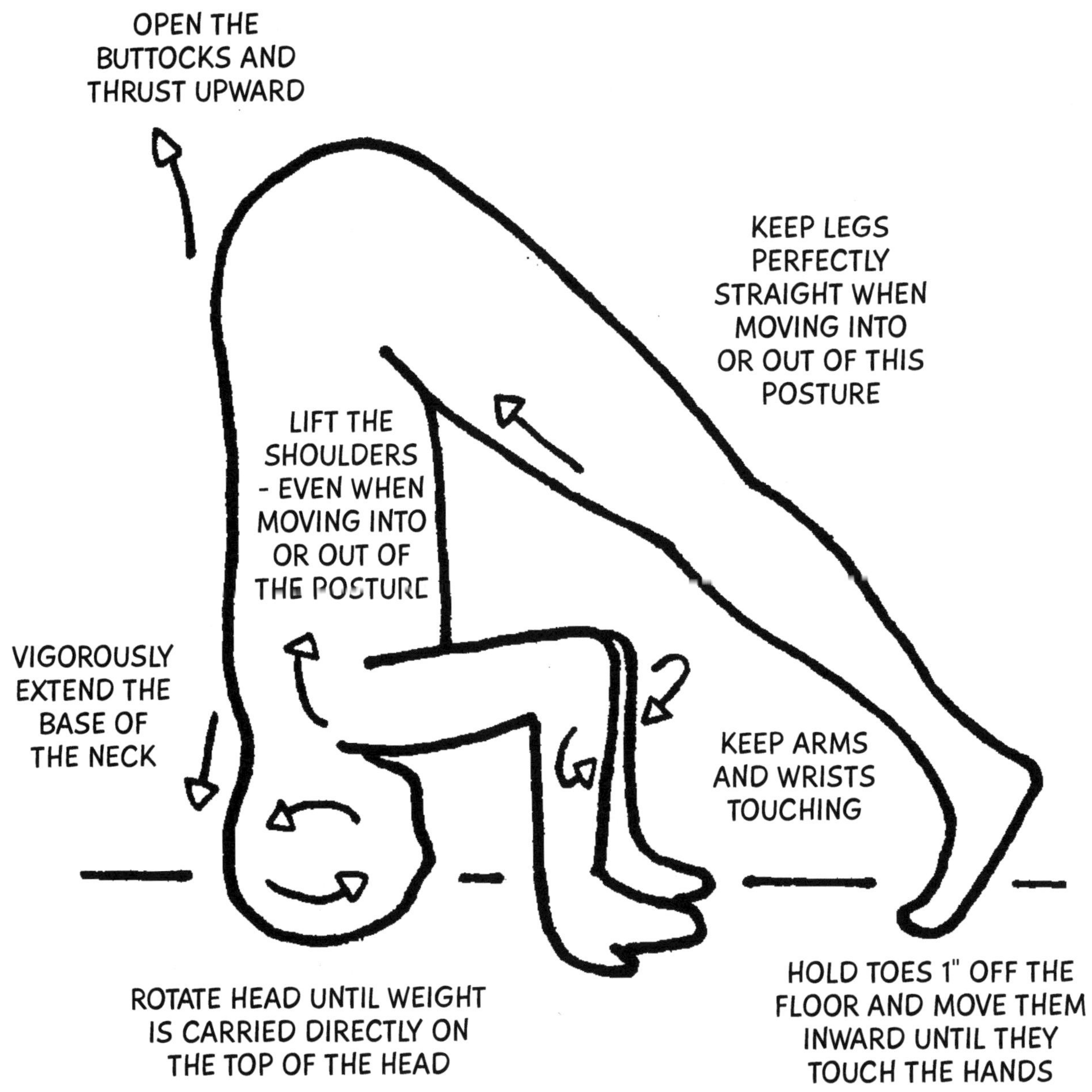
OPEN THE BUTTOCKS AND THRUST UPWARD
KEEP LEGS PERFECTLY STRAIGHT WHEN MOVING INTO OR OUT OF THIS POSTURE
LIFT THE SHOULDERS - EVEN WHEN MOVING INTO OR OUT OF THE POSTURE
VIGOROUSLY EXTEND THE BASE OF THE NECK
KEEP ARMS AND WRISTS TOUCHING
ROTATE HEAD UNTIL WEIGHT IS CARRIED DIRECTLY ON THE TOP OF THE HEAD
HOLD TOES 1" OFF THE FLOOR AND MOVE THEM INWARD UNTIL THEY TOUCH THE HANDS

Sirsasana III 60s (52)

head

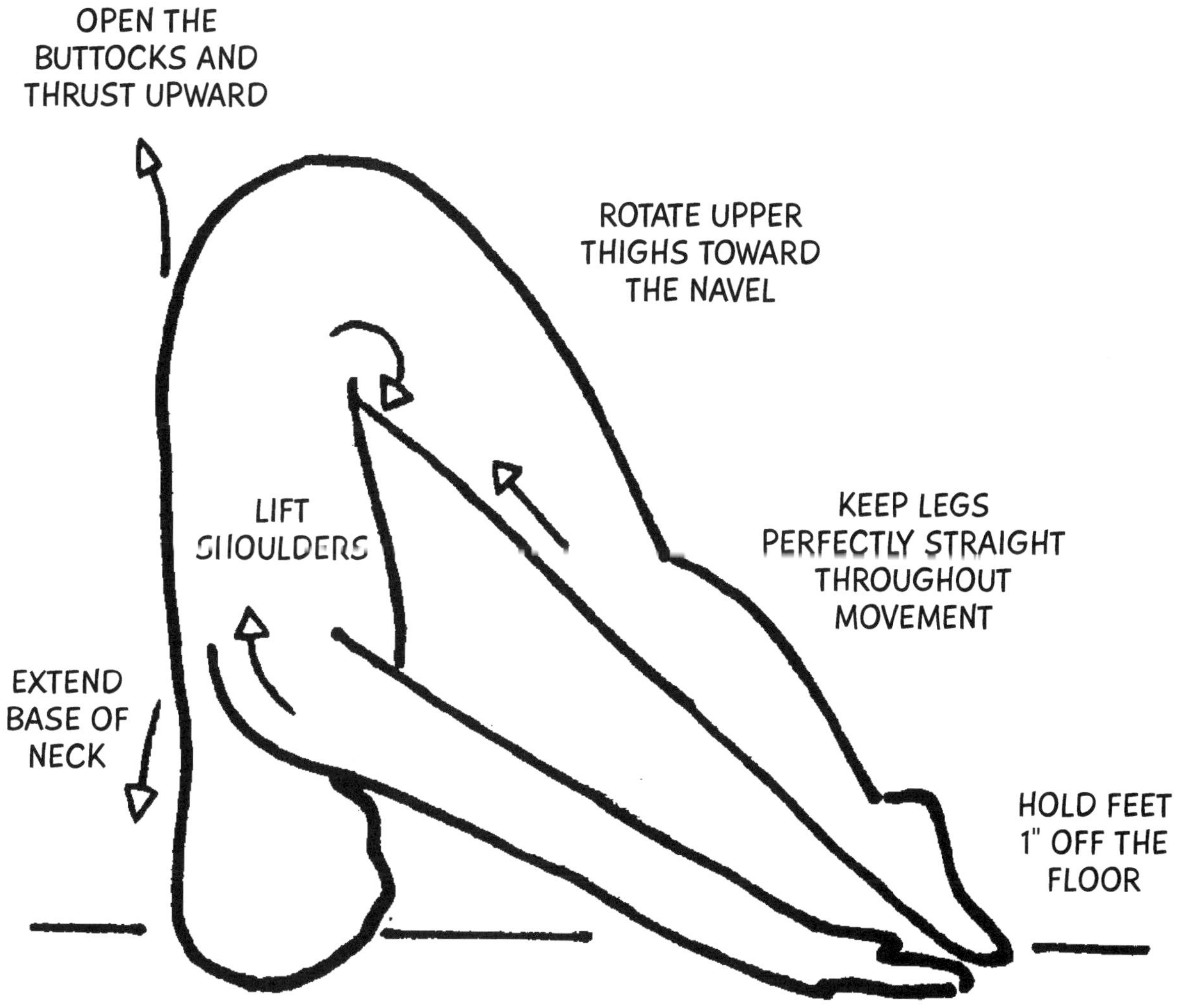
OPEN THE BUTTOCKS AND THRUST UPWARD
ROTATE UPPER THIGHS TOWARD THE NAVEL
LIFT SHOULDERS
KEEP LEGS PERFECTLY STRAIGHT THROUGHOUT MOVEMENT
EXTEND BASE OF NECK
HOLD FEET 1" OFF THE FLOOR

Note: In this and all other head standing postures, you should strive to balance the entire body weight on the top of the head, lifting the shoulders and extending the base of the neck back until the spine is as straight as possible. Only a few ounces of weight should be carried by the elbows, hands— or in the case of this posture, the fingertips of the outstretched hands,.

Parsva Sirsasana 20-30s (53)

side head

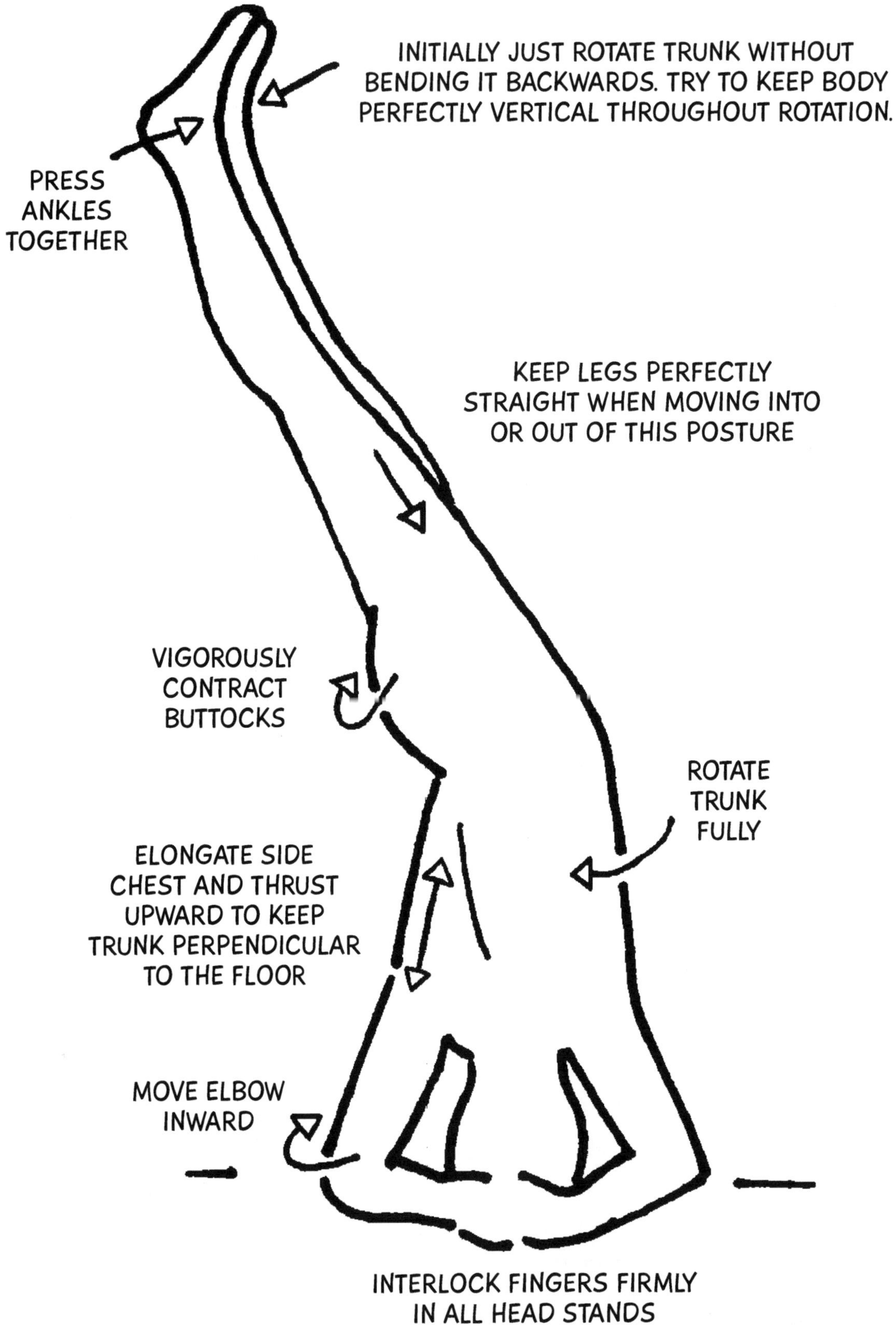
INITIALLY JUST ROTATE TRUNK WITHOUT BENDING IT BACKWARDS. TRY TO KEEP BODY PERFECTLY VERTICAL THROUGHOUT ROTATION.
PRESS ANKLES TOGETHER
KEEP LEGS PERFECTLY STRAIGHT WHEN MOVING INTO OR OUT OF THIS POSTURE
VIGOROUSLY CONTRACT BUTTOCKS
ROTATE TRUNK FULLY
ELONGATE SIDE CHEST AND THRUST UPWARD TO KEEP TRUNK PERPENDICULAR TO THE FLOOR
MOVE ELBOW INWARD
INTERLOCK FINGERS FIRMLY IN ALL HEAD STANDS

Sarvangasana II 60s (54)

whole body

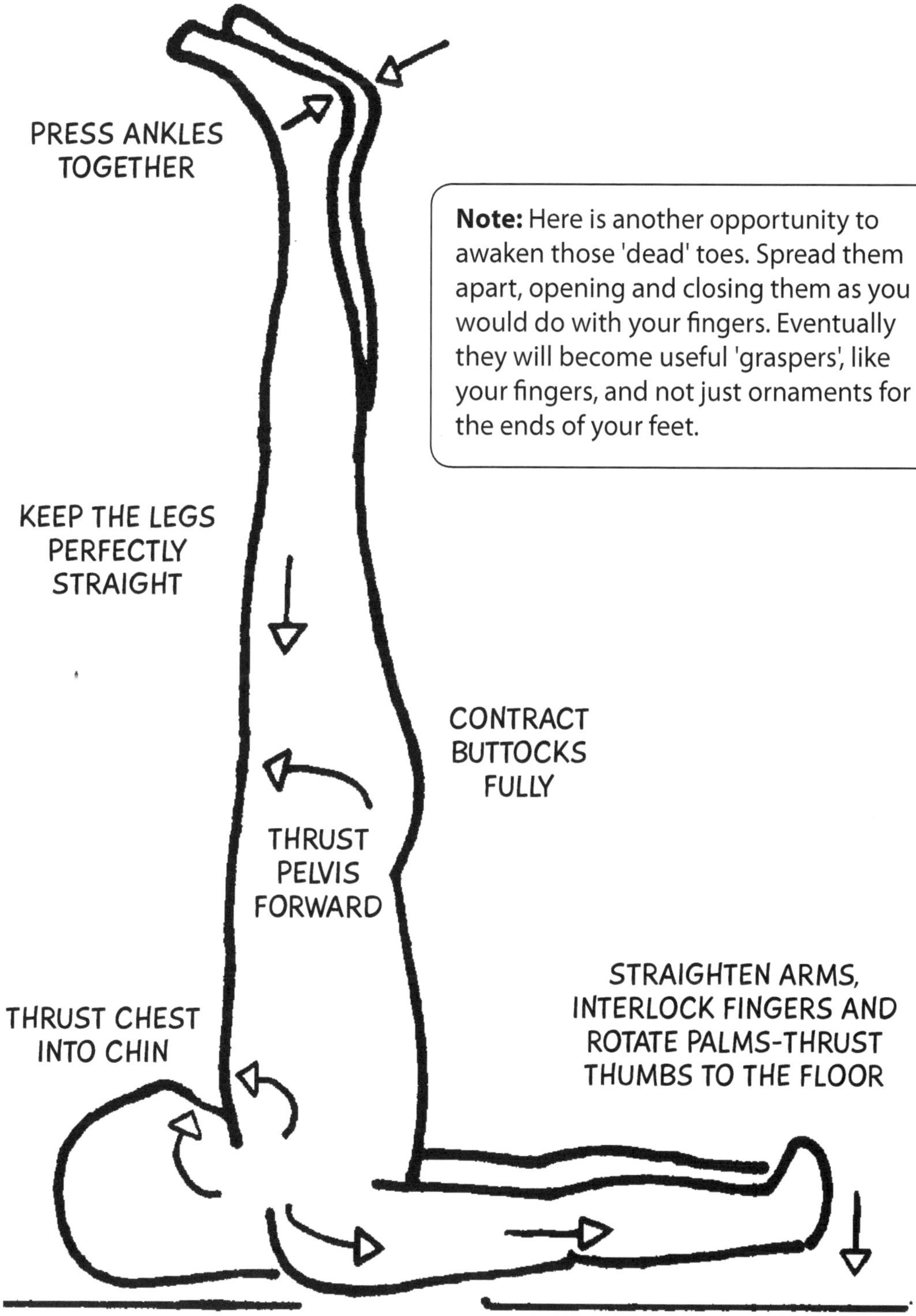
PRESS ANKLES TOGETHER
KEEP THE LEGS PERFECTLY STRAIGHT
CONTRACT BUTTOCKS FULLY
THRUST PELVIS FORWARD
THRUST CHEST INTO CHIN
STRAIGHTEN ARMS, INTERLOCK FINGERS AND ROTATE PALMS-THRUST THUMBS TO THE FLOOR
ROLL SHOULDERS BACK, PULLING THEM TO THE REAR

Note: Here is another opportunity to awaken those 'dead' toes. Spread them apart, opening and closing them as you would do with your fingers. Eventually they will become useful 'graspers', like your fingers, and not just ornaments for the ends of your feet.

Sarvangasana III 60s (55)

whole body

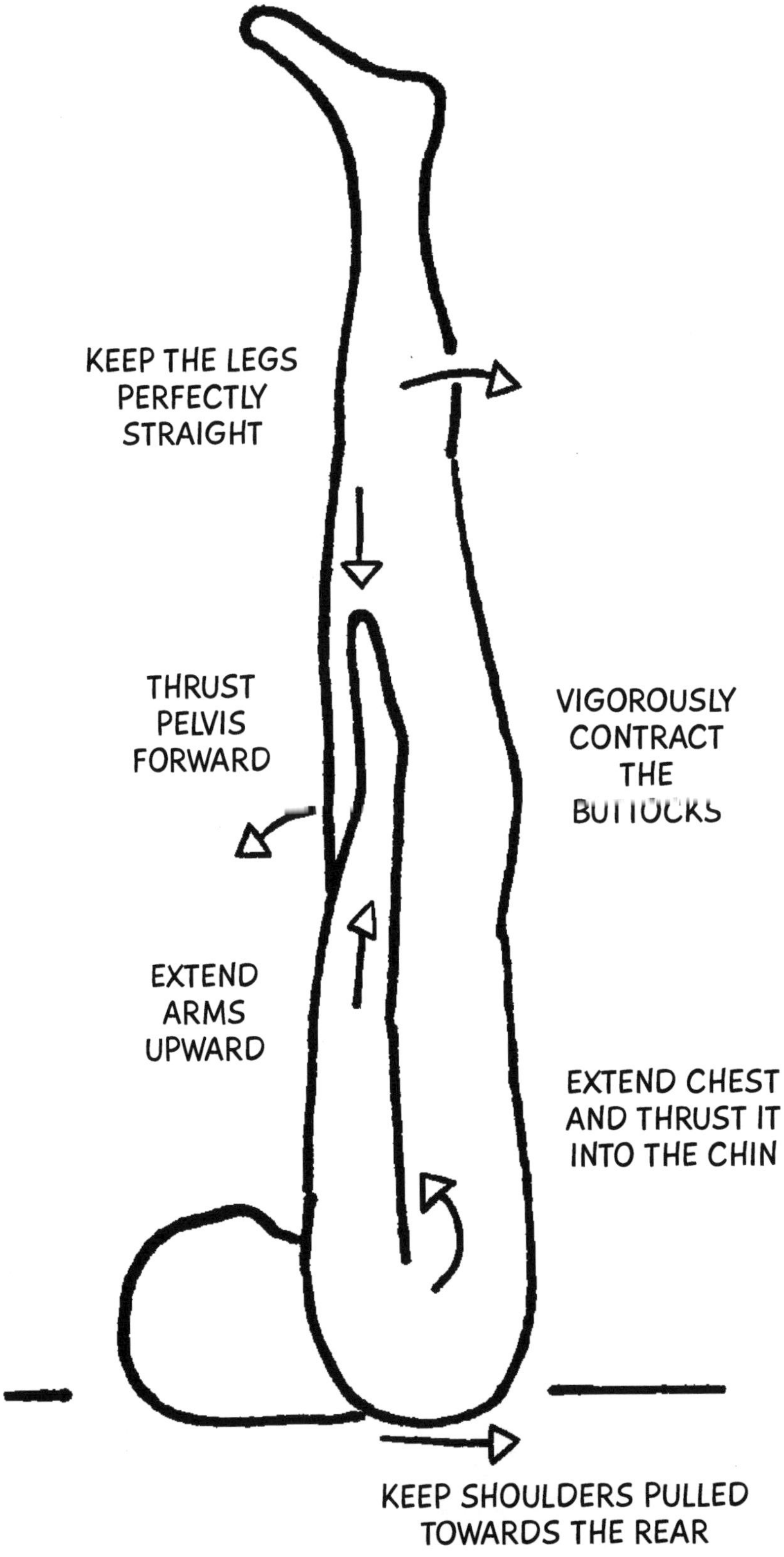

KEEP THE LEGS PERFECTLY STRAIGHT
THRUST PELVIS FORWARD
VIGOROUSLY CONTRACT THE BUTTOCKS
EXTEND ARMS UPWARD
EXTEND CHEST AND THRUST IT INTO THE CHIN
KEEP SHOULDERS PULLED TOWARDS THE REAR

Supta Konasana 20-30s (56)

lying down angle

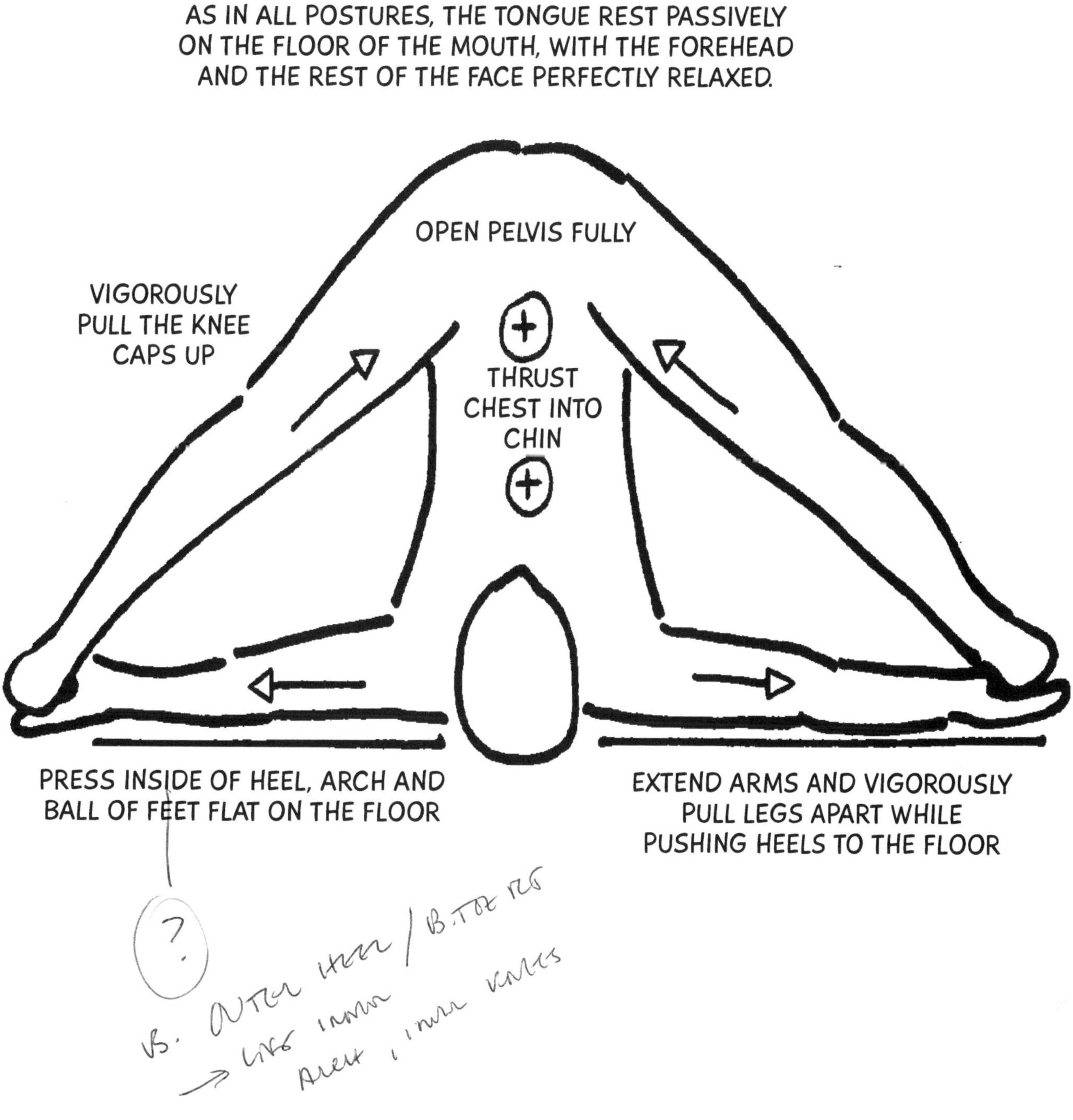
AS IN ALL POSTURES, THE TONGUE REST PASSIVELY ON THE FLOOR OF THE MOUTH, WITH THE FOREHEAD AND THE REST OF THE FACE PERFECTLY RELAXED.
OPEN PELVIS FULLY
VIGOROUSLY PULL THE KNEE CAPS UP
THRUST CHEST INTO CHIN
PRESS INSIDE OF HEEL, ARCH AND BALL OF FEET FLAT ON THE FLOOR
EXTEND ARMS AND VIGOROUSLY PULL LEGS APART WHILE PUSHING HEELS TO THE FLOOR

Parsva Halasana 30s (57)

side plow

Note: In this and in all other shoulder stand postures, you should strive to open the chest and sternum as such as possible and thrust the trunk upward and forward with the palms pressing the top of the sternum firmly into the chin.

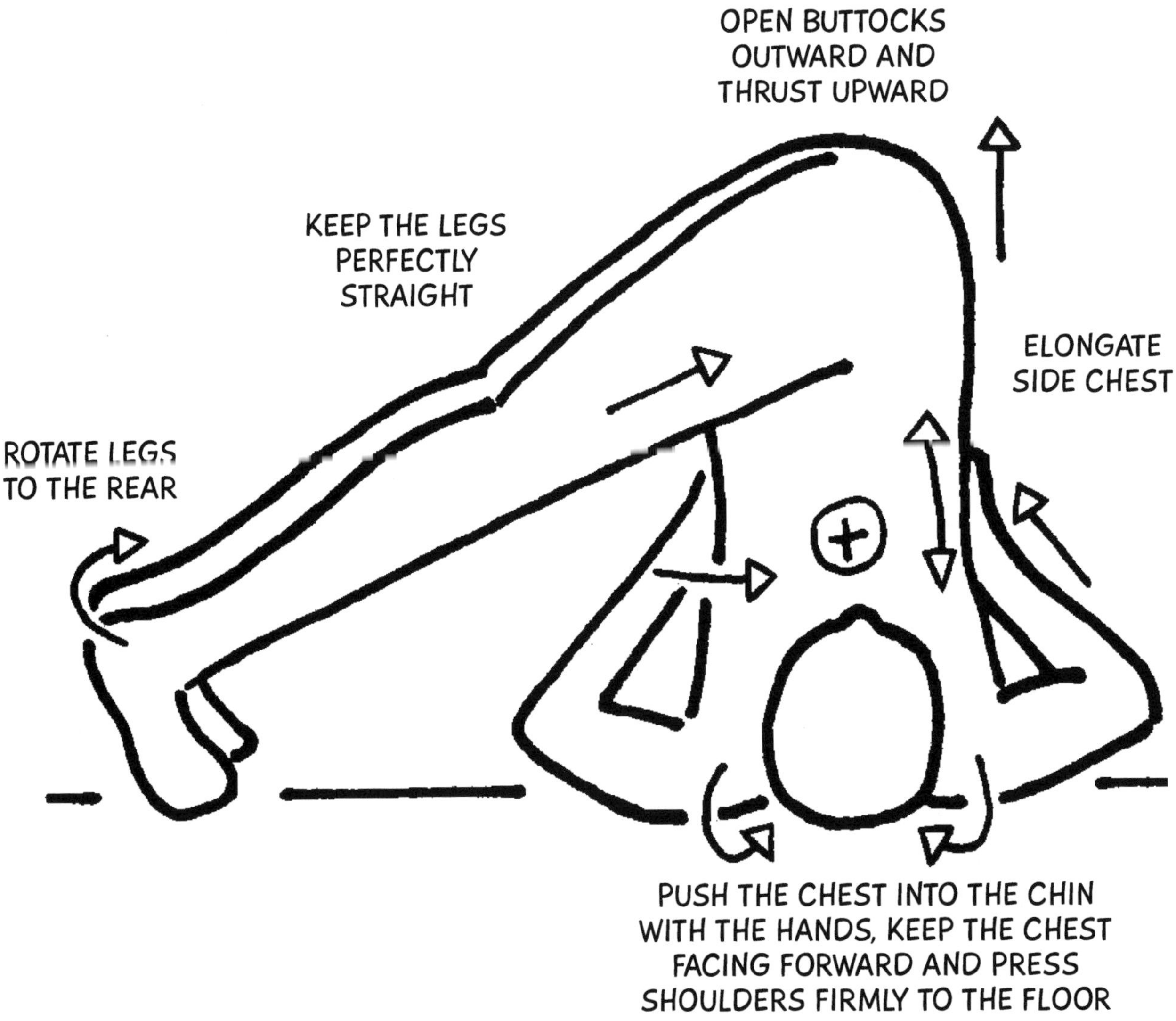
OPEN BUTTOCKS
OUTWARD AND
THRUST UPWARD
KEEP THE LEGS
PERFECTLY
STRAIGHT
ELONGATE
SIDE CHEST
ROTATE LEGS
TO THE REAR
PUSH THE CHEST INTO THE CHIN
WITH THE HANDS, KEEP THE CHEST
FACING FORWARD AND PRESS
SHOULDERS FIRMLY TO THE FLOOR

Eka Pada Sarvangasana 20s (58)

one foot whole body

> **Note:** Remember the toes. Are they alive yet?

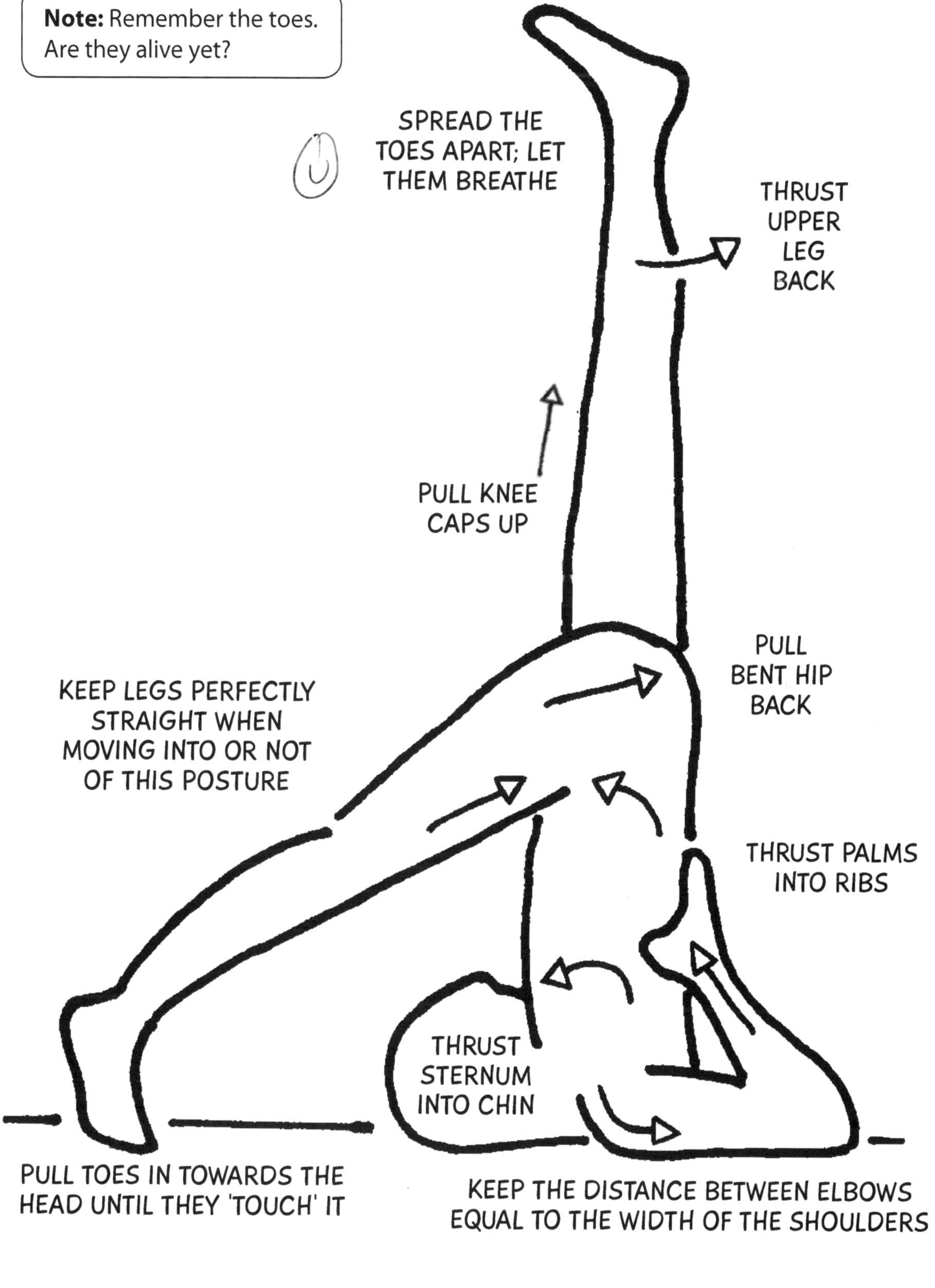
SPREAD THE TOES APART; LET THEM BREATHE
THRUST UPPER LEG BACK
PULL KNEE CAPS UP
PULL BENT HIP BACK
KEEP LEGS PERFECTLY STRAIGHT WHEN MOVING INTO OR NOT OF THIS POSTURE
THRUST PALMS INTO RIBS
THRUST STERNUM INTO CHIN
PULL TOES IN TOWARDS THE HEAD UNTIL THEY 'TOUCH' IT
KEEP THE DISTANCE BETWEEN ELBOWS EQUAL TO THE WIDTH OF THE SHOULDERS

Parsva Eka Papa Sarvangasana 20s (59)

side one foot whole body

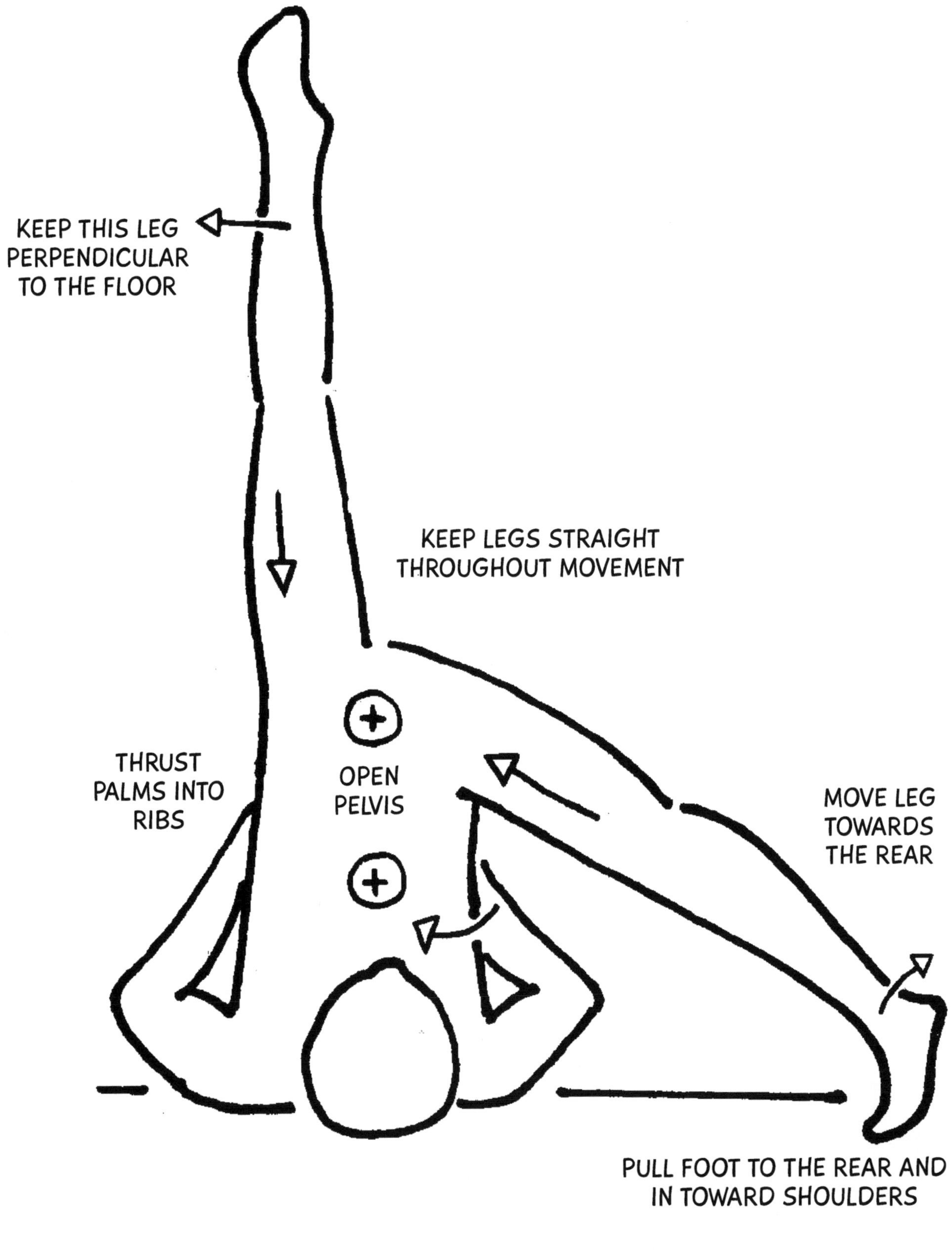
KEEP THIS LEG
PERPENDICULAR
TO THE FLOOR
KEEP LEGS STRAIGHT
THROUGHOUT MOVEMENT
THRUST
PALMS INTO
RIBS
OPEN
PELVIS
MOVE LEG
TOWARDS
THE REAR
PULL FOOT TO THE REAR AND
IN TOWARD SHOULDERS

Padma Sarvangasana 20-30s (60)

lotus whole body

Note: In this and all shoulder-stand postures, thrust the fingers (forefinger and thumb) into the ribs- as high up on the back as possible toward the shoulder blades. Then push the chest forward and upward until the sternum presses firmly into the chin.

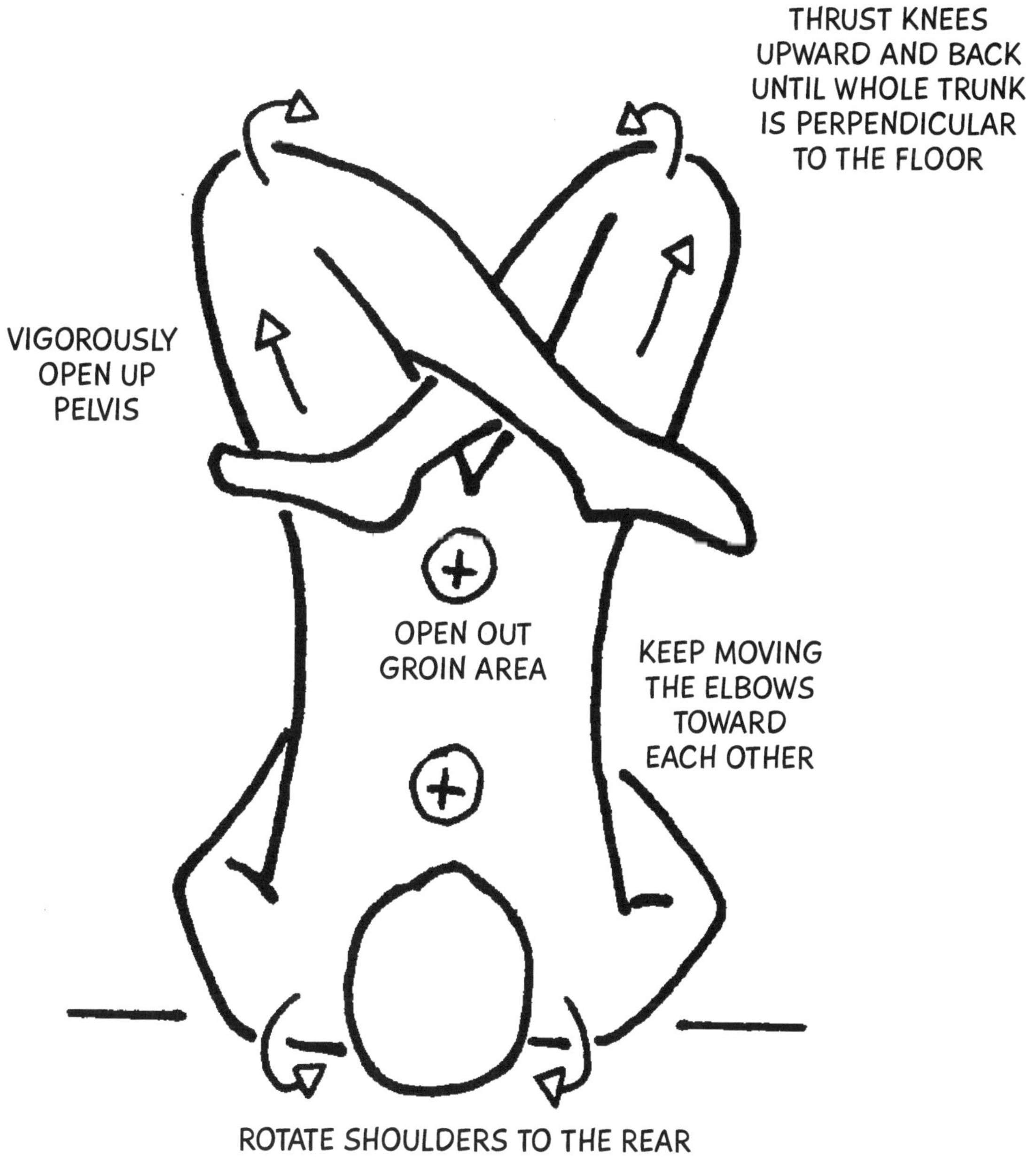
THRUST KNEES UPWARD AND BACK UNTIL WHOLE TRUNK IS PERPENDICULAR TO THE FLOOR
VIGOROUSLY OPEN UP PELVIS
OPEN OUT GROIN AREA
KEEP MOVING THE ELBOWS TOWARD EACH OTHER
ROTATE SHOULDERS TO THE REAR

Parsva Padma Sarvangasana 10-15s (61)

side lotus whole body

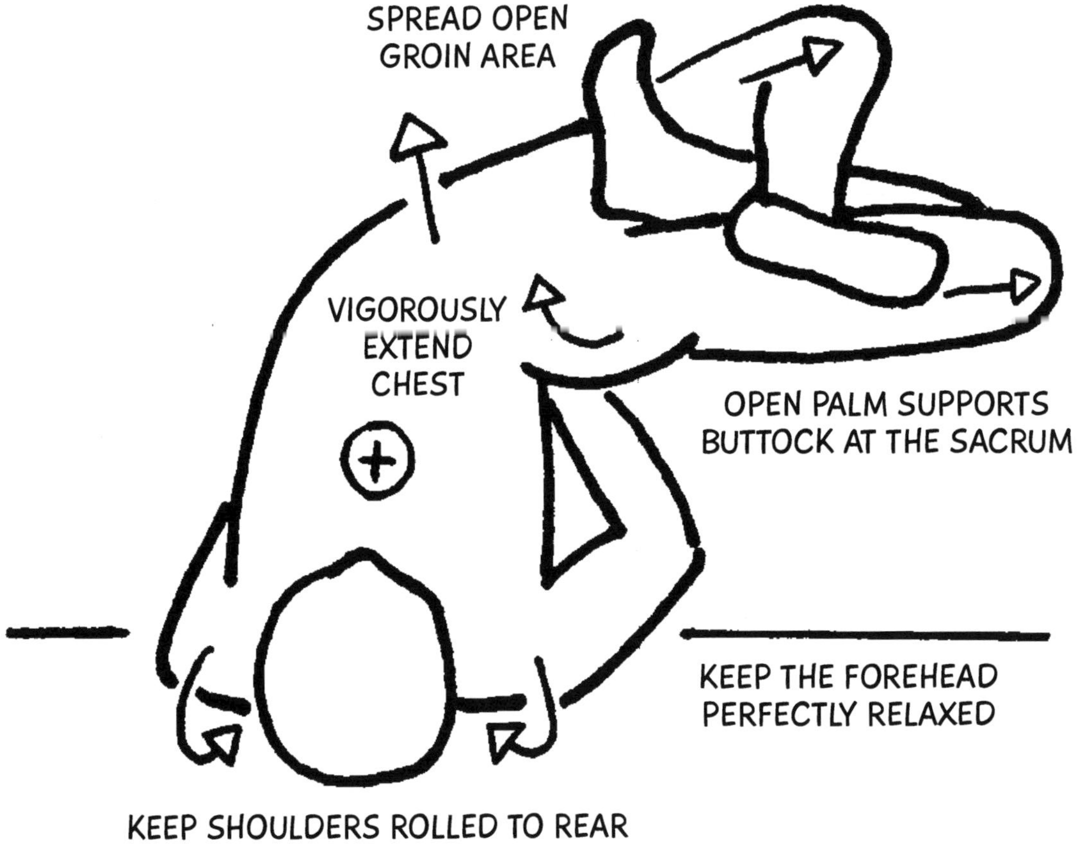
SPREAD OPEN
GROIN AREA
VIGOROUSLY
EXTEND
CHEST
OPEN PALM SUPPORTS
BUTTOCK AT THE SACRUM
KEEP THE FOREHEAD
PERFECTLY RELAXED
KEEP SHOULDERS ROLLED TO REAR

Pinda Sarvangasna 20-30s (62)

embryo whole body

Var: Continue supporting the trunk with palms as in previous posture, bend legs down and draw them toward the chest.

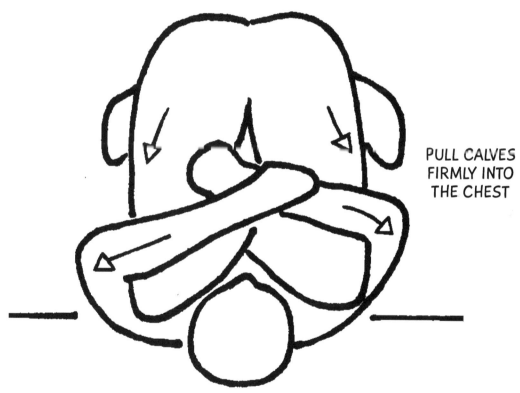

INTERLOCK THE LEGS WITH AS MUCH OF THE ANKLE CROSSING OVER THE THIGH AS POSSIBLE.
PULL CALVES FIRMLY INTO THE CHEST
TONGUES RESTS PASSIVELY ON FLOOR OF MOUTH WITH MOUTH SHUT AND FACE RELAXED.

Parsva Pinda Sarvangasana 20-30s (63)

side embryo whole body

Note: When you return to the floor from SARVANGASANA lower the legs over the head, extend the arms straight back on the floor, and lower the body very slowly. Keep the back of the neck thrust toward the floor throughout this transition, i.e. don't allow the chin to rise,

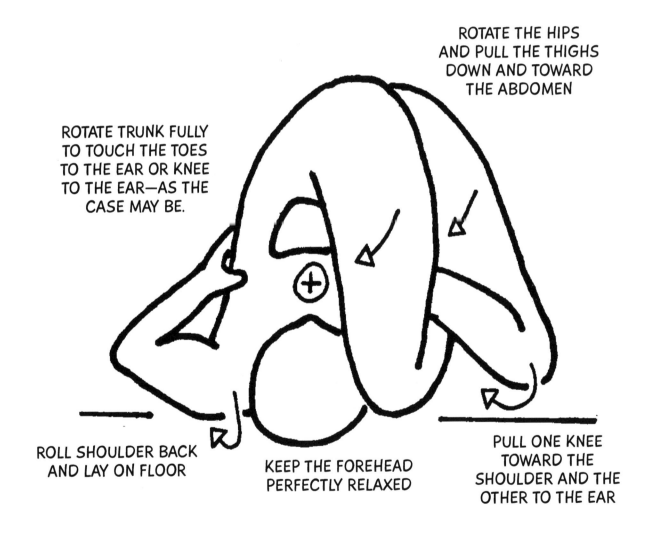

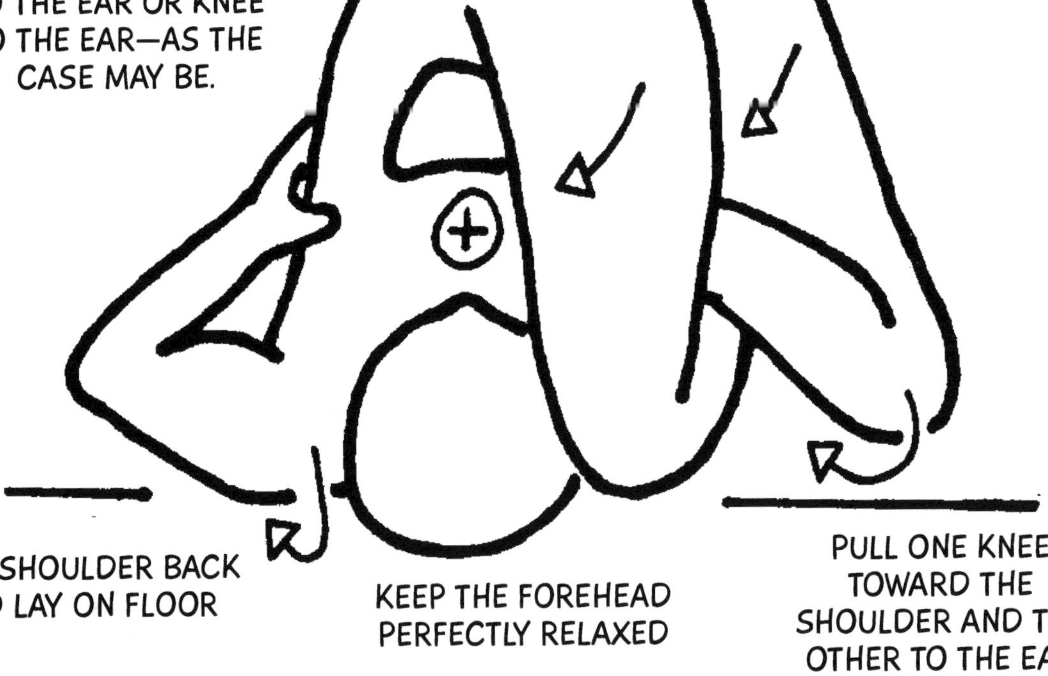
ROTATE THE HIPS AND PULL THE THIGHS DOWN AND TOWARD THE ABDOMEN
ROTATE TRUNK FULLY TO TOUCH THE TOES TO THE EAR OR KNEE TO THE EAR—AS THE CASE MAY BE.
ROLL SHOULDER BACK AND LAY ON FLOOR
KEEP THE FOREHEAD PERFECTLY RELAXED
PULL ONE KNEE TOWARD THE SHOULDER AND THE OTHER TO THE EAR

Parivrtta Janu Sirsasana 20s (64)

revolved knee head

Note: In this and other postures, never use strained exhalations. Instead, allow diaphragm to return to a completely relaxed and natural state while still keeping chest fully extended.

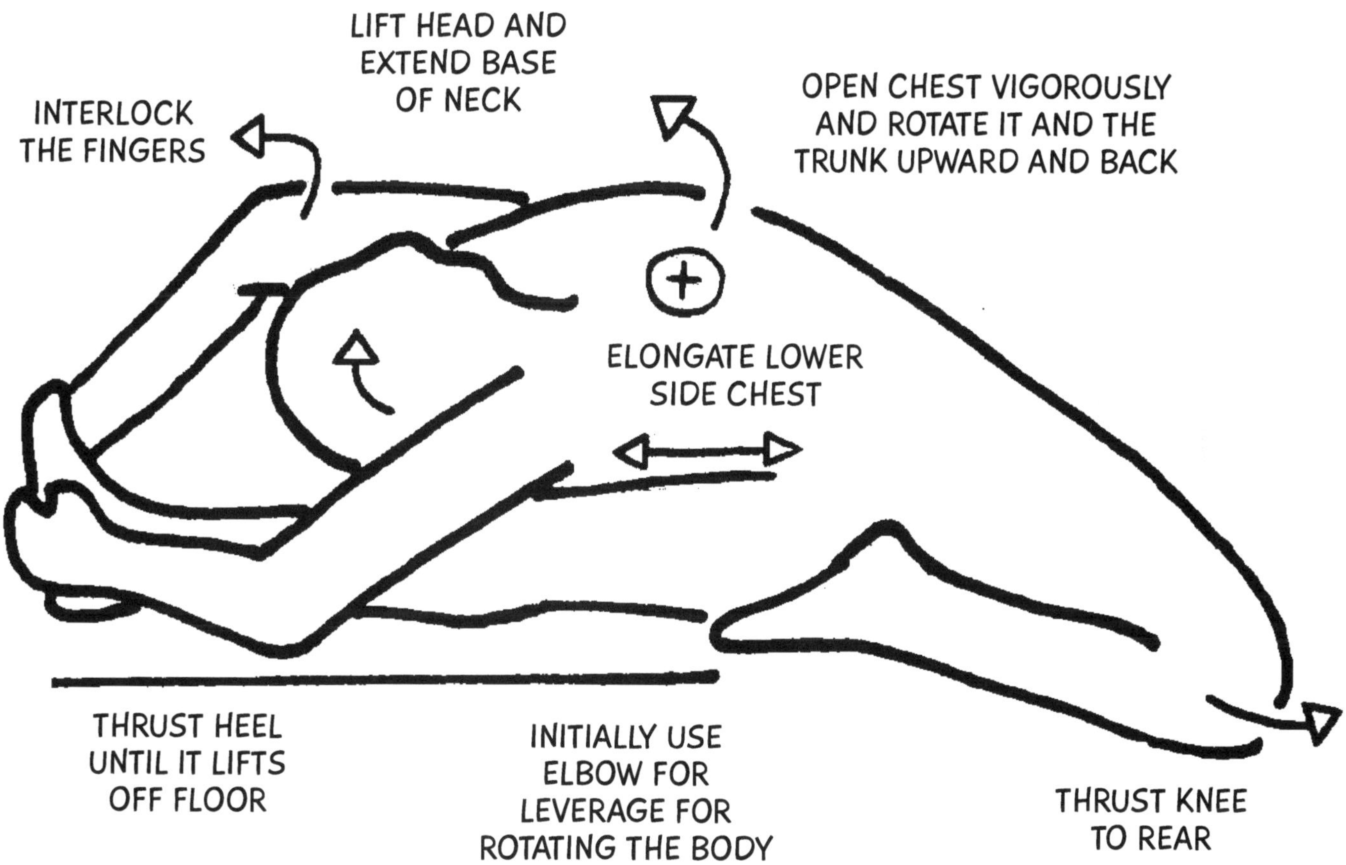

INTERLOCK THE FINGERS
LIFT HEAD AND EXTEND BASE OF NECK
OPEN CHEST VIGOROUSLY AND ROTATE IT AND THE TRUNK UPWARD AND BACK
ELONGATE LOWER SIDE CHEST
THRUST HEEL UNTIL IT LIFTS OFF FLOOR
INITIALLY USE ELBOW FOR LEVERAGE FOR ROTATING THE BODY
THRUST KNEE TO REAR

Triang Mukhaika Pada Paschimottanasana 30-60s (65)

3 parts, face, one foot stretch

Note: In this and all other forward bends, your primary effort is directed toward vigorously extending the chest and thrusting it forward. As your flexibility improves you will strive to press the entire length of the trunk (chest and abdomen) onto the thigh. You then thrust the trunk along the thigh, rubbing it as you thrust the trunk forward on each inhalation.

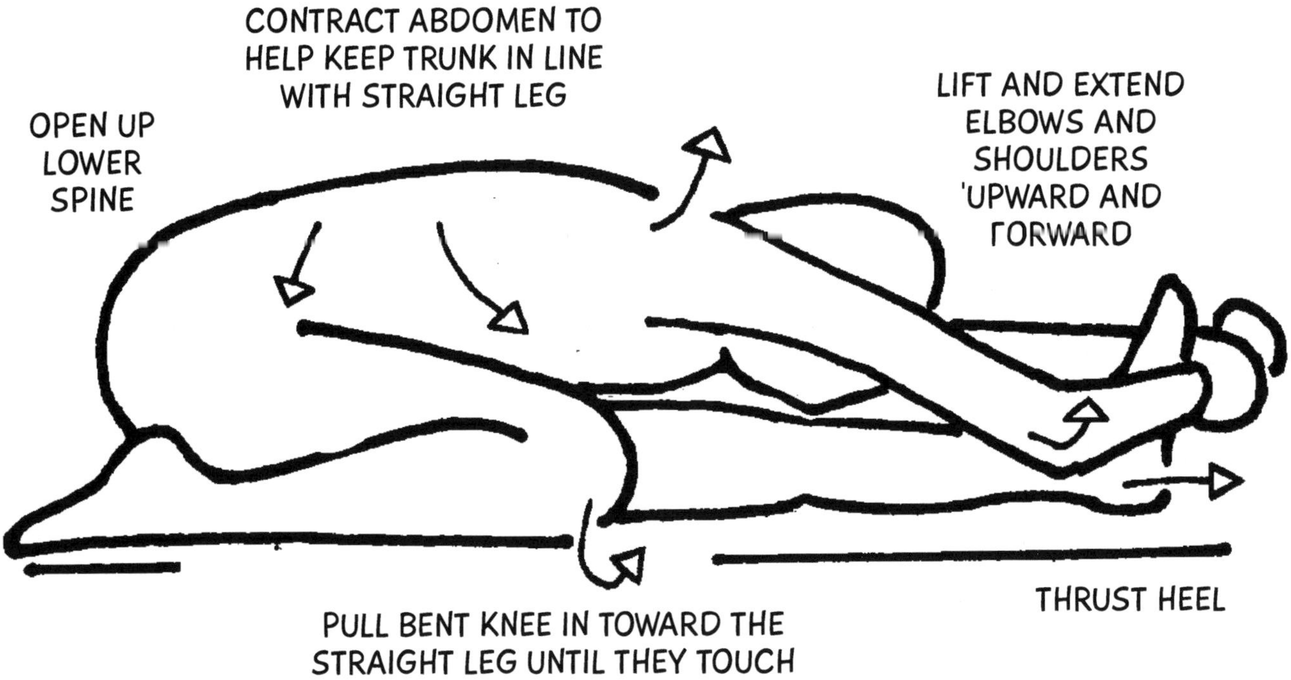

CONTRACT ABDOMEN TO HELP KEEP TRUNK IN LINE WITH STRAIGHT LEG
OPEN UP LOWER SPINE
LIFT AND EXTEND ELBOWS AND SHOULDERS 'UPWARD AND FORWARD
PULL BENT KNEE IN TOWARD THE STRAIGHT LEG UNTIL THEY TOUCH
THRUST HEEL

Upavistha Konasana 30-60s (66)

seated angle

Note: In this and most forward bending postures, begin by pulling the fleshy part of the buttocks outward from under the pelvis. This allows you to bring more of the lower front of the pelvic bone in firm contact with the floor.

As a variation, keep your hands extended above your toes and thrust them outward as you lift them upward.

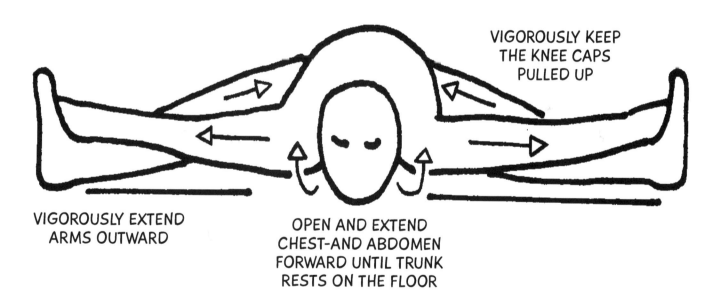

VIGOROUSLY KEEP THE KNEE CAPS PULLED UP
VIGOROUSLY EXTEND ARMS OUTWARD
OPEN AND EXTEND CHEST-AND ABDOMEN FORWARD UNTIL TRUNK RESTS ON THE FLOOR

Baddha Padmasana 30-60s (67)

bound lotus

Note: To make grasping the feet easier, pass the right arm over the left when the left leg passes over the right, and visa versa.

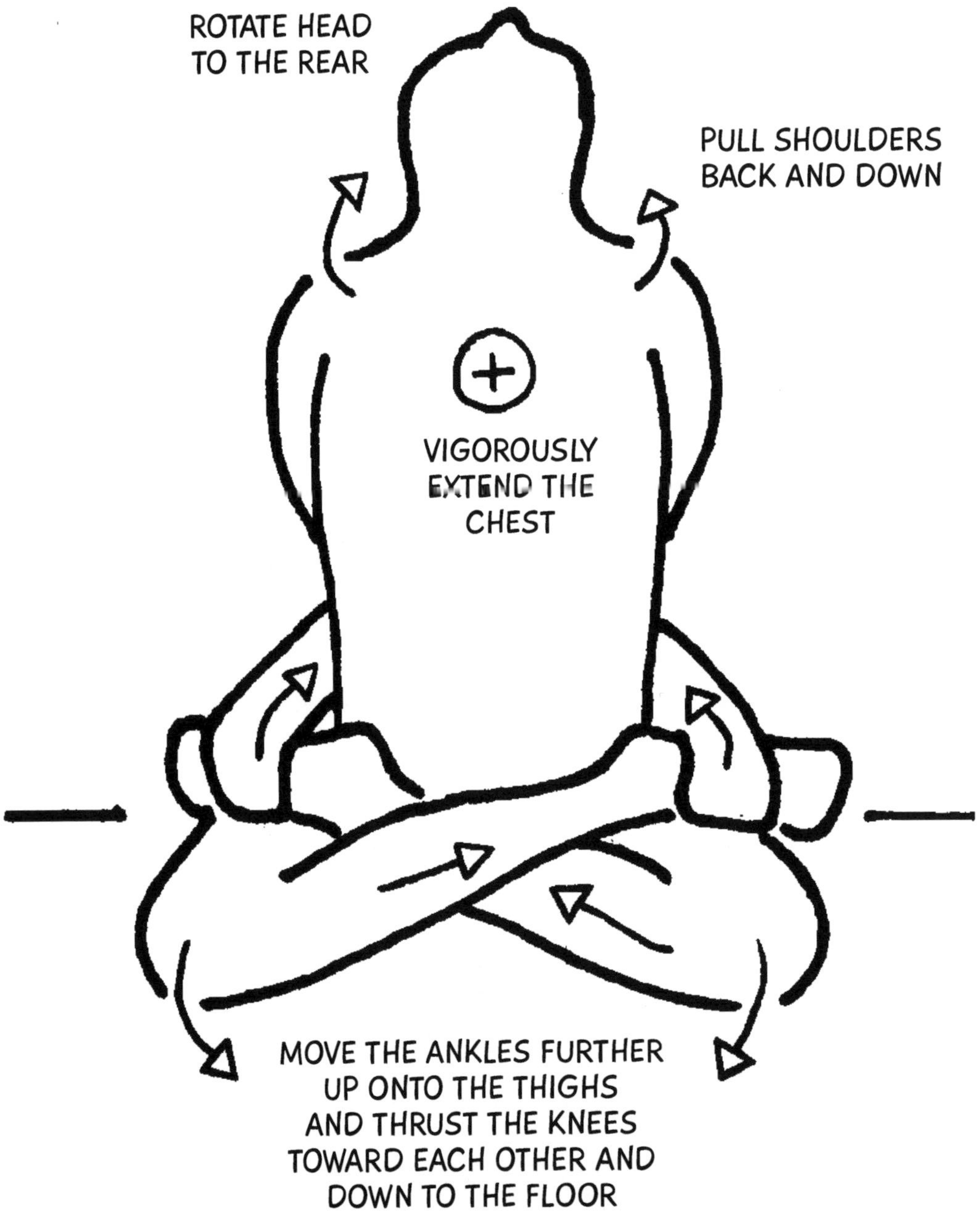
ROTATE HEAD
TO THE REAR
PULL SHOULDERS
BACK AND DOWN
VIGOROUSLY
EXTEND THE
CHEST
MOVE THE ANKLES FURTHER
UP ONTO THE THIGHS
AND THRUST THE KNEES
TOWARD EACH OTHER AND
DOWN TO THE FLOOR

Yoga Mudrasana 60s (68)

Yoga sealing

> **Var:** If you can't grasp the toes, press the palms together as in Parsvottanasana or interlock fingers and rotate palms upward over the head as in Halasana. Then bend forward.

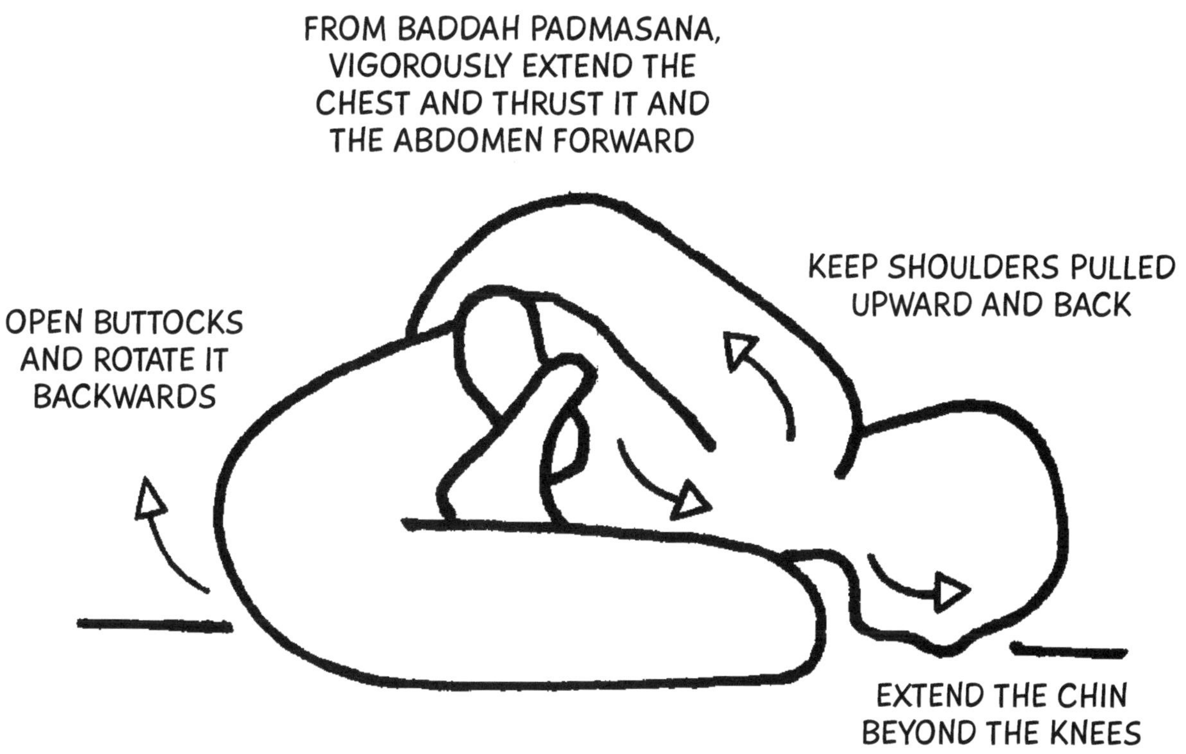
FROM BADDAH PADMASANA, VIGOROUSLY EXTEND THE CHEST AND THRUST IT AND THE ABDOMEN FORWARD
KEEP SHOULDERS PULLED UPWARD AND BACK
OPEN BUTTOCKS AND ROTATE IT BACKWARDS
EXTEND THE CHIN BEYOND THE KNEES

> **Note:** In this and in all other lotus postures, you should strive to bring the feet up onto the thigh as high as possible, until the ankles rest on the upper part of the thighs. This produces a very firm interlocking of the legs.

Simhasana 30-60s

lion

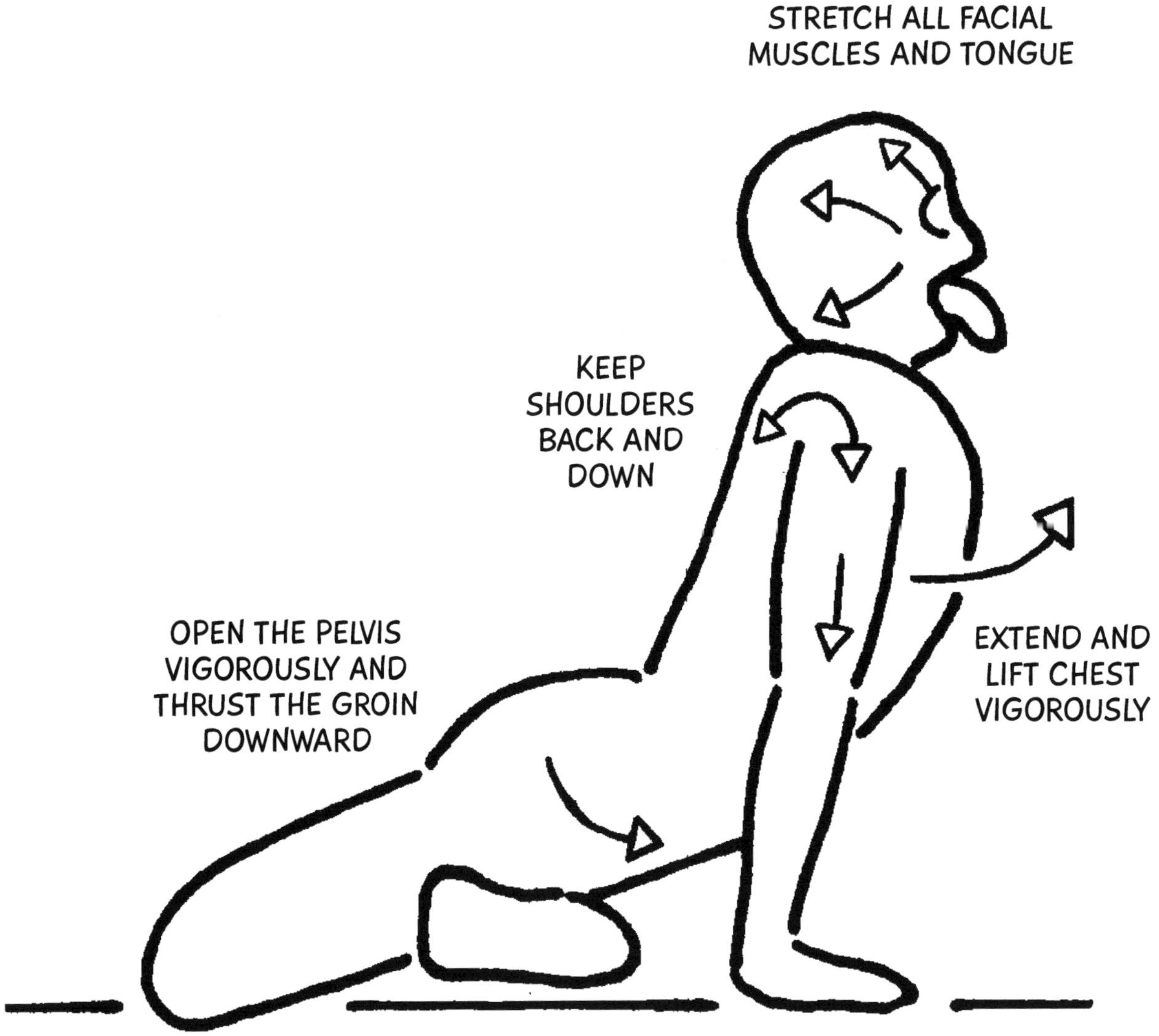
STRETCH ALL FACIAL MUSCLES AND TONGUE
KEEP SHOULDERS BACK AND DOWN
EXTEND AND LIFT CHEST VIGOROUSLY
OPEN THE PELVIS VIGOROUSLY AND THRUST THE GROIN DOWNWARD

Note: You can also lower the body until the chest nearly touches the floor.

Garbha Pindasana 15-30s (70)

embryo lotus

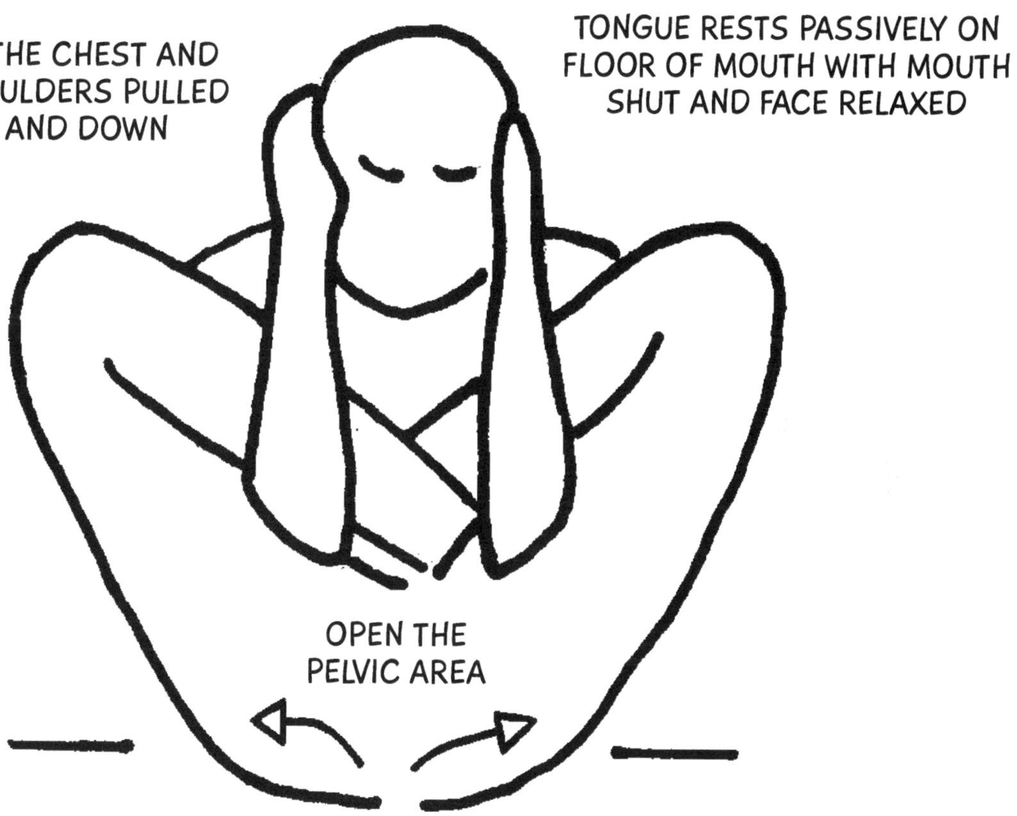

EXTEND THE CHEST AND KEEP SHOULDERS PULLED BACK AND DOWN
TONGUE RESTS PASSIVELY ON FLOOR OF MOUTH WITH MOUTH SHUT AND FACE RELAXED
OPEN THE PELVIC AREA

Note: When the left leg crosses over the right, first slip the right arm thru the interlocked legs between the left ankle and the back of the right knee. Now slip the left arm through between the right ankle and the back of the left knee.

Goraksasana a few seconds (71)

cowhead

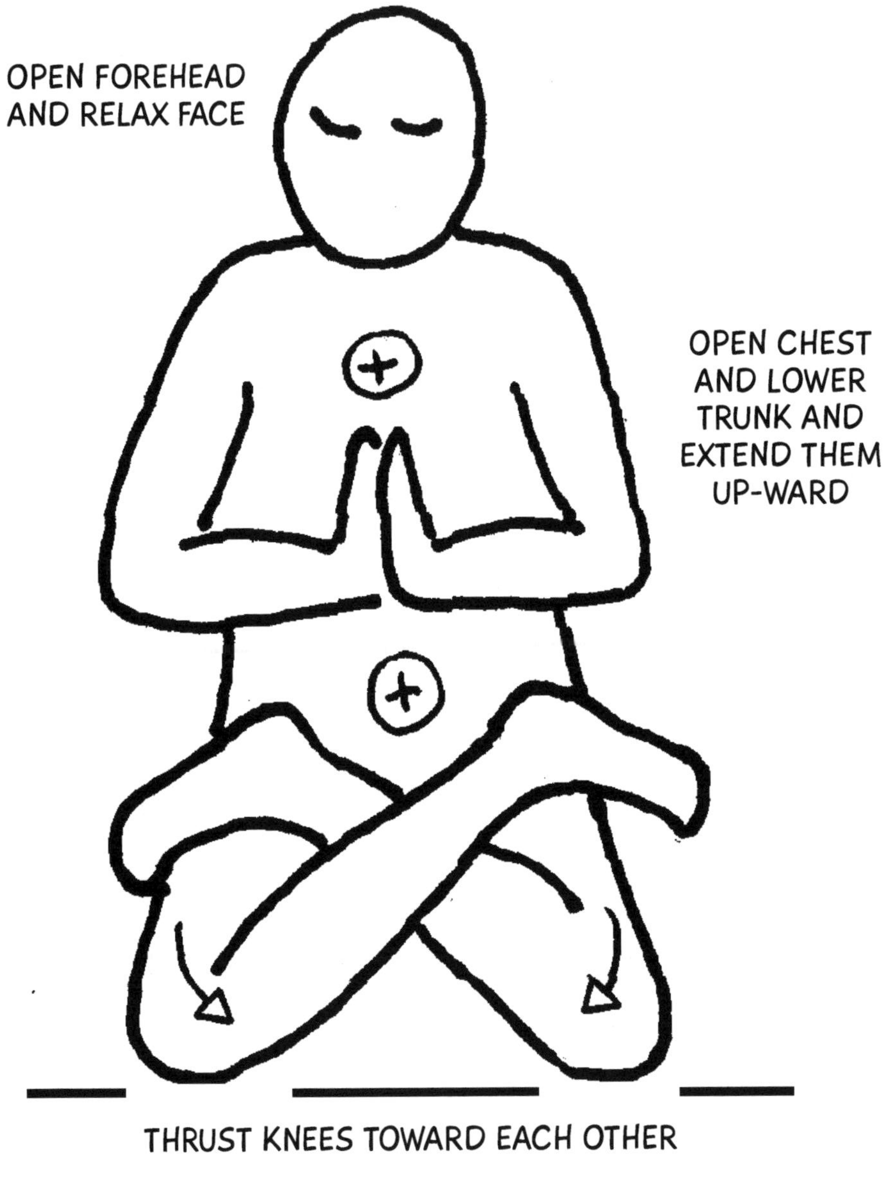

OPEN FOREHEAD
AND RELAX FACE
OPEN CHEST
AND LOWER
TRUNK AND
EXTEND THEM
UP-WARD
THRUST KNEES TOWARD EACH OTHER

Note: It can take years to be able to maintain the balance in this posture. For one thing, balance depends on pelic flexibility. The more upright you are the longer you can keep balance.

Vatayanasana 30s (72)

horse

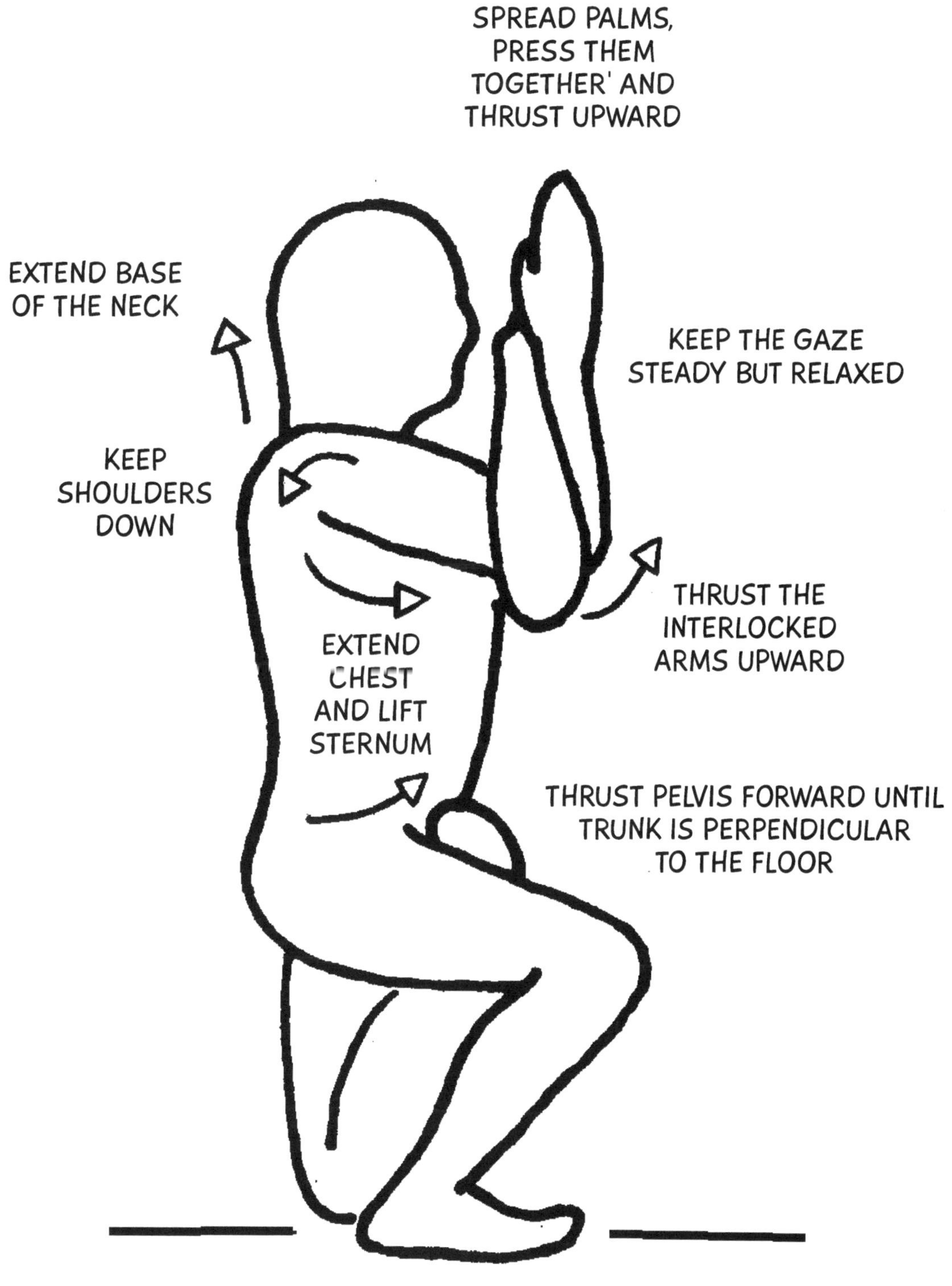
SPREAD PALMS,
PRESS THEM
TOGETHER' AND
THRUST UPWARD
EXTEND BASE
OF THE NECK
KEEP THE GAZE
STEADY BUT RELAXED
KEEP
SHOULDERS
DOWN
THRUST THE
INTERLOCKED
ARMS UPWARD
EXTEND
CHEST
AND LIFT
STERNUM
THRUST PELVIS FORWARD UNTIL
TRUNK IS PERPENDICULAR
TO THE FLOOR

Note: When the right ankle rest on the left thigh wrap the right arm around the left.

Urdhva Dhanurasana 6 times @30s each (73)

up bow

Var.: You may keep legs bent and move feet closer in toward the hands for first few years. Try this posture with hands next to a wall. Later go up to or down from standing position by walking hands up or down the wall.

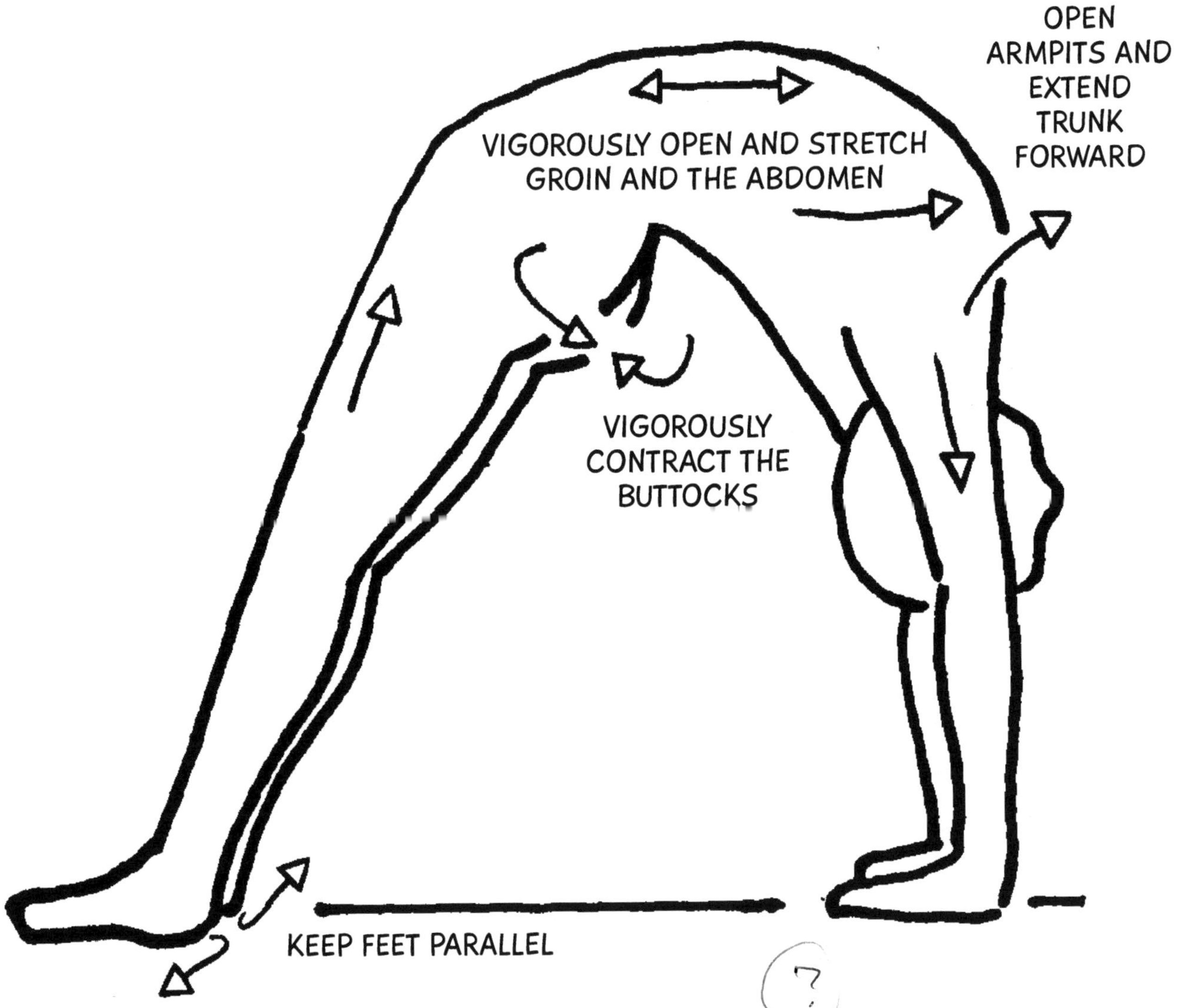

OPEN ARMPITS AND EXTEND TRUNK FORWARD
VIGOROUSLY OPEN AND STRETCH GROIN AND THE ABDOMEN
VIGOROUSLY CONTRACT THE BUTTOCKS
KEEP FEET PARALLEL

Note: In this and in all other back bending postures, you should vigorously contract the buttocks and the anal sphincter muscle. Also stretch and open the groin outward as much as possible. Allow diaphragm to relax naturally - while still keeping chest fully extended.

Move into this posture slowly, bending from the lower lumbar area of the spine. Try to imagine space being created between these vertebrae which allows them to bend more fully.

Bakasana 15-30s (74)

crane

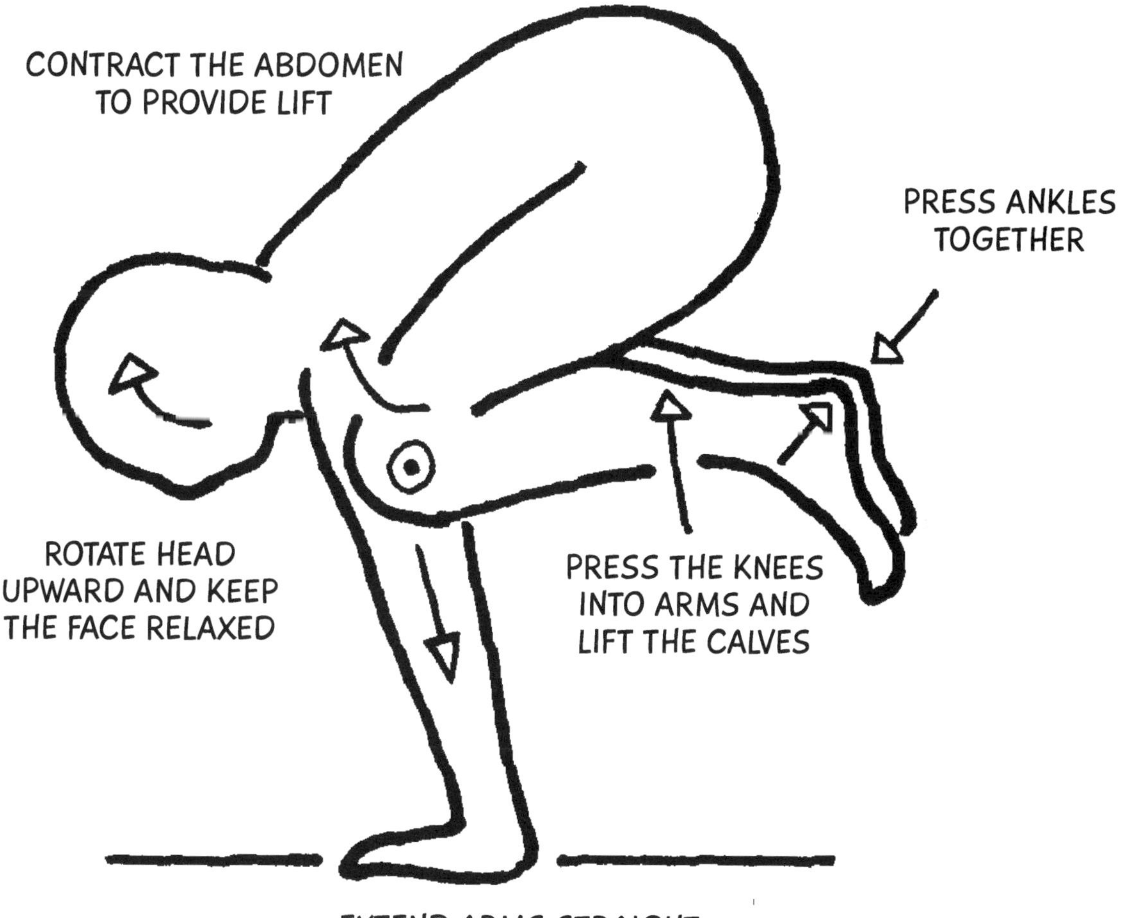
CONTRACT THE ABDOMEN
TO PROVIDE LIFT
PRESS ANKLES
TOGETHER
ROTATE HEAD
UPWARD AND KEEP
THE FACE RELAXED
PRESS THE KNEES
INTO ARMS AND
LIFT THE CALVES
EXTEND ARMS STRAIGHT

Keep the wrists firm and feel them rooted to the floor. This helps stabilize balance.

Bhujapidasana 30-60s (75)

arm pressure

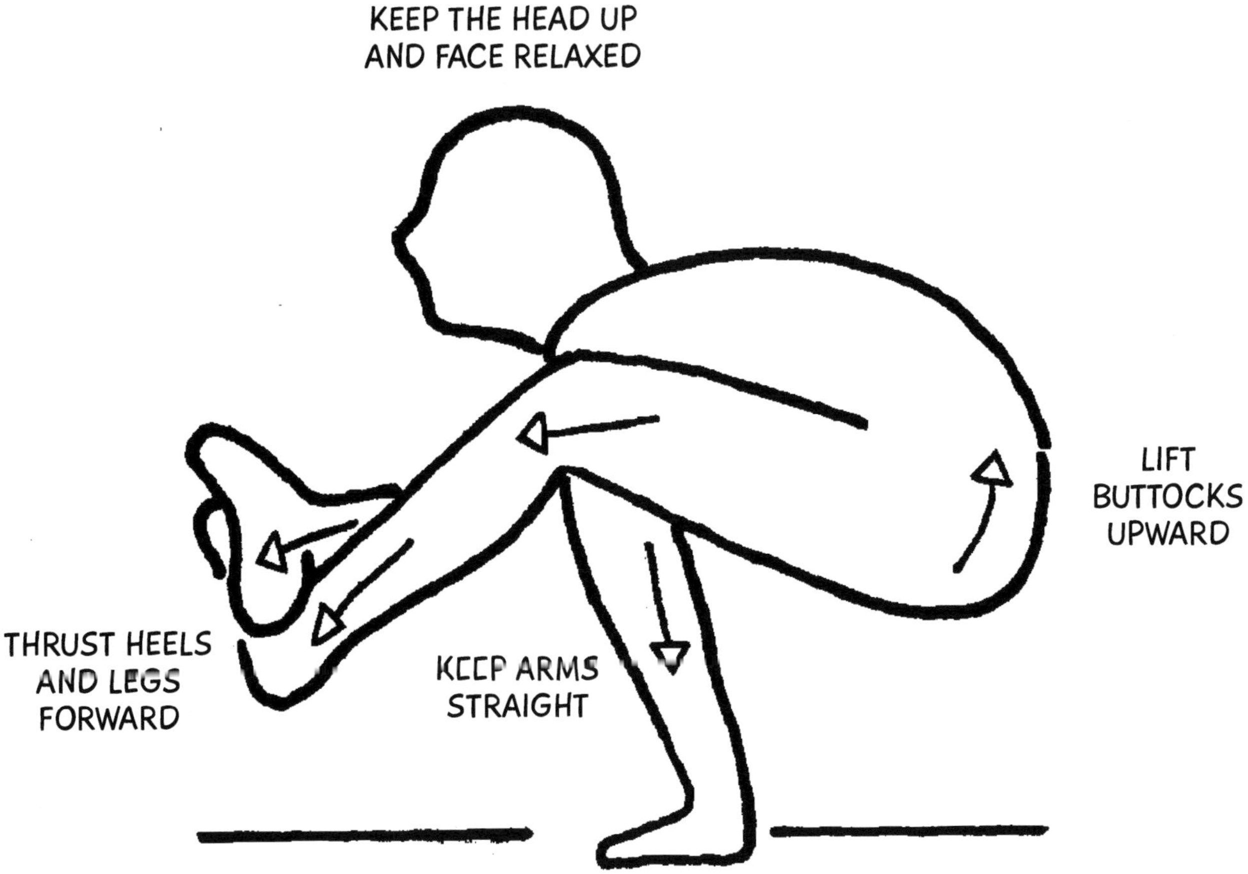
KEEP THE HEAD UP
AND FACE RELAXED
LIFT
BUTTOCKS
UPWARD
THRUST HEELS
AND LEGS
FORWARD
KEEP ARMS
STRAIGHT

Note: It helps to get the knees as high up on the shoulder as possible before lifting the feet off the ground. In this and other postures, never use strained exhalations. Instead, allow diaphragm to relax naturally - while still keeping chest fully extended. However, to move into the posture fully, initially pull your trunk between your arms using vigorous, repeated exhalations.

Again, for help in learning how to move into or out of the Yoga postures, take a Hatha Yoga class from a competent teacher and/or refer to B.K.S, Iyengars' most excellent book - ***Light on Yoga.***

Mayurasana 30-60s (76)

peacock

Var: Keep the toes on the floor, keep the body straight, extend the chest and lift the upper trunk. Then keeping the body straight, gradually move the body forward until toes leave the floor.

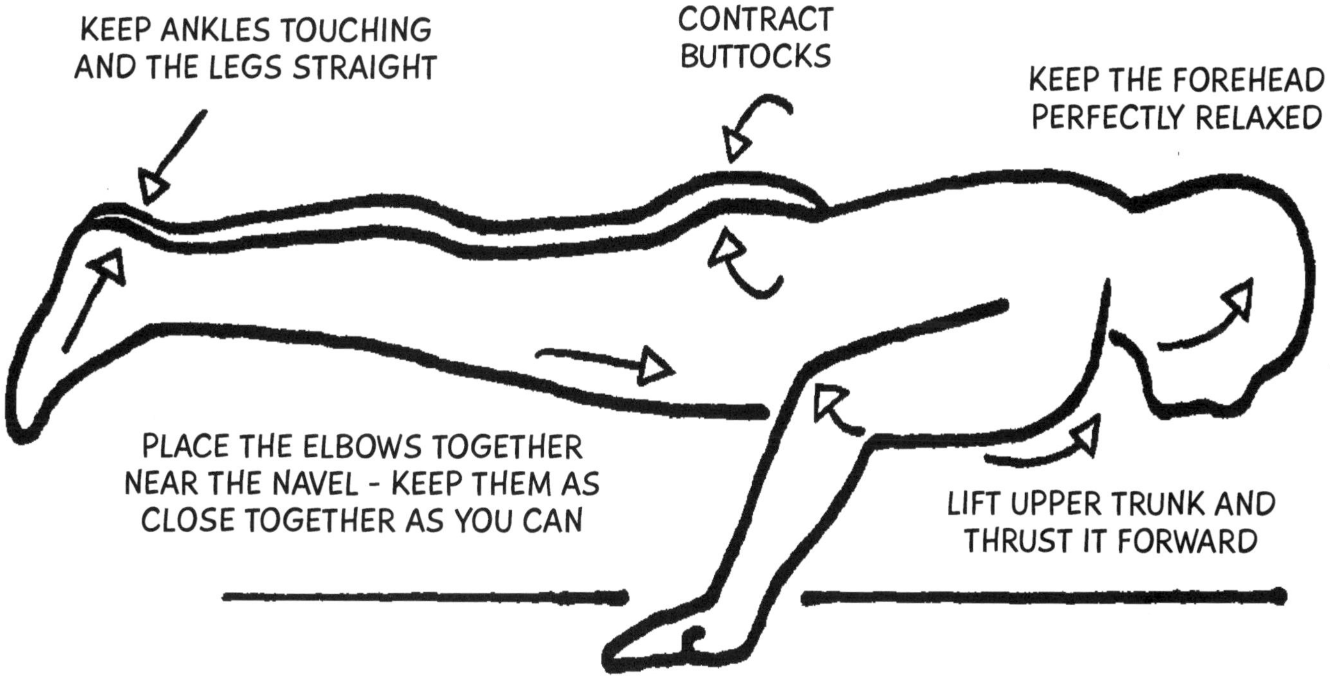
KEEP ANKLES TOUCHING AND THE LEGS STRAIGHT
CONTRACT BUTTOCKS
KEEP THE FOREHEAD PERFECTLY RELAXED
PLACE THE ELBOWS TOGETHER NEAR THE NAVEL - KEEP THEM AS CLOSE TOGETHER AS YOU CAN
LIFT UPPER TRUNK AND THRUST IT FORWARD

Parsva Dhanurasana 20-30s (77)

side bow

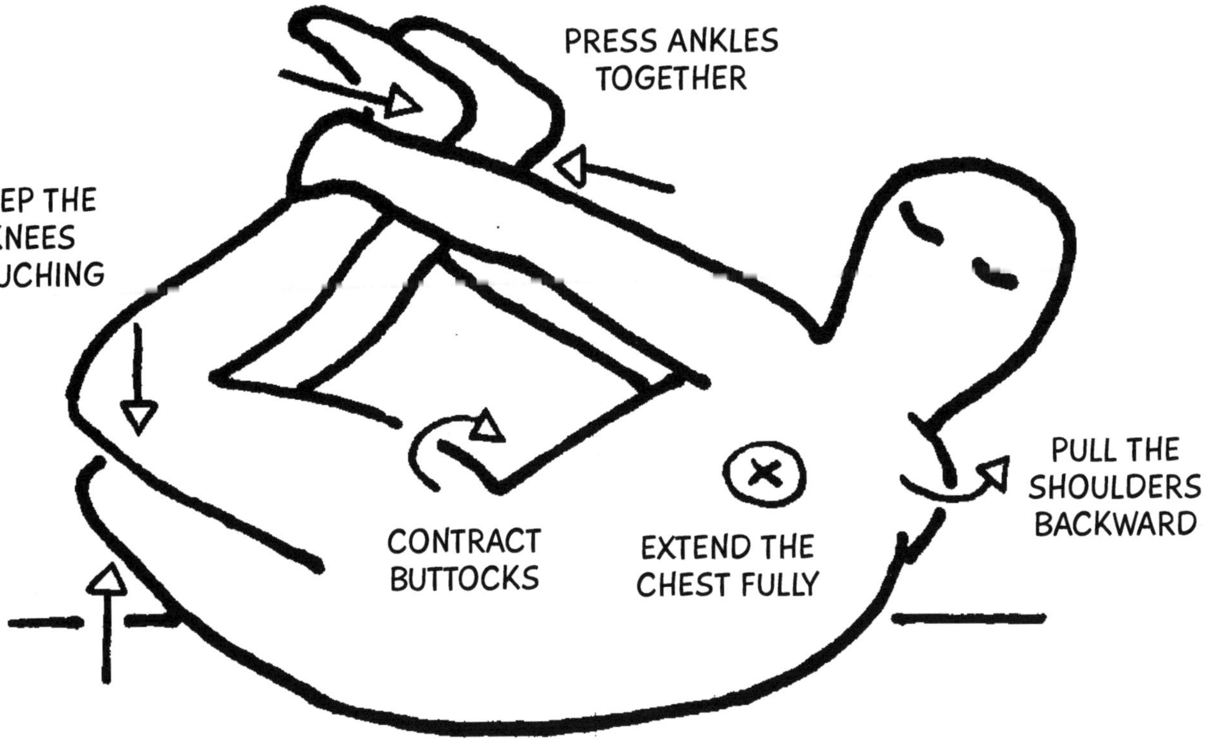
PRESS ANKLES TOGETHER
KEEP THE KNEES TOUCHING
PULL THE SHOULDERS BACKWARD
CONTRACT BUTTOCKS
EXTEND THE CHEST FULLY

Bhekasana 30s (78)

frog

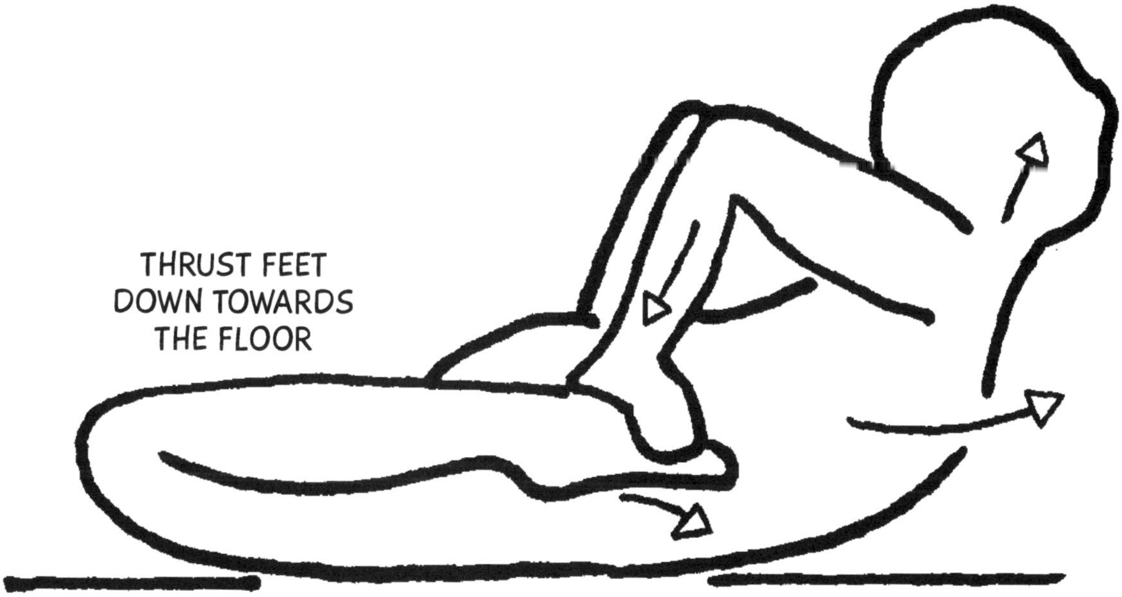
ROTATE HEAD
UPWARD
THRUST FEET
DOWN TOWARDS
THE FLOOR
VIGOROUSLY EXTEND
CHEST AND CONTRACT
ABDOMEN TO PROVIDE LIFT

Program 5

First Day: Begin with the **Headstand Cycle (page 103)**. Half of the postures will be new to you. Add those you feel ready for. Skip those you don't, and return to them later when you feel ready. Be patient. You have a lifetime to incorporate these into your practice. Consistency of practice is the key, not which postures you do, or don't do.

Next do the **Forward Cycle (page 73)**. Here also, half of them will be new to you. Again, add those you feel ready for and skip those you don't. Finish up with the **Lotus Cycle (page 72)** and then these twists postures and Urdhva Dhanurasana below. Finally, treat yourself to a few minute of Savasana. You have earned it!

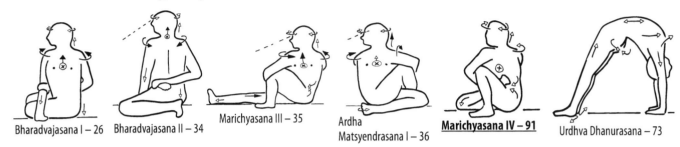

Bharadvajasana I – 26

Bharadvajasana II – 34

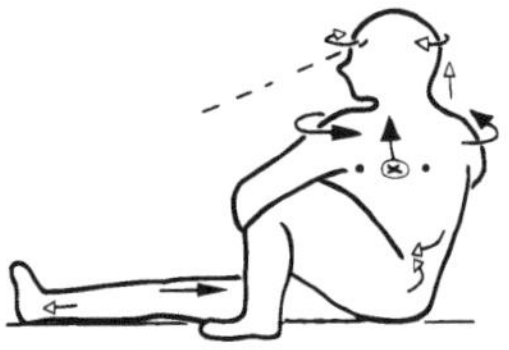
Marichyasana III – 35

Ardha Matsyendrasana I – 36

Marichyasana IV – 91

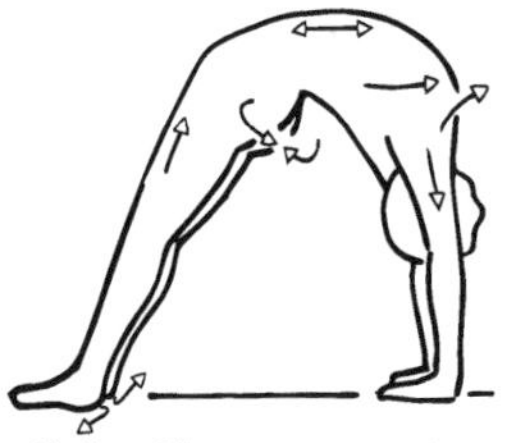
Urdhva Dhanurasana – 73

Second Day: Begin with the Sirsasana, Urdhva Danadasana and the arm balances below. Next do the **Shoulderstand Cycle (page 103)**. Here, there are only a few new postures to add. Afterward, do the **Forward Cycle (page 73)**. Finish up with the twists and Urdhva Dhanurasana above, and then with a few minute of Savasana.

Sirsasana I – 27

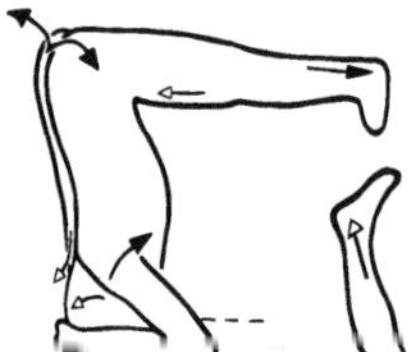
Urdhva Dandasana – 28

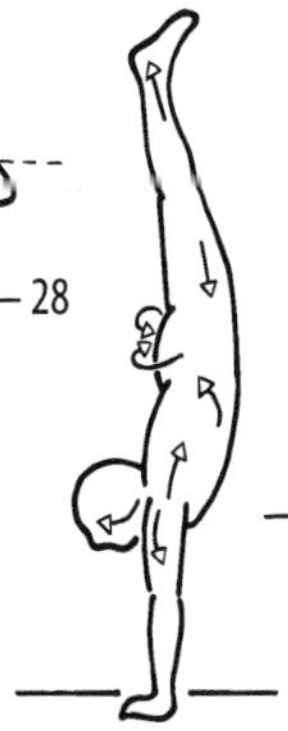
Adho Mukha Vrksasana – 92

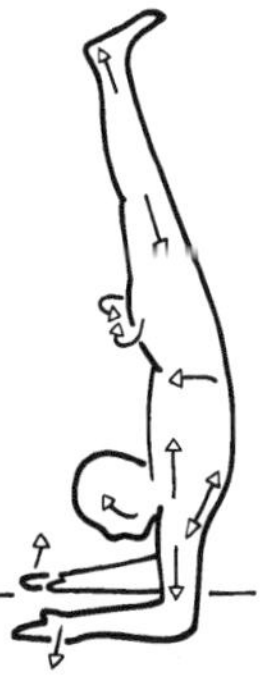
Pincha Mayurasana – 93

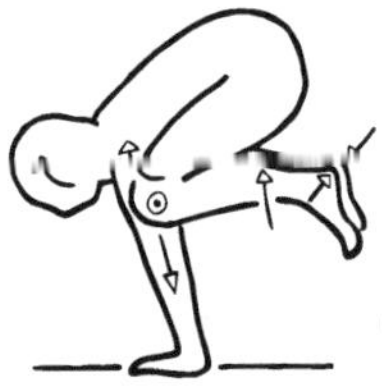
Bakasana – 74

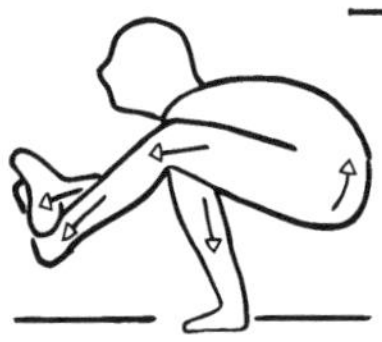
Bhujapidasana – 75

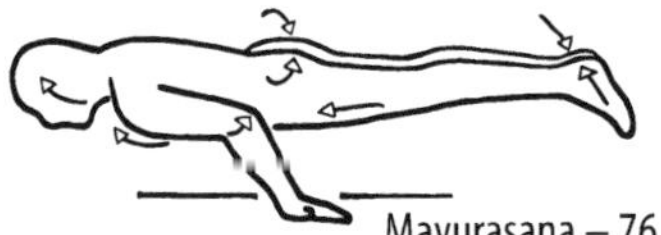
Mayurasana – 76

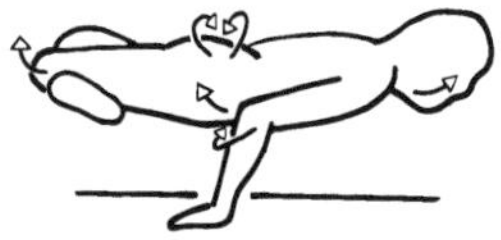

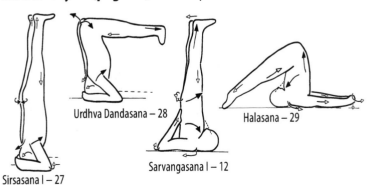
Padma Mayurasana – 94

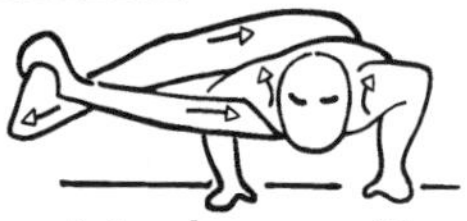
Astavakrasana – 95

Review (or Third) Day: Begin with the Sirsasana, Urdhva Danadasana, Sarvangasana and Halasana below. Hold these longer - up to 10 minutes for Sirsasana and Sarvangasana. Next do the **Standing Cycle (page 72)** followed by the **Basic Cycle (page 73)**. Finish up with a few minute of Savasana, Pranayama in Savasana, and Meditation (to suit).

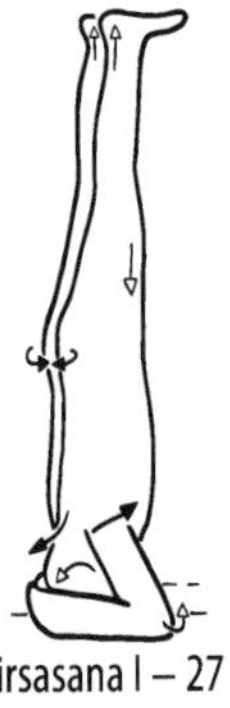
Sirsasana I – 27

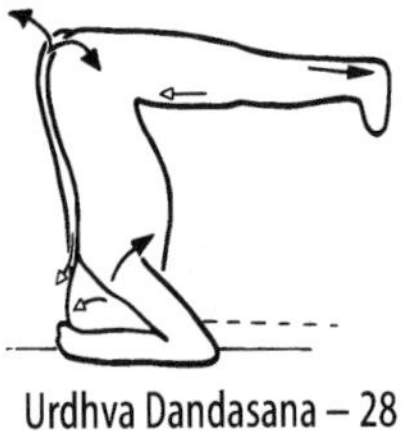
Urdhva Dandasana – 28

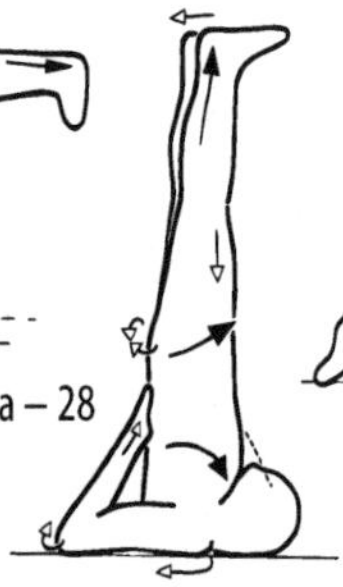
Sarvangasana I – 12

Halasana – 29

Note: Mentally explore your body and all the aspects of each posture to find more subtle ways to increase the challenge. The arrows only show the basic and easily defined dynamics of the posture. By conscientious practice you will continually find subtler and more personal aspects to work on - especially if you build a solid foundation in the basics.

With postures you find too difficult, you can invent your own variation if you need to. You will progress steadily, even without a teacher, as long as you are working and watchful.

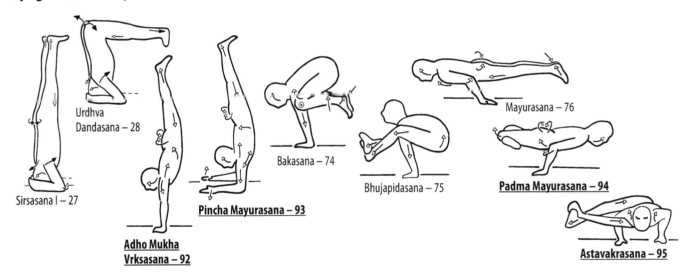

Headstand Cycle (About 11 minutes)

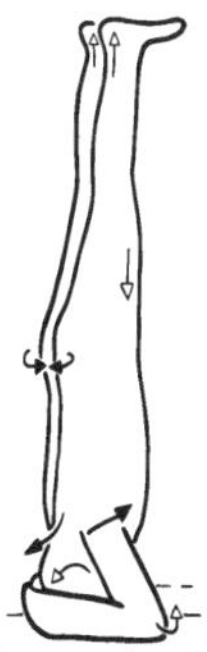

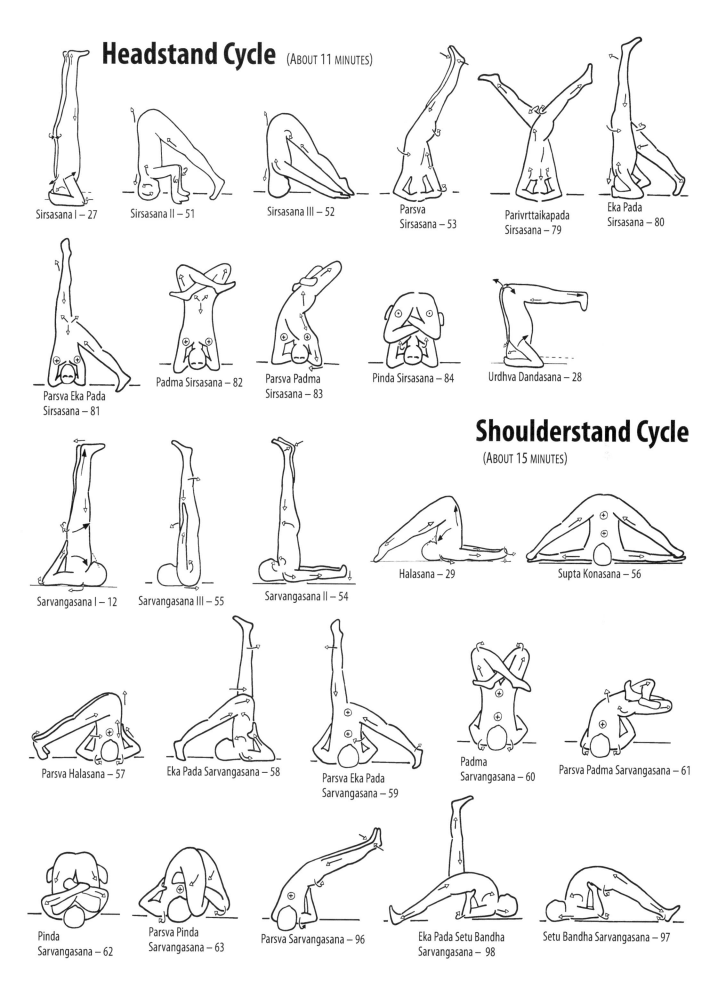

Sirsasana I – 27

Sirsasana II – 51

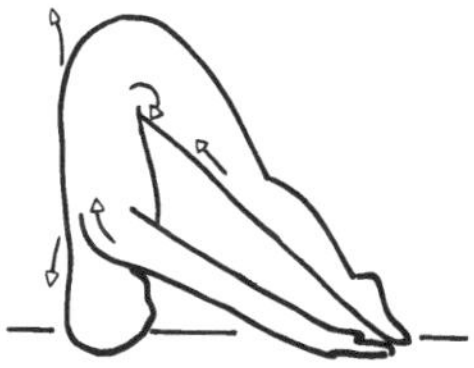

Sirsasana III – 52

Parsva Sirsasana – 53

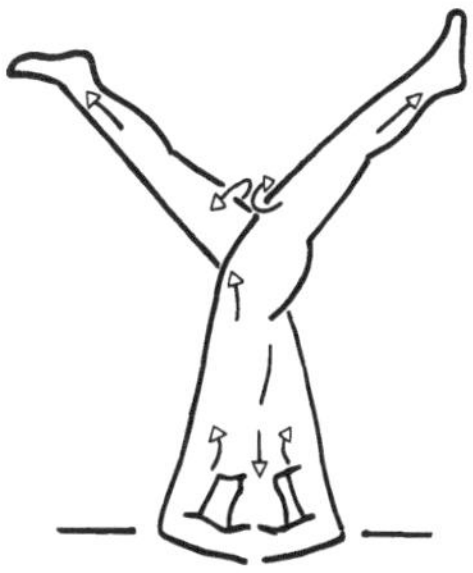

Parivrttaikapada Sirsasana – 79

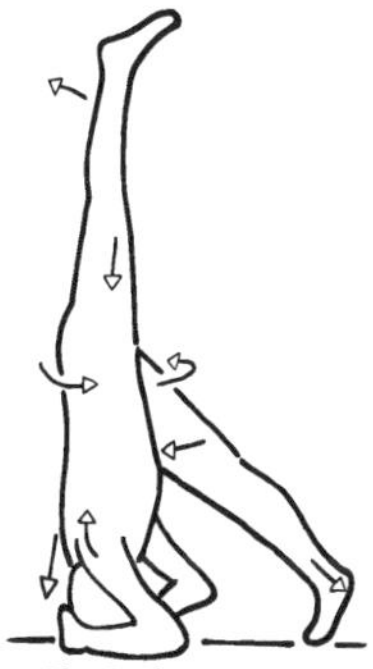

Eka Pada Sirsasana – 80

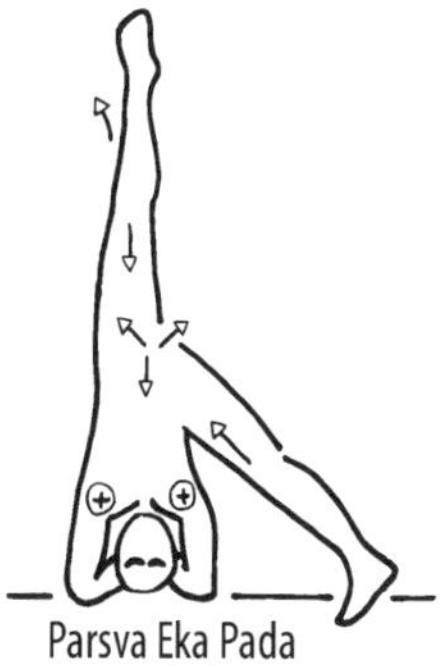

Parsva Eka Pada Sirsasana – 81

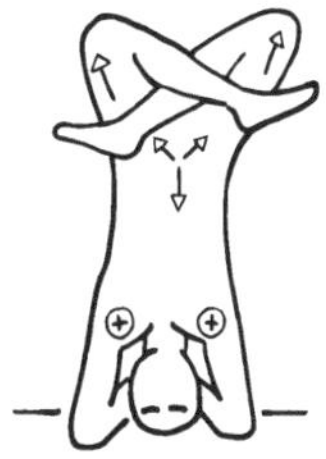

Padma Sirsasana – 82

Parsva Padma Sirsasana – 83

Pinda Sirsasana – 84

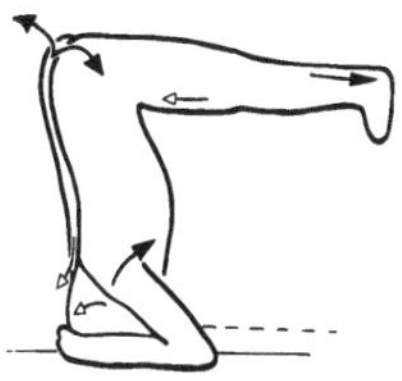

Urdhva Dandasana – 28

Shoulderstand Cycle (About 15 minutes)

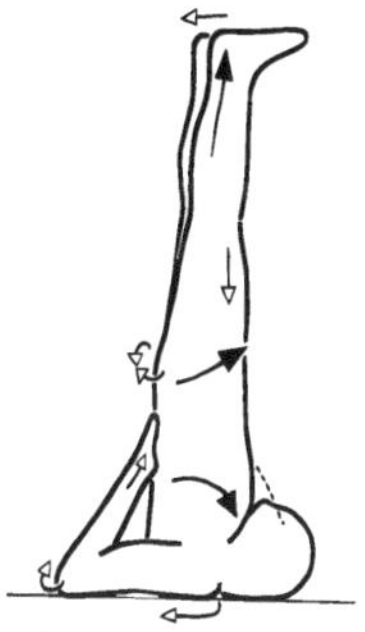

Sarvangasana I – 12

Sarvangasana III – 55

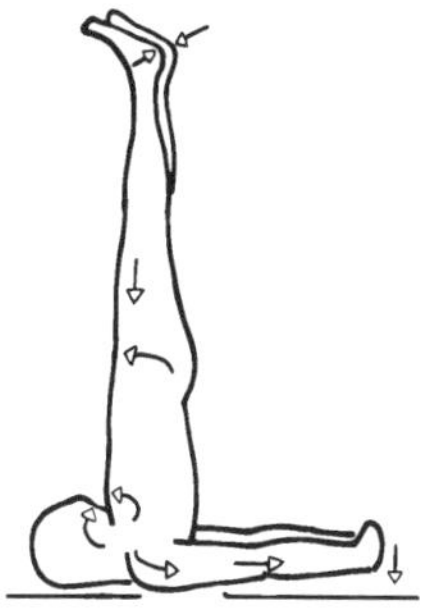

Sarvangasana II – 54

Halasana – 29

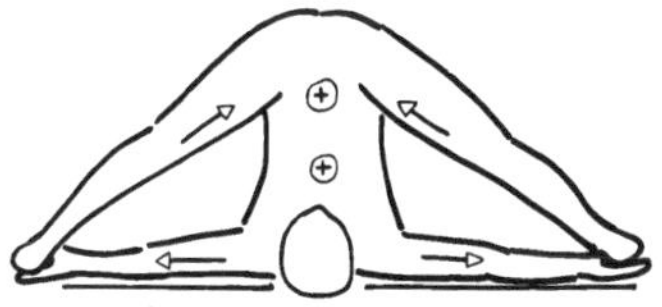

Supta Konasana – 56

Parsva Halasana – 57

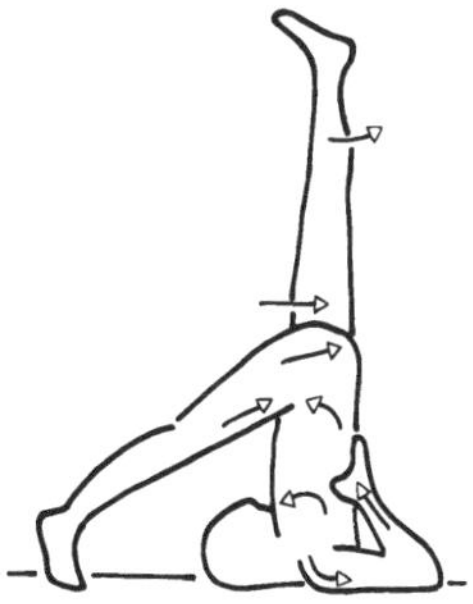

Eka Pada Sarvangasana – 58

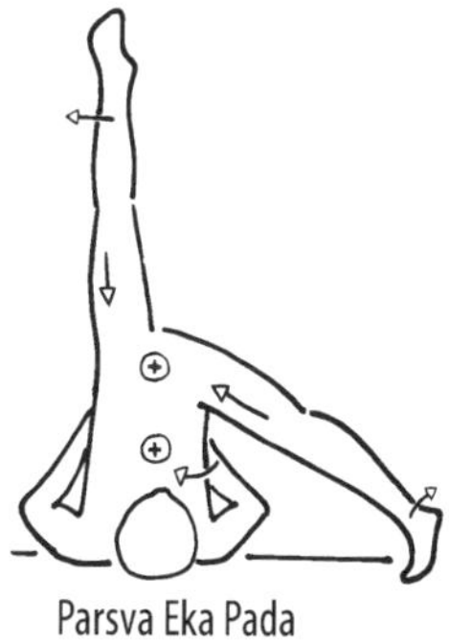

Parsva Eka Pada Sarvangasana – 59

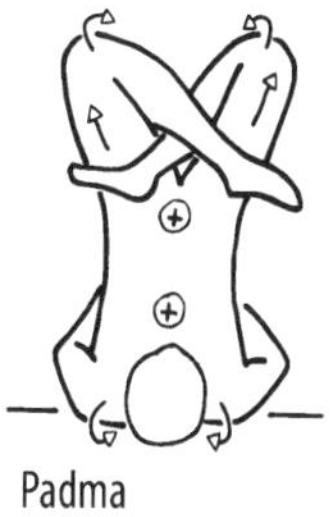

Padma Sarvangasana – 60

Parsva Padma Sarvangasana – 61

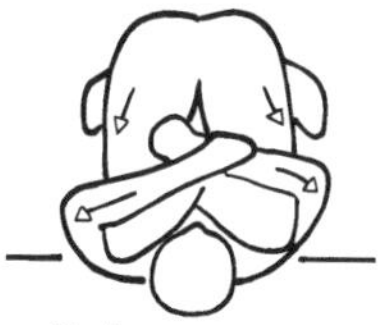

Pinda Sarvangasana – 62

Parsva Pinda Sarvangasana – 63

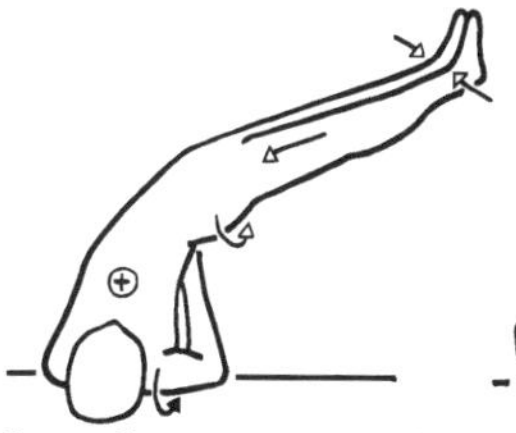

Parsva Sarvangasana – 96

Eka Pada Setu Bandha Sarvangasana – 98

Setu Bandha Sarvangasana – 97

Parivrttaikapada Sirsasana 20s (79)

revolved one leg head

Note: In this and most headstand postures, interlock the fingers firmly and place the head firmly into the cup formed by the hands. This aids stability.

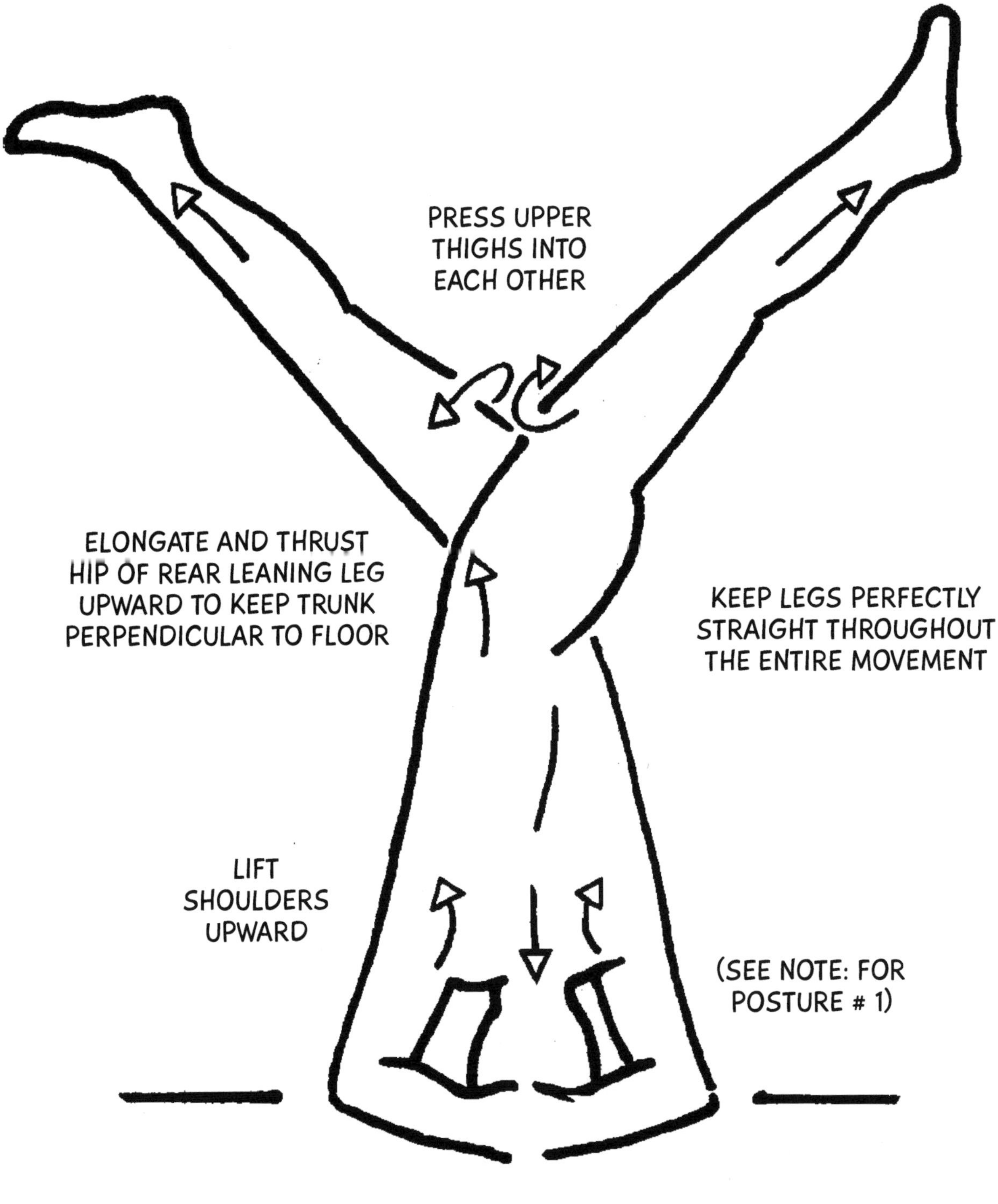

PRESS UPPER THIGHS INTO EACH OTHER
ELONGATE AND THRUST HIP OF REAR LEANING LEG UPWARD TO KEEP TRUNK PERPENDICULAR TO FLOOR
KEEP LEGS PERFECTLY STRAIGHT THROUGHOUT THE ENTIRE MOVEMENT
LIFT SHOULDERS UPWARD
(SEE NOTE: FOR POSTURE # 1)

Eka Pada Sirsasana 10-30s (80)

one leg head

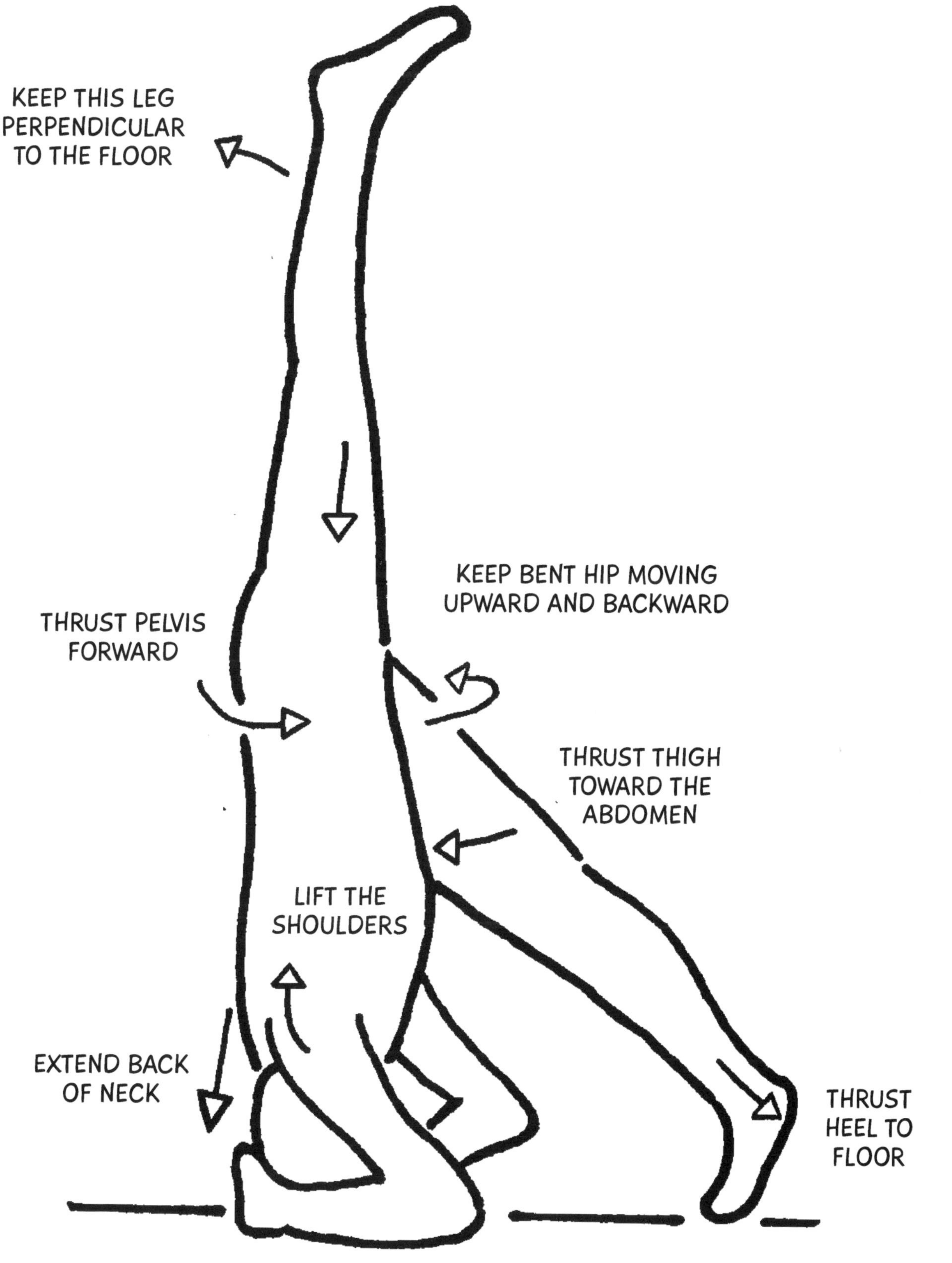

KEEP THIS LEG PERPENDICULAR TO THE FLOOR
KEEP BENT HIP MOVING UPWARD AND BACKWARD
THRUST PELVIS FORWARD
THRUST THIGH TOWARD THE ABDOMEN
LIFT THE SHOULDERS
EXTEND BACK OF NECK
THRUST HEEL TO FLOOR

Parsva Eka Pada Sirsasana 10-30s (81)

side one leg head

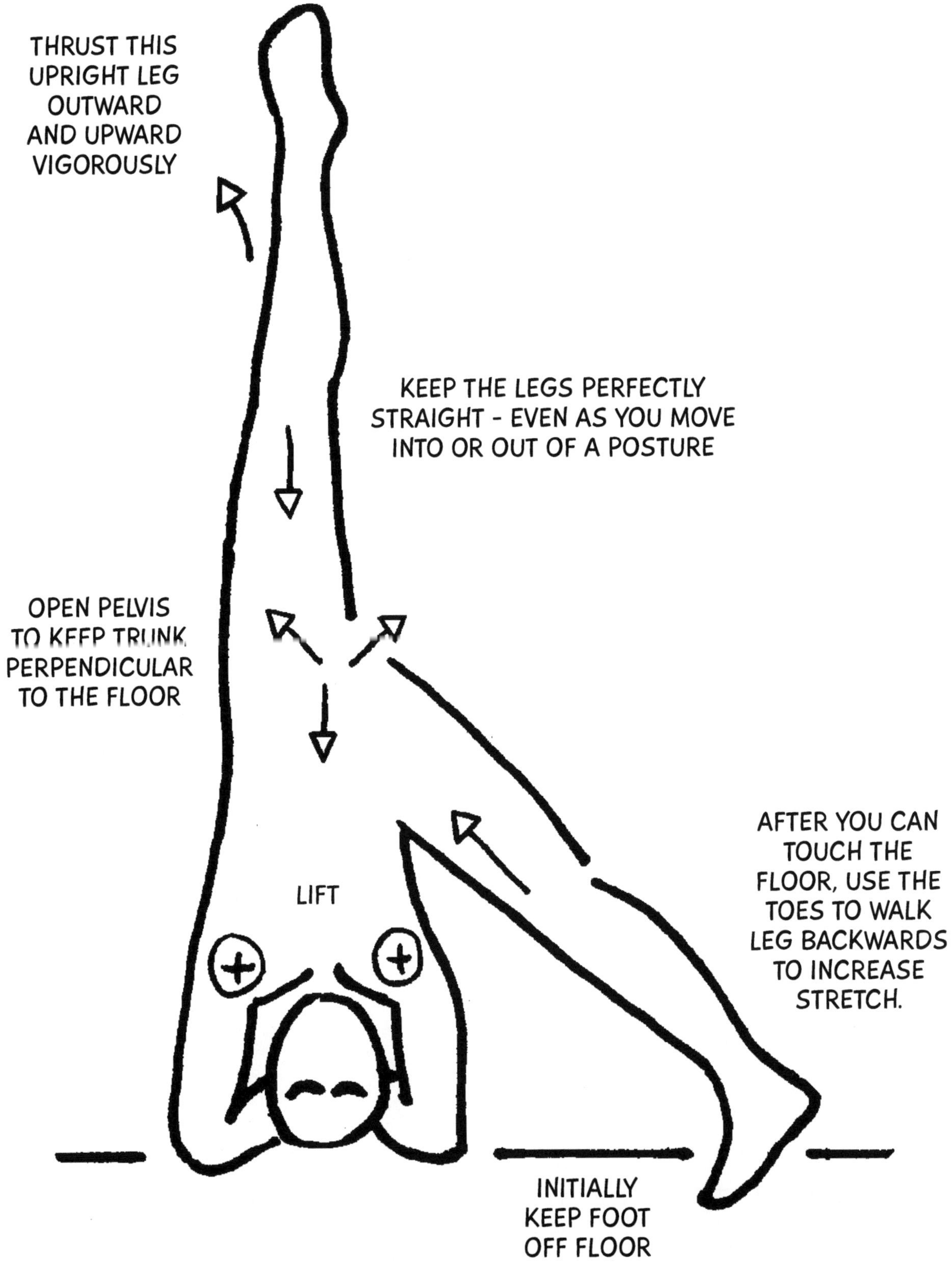
THRUST THIS UPRIGHT LEG OUTWARD AND UPWARD VIGOROUSLY
KEEP THE LEGS PERFECTLY STRAIGHT - EVEN AS YOU MOVE INTO OR OUT OF A POSTURE
OPEN PELVIS TO KEEP TRUNK PERPENDICULAR TO THE FLOOR
LIFT
AFTER YOU CAN TOUCH THE FLOOR, USE THE TOES TO WALK LEG BACKWARDS TO INCREASE STRETCH.
INITIALLY KEEP FOOT OFF FLOOR

Padma Sirsasana 30s (82)

lotus head

Var: If unable to do a full Padmasana, do a Siddhasana [39] instead. Or warms up with a Siddhasana and then work your legs and feet into Padmasana.

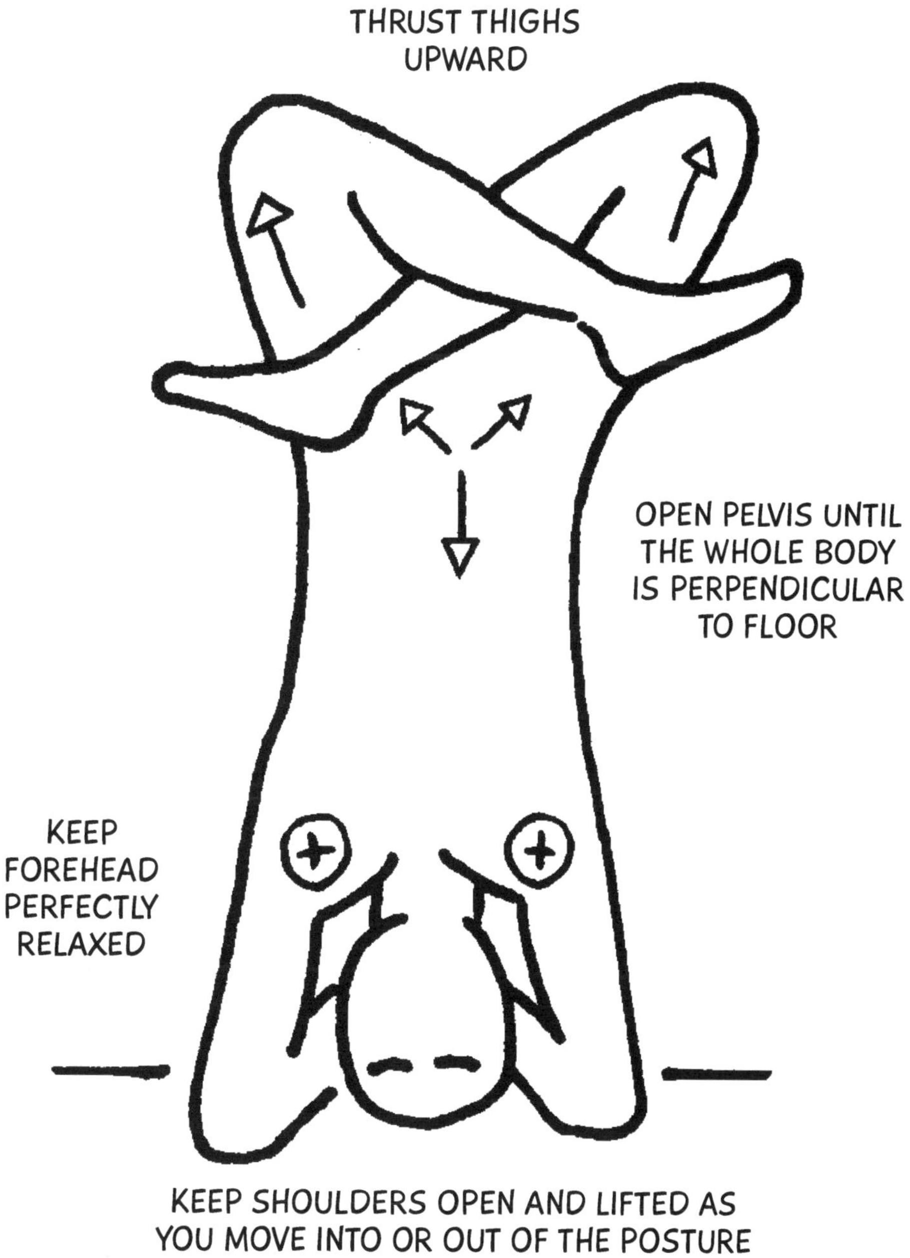
THRUST THIGHS UPWARD
OPEN PELVIS UNTIL THE WHOLE BODY IS PERPENDICULAR TO FLOOR
KEEP FOREHEAD PERFECTLY RELAXED
KEEP SHOULDERS OPEN AND LIFTED AS YOU MOVE INTO OR OUT OF THE POSTURE

Parsva Padma Sirsasana 15s (83)

side lotus head

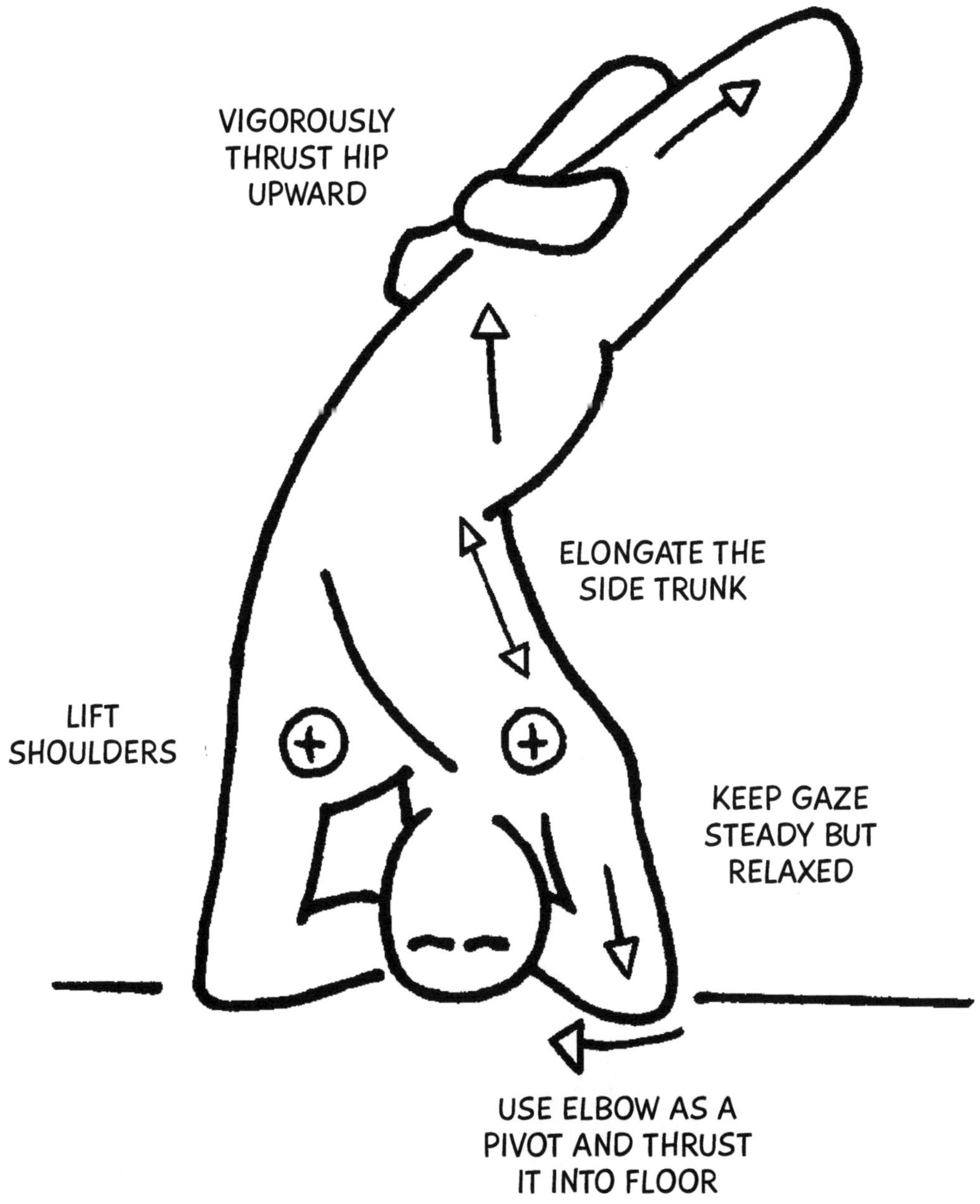

VIGOROUSLY
THRUST HIP
UPWARD
ELONGATE THE
SIDE TRUNK
LIFT
SHOULDERS
KEEP GAZE
STEADY BUT
RELAXED
USE ELBOW AS A
PIVOT AND THRUST
IT INTO FLOOR

Pinda Sirsasana 20-30s

embryo head

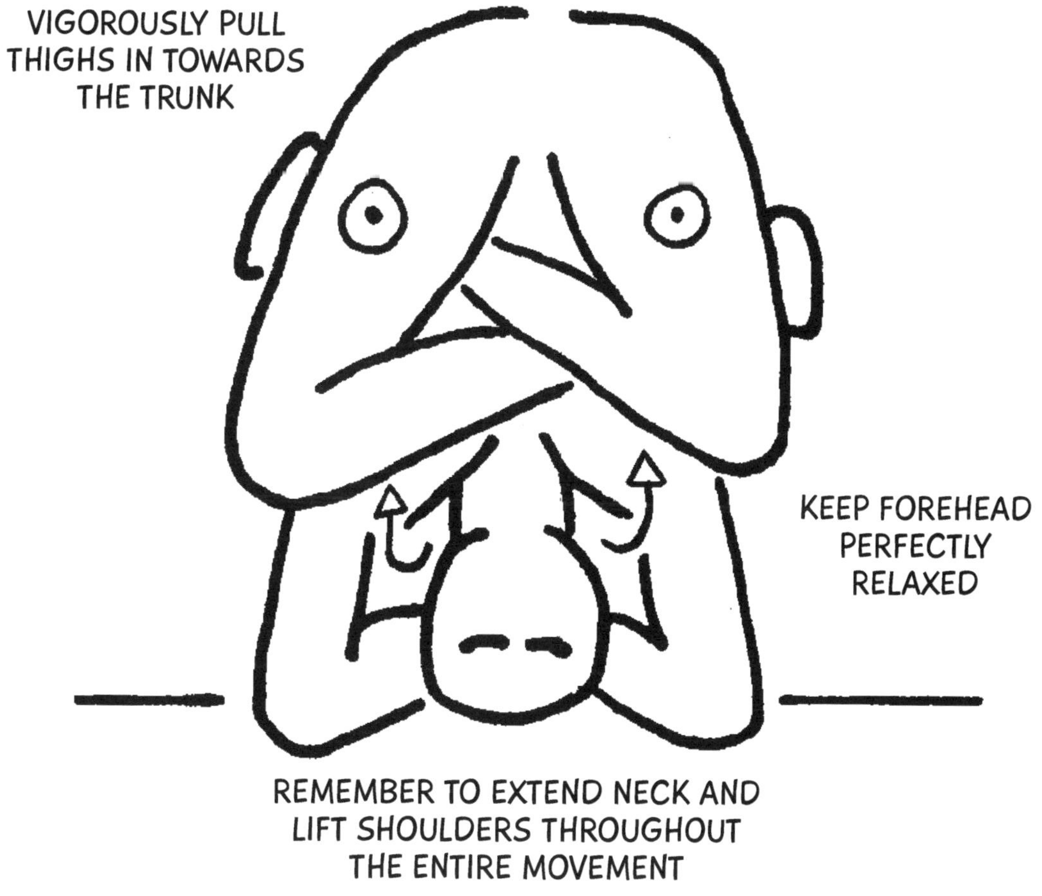
VIGOROUSLY PULL THIGHS IN TOWARDS THE TRUNK
KEEP FOREHEAD PERFECTLY RELAXED
REMEMBER TO EXTEND NECK AND LIFT SHOULDERS THROUGHOUT THE ENTIRE MOVEMENT

Parivrtta Paschimottanasana 20s (85)

revolved west stretch

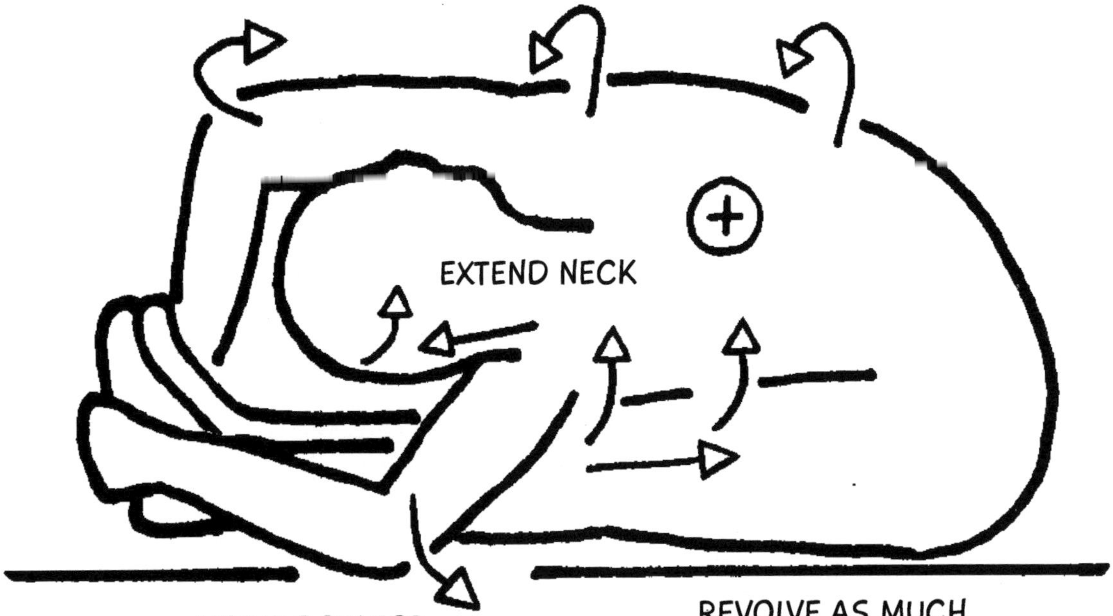

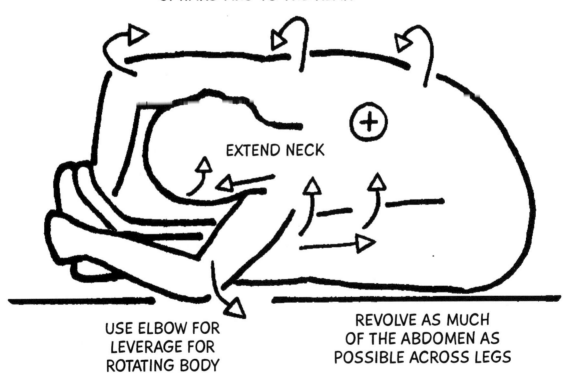

THRUST UPPER SIDE OF TRUNK
UPWARD AND TO THE REAR
EXTEND NECK
USE ELBOW FOR
LEVERAGE FOR
ROTATING BODY
REVOLVE AS MUCH
OF THE ABDOMEN AS
POSSIBLE ACROSS LEGS

Krounchasana 20-30s (86)

heron

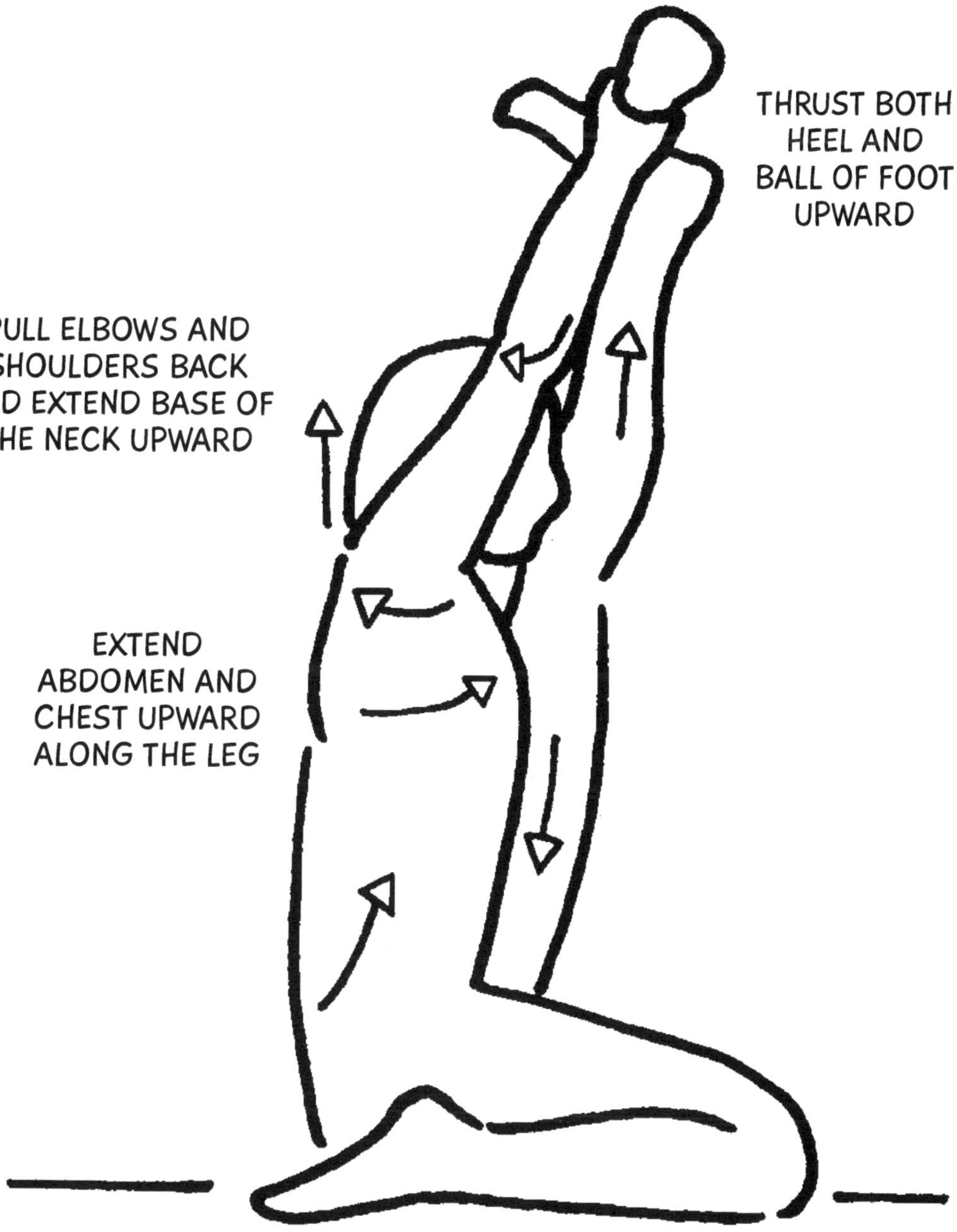
THRUST BOTH
HEEL AND
BALL OF FOOT
UPWARD
PULL ELBOWS AND
SHOULDERS BACK
AND EXTEND BASE OF
THE NECK UPWARD
EXTEND
ABDOMEN AND
CHEST UPWARD
ALONG THE LEG

Note: In this and all forward bends where the hands extend toward the foot, first strive to grasp the toes, then interlock the fingers beyond the toes, then grasp the palms. After you can grasp the wrist, work upward to grasp the lower forearm. Eventually you will be able to touch the elbow to the toe... more or less.

In bending postures where the hands and wrists are grasped, use the hand running next to the instep on the inner side of the leg to grasp the wrist of the other arm.

Akarna Dhanurasana 15-20s (87)

near to ear bow

Var: Try your hand at a little archery using a high tension bow. This gives you the sense of what you're looking for in this posture.

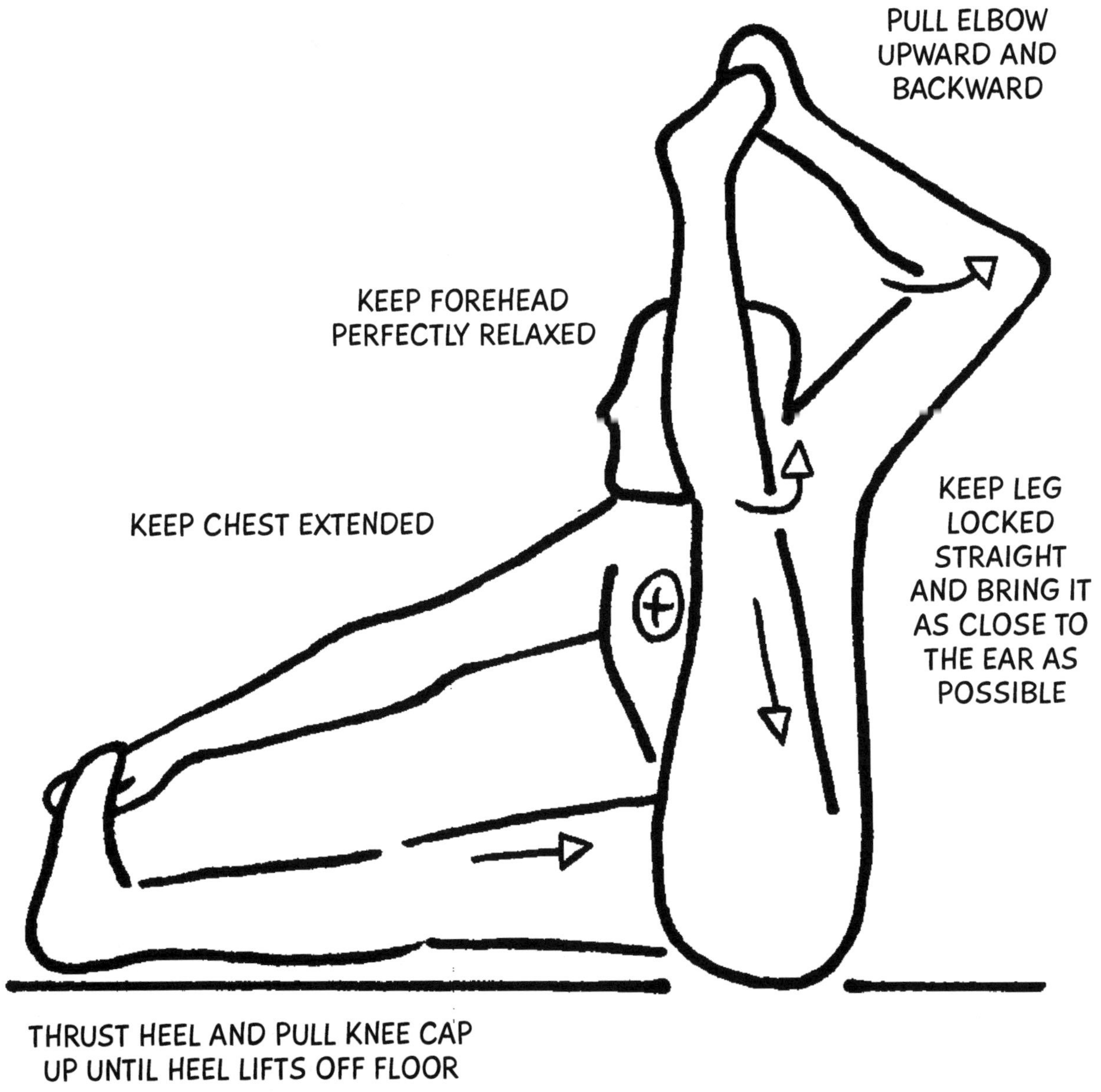

PULL ELBOW UPWARD AND BACKWARD
KEEP FOREHEAD PERFECTLY RELAXED
KEEP CHEST EXTENDED
KEEP LEG LOCKED STRAIGHT AND BRING IT AS CLOSE TO THE EAR AS POSSIBLE
THRUST HEEL AND PULL KNEE CAP UP UNTIL HEEL LIFTS OFF FLOOR

Supta Padangusthasana 20s each (88)

lying big toe

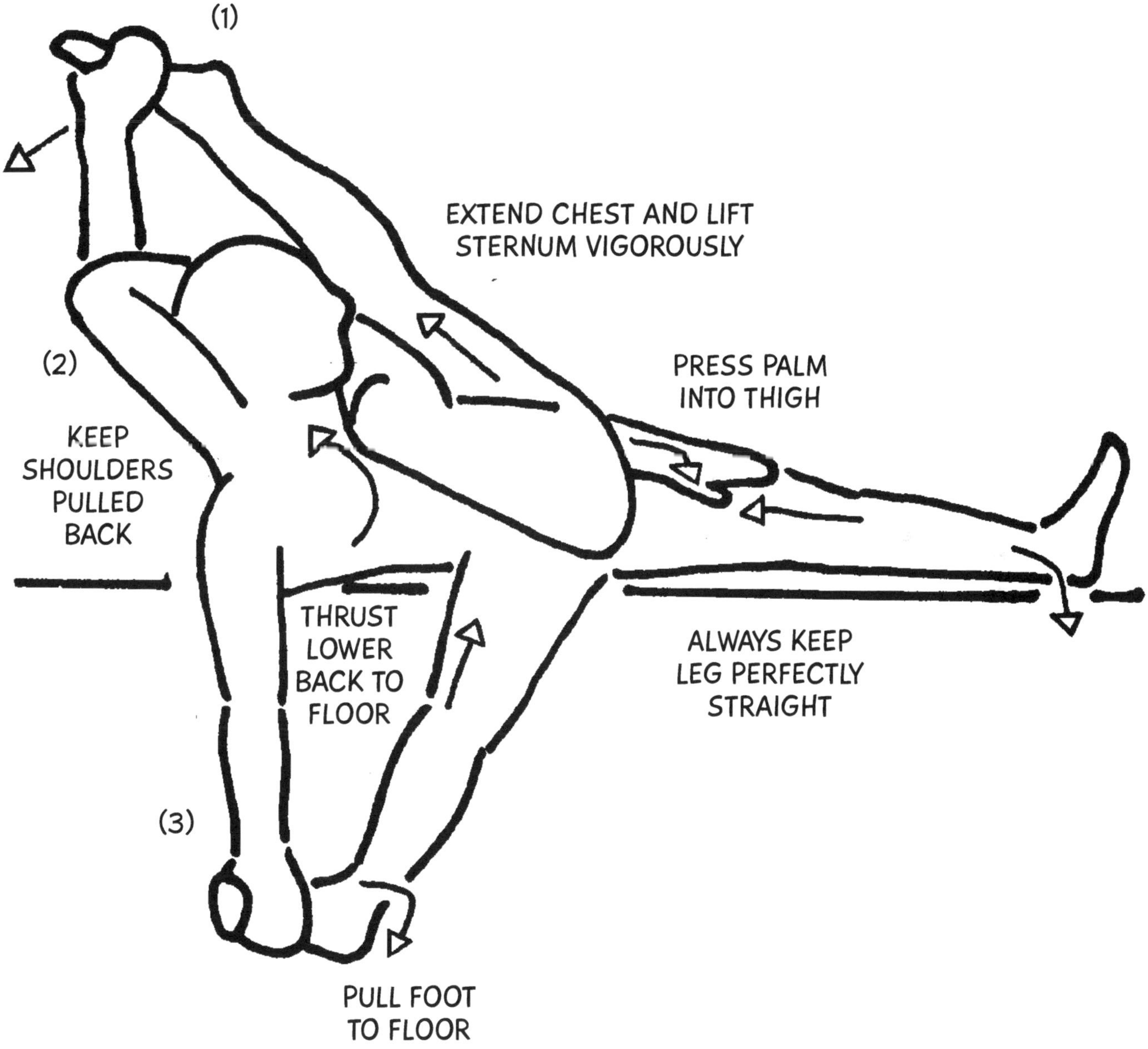

(1)
EXTEND CHEST AND LIFT STERNUM VIGOROUSLY
PRESS PALM INTO THIGH
(2)
KEEP SHOULDERS PULLED BACK
THRUST LOWER BACK TO FLOOR
ALWAYS KEEP LEG PERFECTLY STRAIGHT
(3)
PULL FOOT TO FLOOR

Kurmasana 30-60s (89)

turtle

Note: Before doing this posture, reach around with the hands and pull the fleshy part of the buttocks out from under the pelvis.

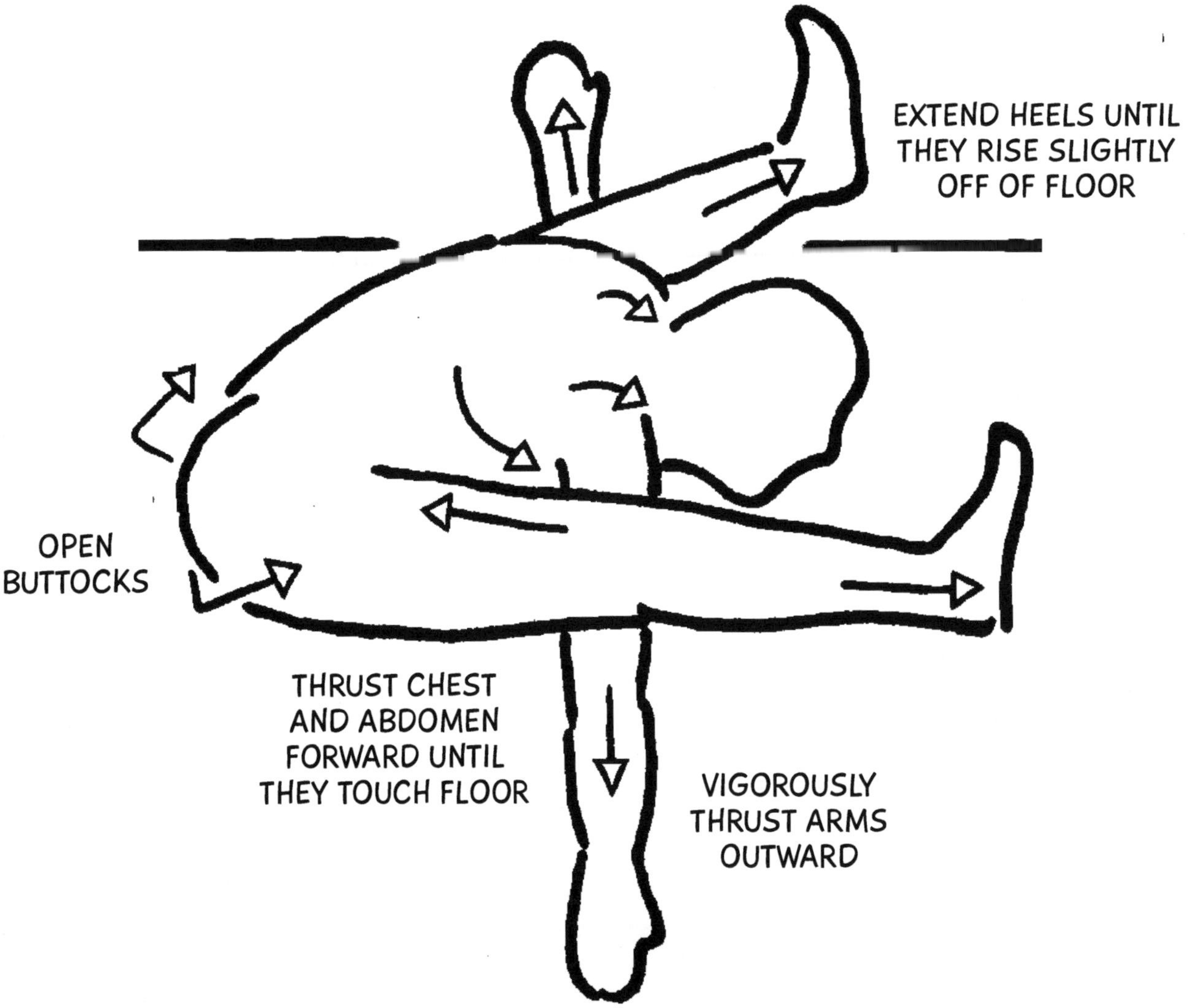
EXTEND HEELS UNTIL
THEY RISE SLIGHTLY
OFF OF FLOOR
OPEN
BUTTOCKS
THRUST CHEST
AND ABDOMEN
FORWARD UNTIL
THEY TOUCH FLOOR
VIGOROUSLY
THRUST ARMS
OUTWARD

Supta Kurmasana 1-2 min (90)

lying turtle

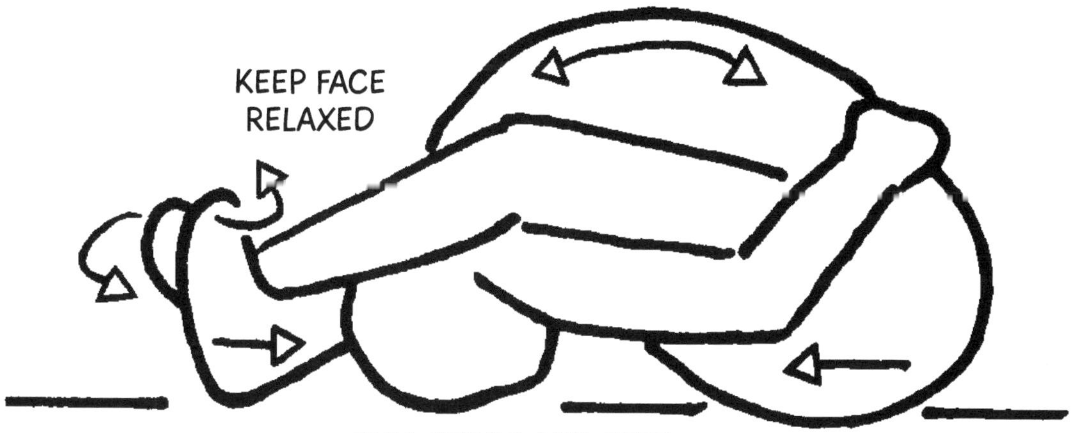
PULL SPINE
INTO AN ARCH
KEEP FACE
RELAXED
PULL PELVIS AND FEET
TOWARD EACH OTHER

Var: Leave the feet unlocked but touching each other at the heels. Pull the legs as high up on to the arms /shoulders as possible.

Note: In this or in any other variation you do, try to eliminate the variation as soon as possible and do the posture as near to what is shown as possible.

Marichyasana IV 30s (91)

son of Brahma

Var: Grasp the foot instead of reaching around to grasp the other hand.

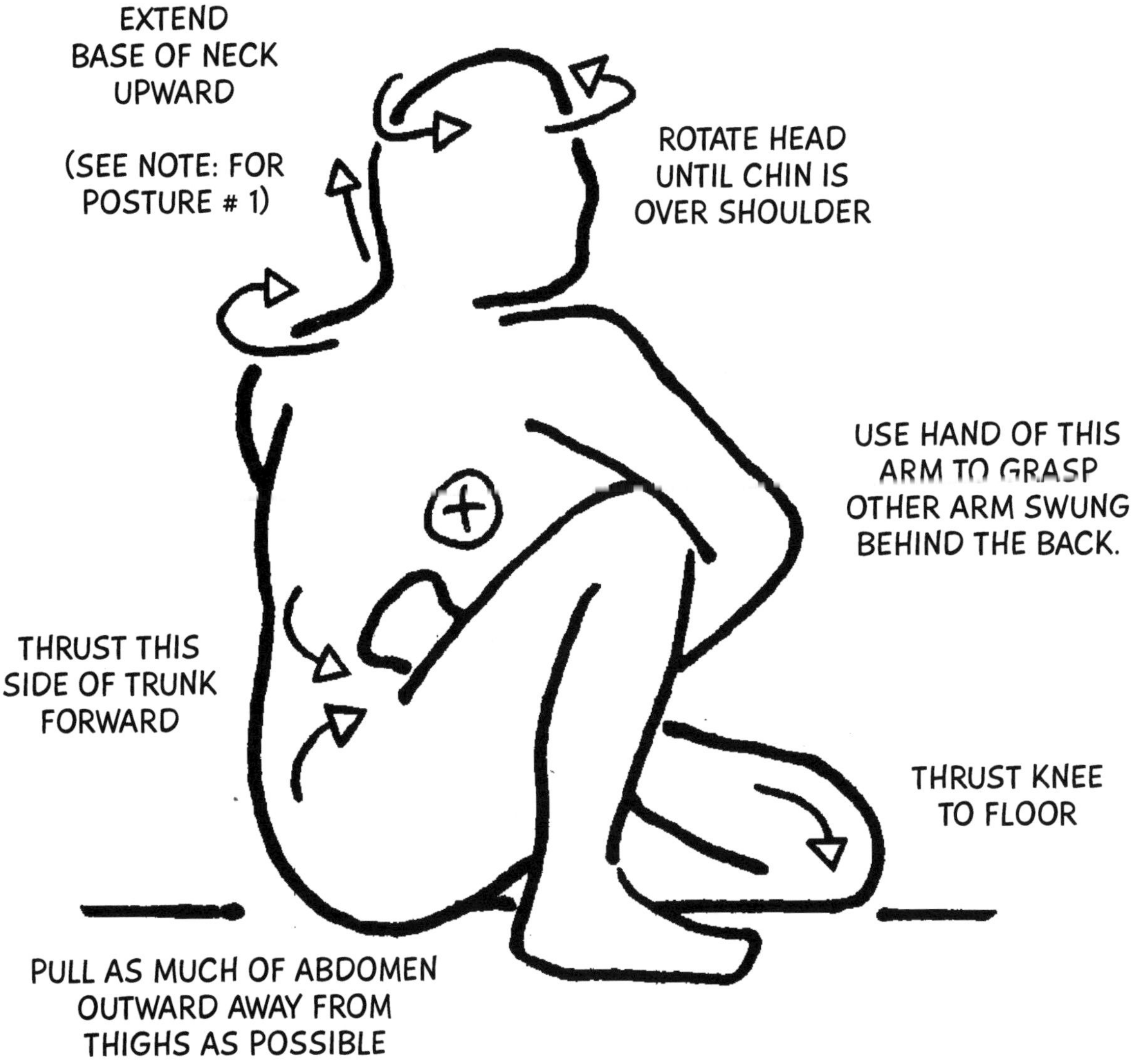
EXTEND BASE OF NECK UPWARD
(SEE NOTE: FOR POSTURE # 1)
ROTATE HEAD UNTIL CHIN IS OVER SHOULDER
USE HAND OF THIS ARM TO GRASP OTHER ARM SWUNG BEHIND THE BACK.
THRUST THIS SIDE OF TRUNK FORWARD
THRUST KNEE TO FLOOR
PULL AS MUCH OF ABDOMEN OUTWARD AWAY FROM THIGHS AS POSSIBLE

Note: In this as in all other twisting postures, you should try to bring as much of the trunk (chest and abdomen) to one side of the leg (or body) as possible.

Adho Mukha Vrksasana 60s (92)

down face tree

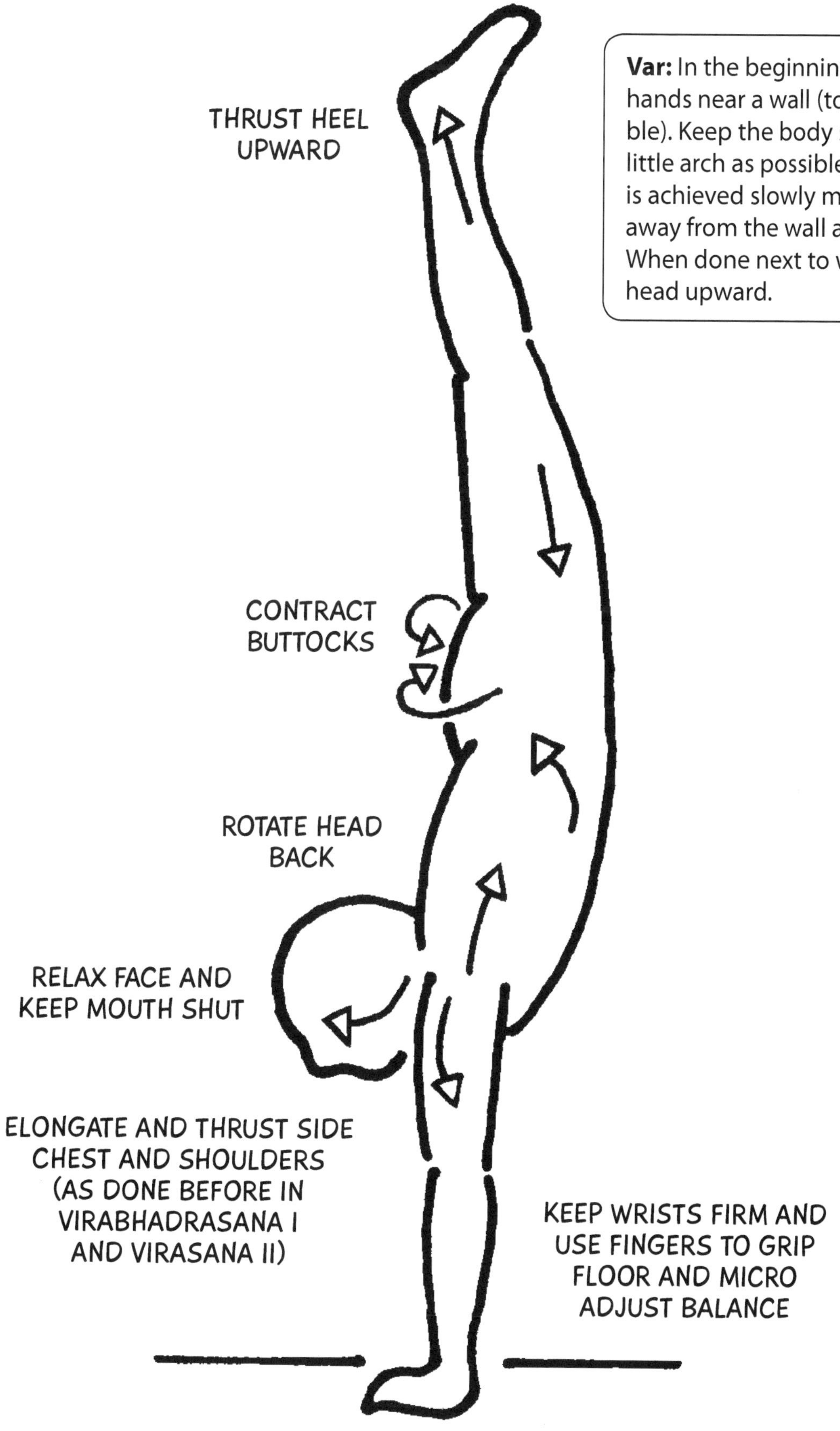

THRUST HEEL UPWARD
CONTRACT BUTTOCKS
ROTATE HEAD BACK
RELAX FACE AND KEEP MOUTH SHUT
ELONGATE AND THRUST SIDE CHEST AND SHOULDERS (AS DONE BEFORE IN VIRABHADRASANA I AND VIRASANA II)
KEEP WRISTS FIRM AND USE FINGERS TO GRIP FLOOR AND MICRO ADJUST BALANCE

Var: In the beginning, place the hands near a wall (touching if possible). Keep the body straight with as little arch as possible. When balance is achieved slowly move the heels away from the wall a few inches. When done next to wall, don't rotate head upward.

Pincha Mayurasana 60s (93)

feather peacock

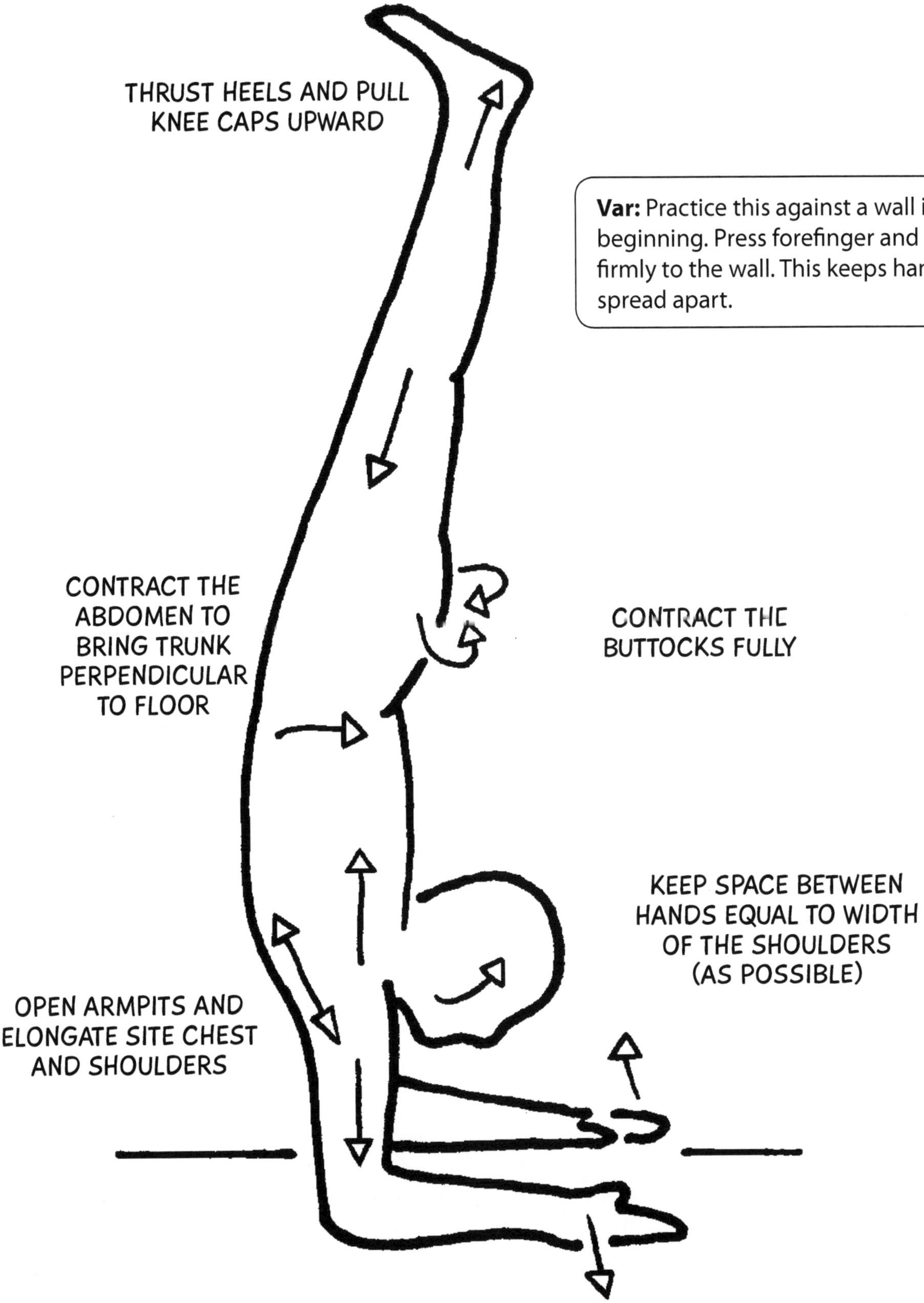
THRUST HEELS AND PULL KNEE CAPS UPWARD
CONTRACT THE ABDOMEN TO BRING TRUNK PERPENDICULAR TO FLOOR
CONTRACT THE BUTTOCKS FULLY
KEEP SPACE BETWEEN HANDS EQUAL TO WIDTH OF THE SHOULDERS (AS POSSIBLE)
OPEN ARMPITS AND ELONGATE SITE CHEST AND SHOULDERS

Var: Practice this against a wall in the beginning. Press forefinger and thumb firmly to the wall. This keeps hands spread apart.

Padma Mayurasana 60s (94)

lotus peacock

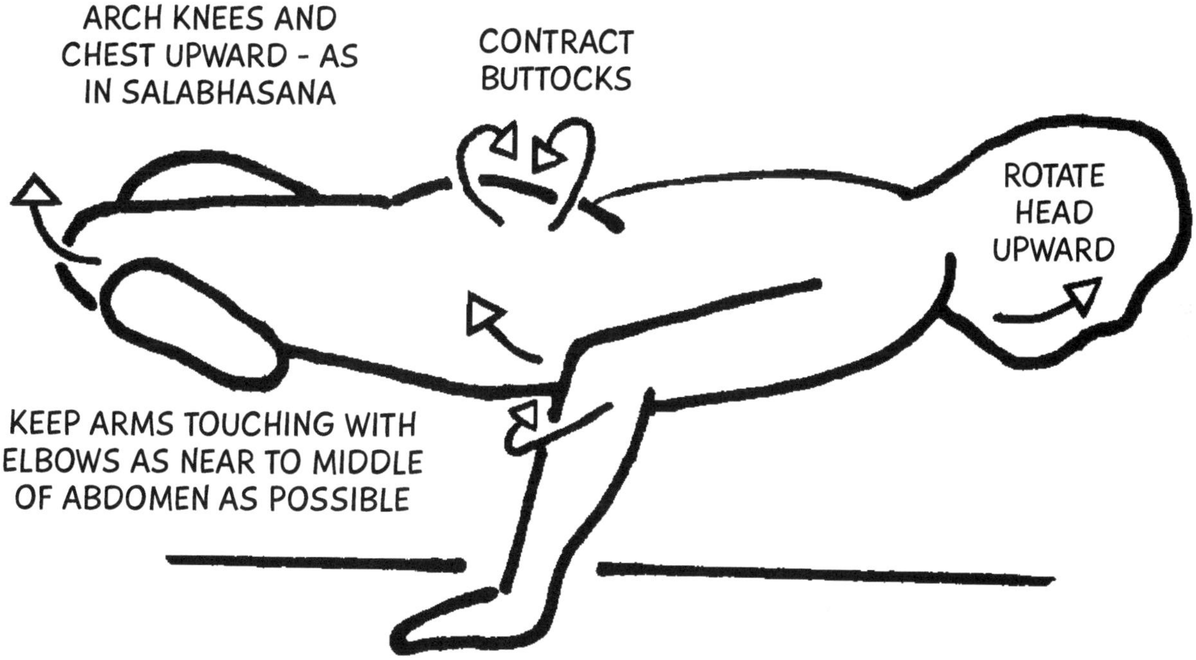

ARCH KNEES AND
CHEST UPWARD - AS
IN SALABHASANA
CONTRACT
BUTTOCKS
ROTATE
HEAD
UPWARD
KEEP ARMS TOUCHING WITH
ELBOWS AS NEAR TO MIDDLE
OF ABDOMEN AS POSSIBLE

Note: First do Mayurasana, then with the legs held off the floor, interlock them in Padmasana. As always be sure to do posture twice - with right leg over left and visa versa.

Astavakrasanasana 20-30s

eight bends

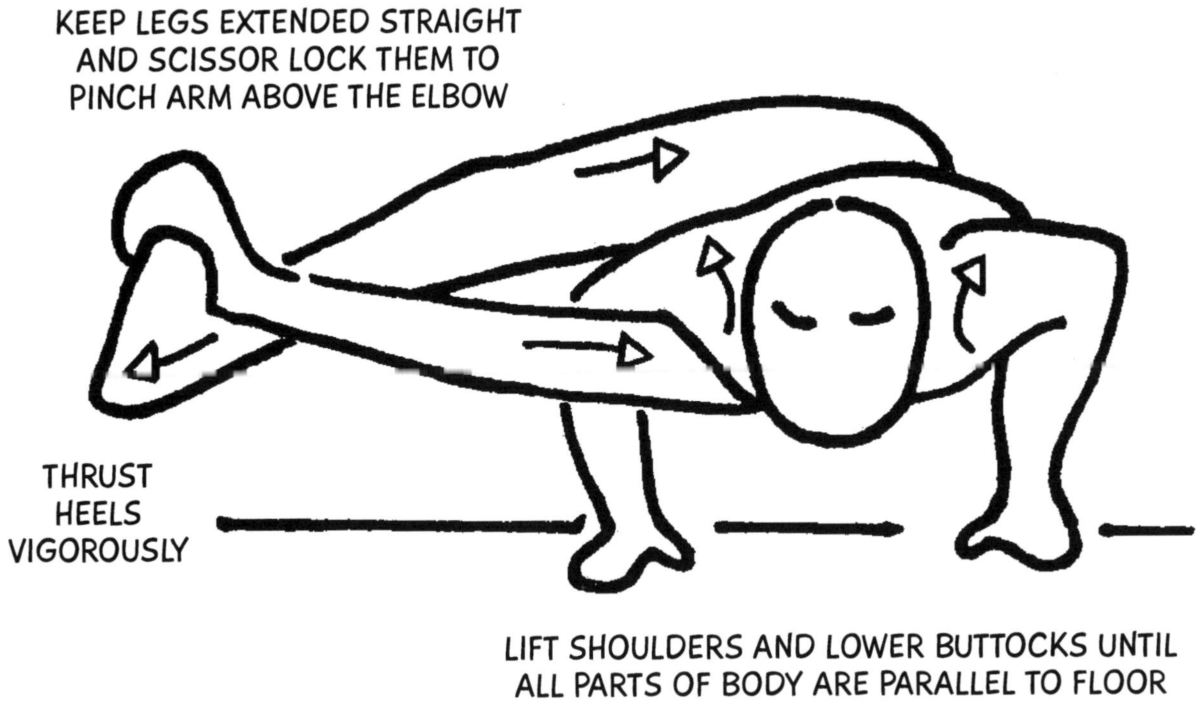
KEEP LEGS EXTENDED STRAIGHT AND SCISSOR LOCK THEM TO PINCH ARM ABOVE THE ELBOW
THRUST HEELS VIGOROUSLY
LIFT SHOULDERS AND LOWER BUTTOCKS UNTIL ALL PARTS OF BODY ARE PARALLEL TO FLOOR

Note: There is some excellent twisting motion in this posture which was hard to illustrate. Think about keeping the body as parallel to the floor as possible.

Parsva Sarvangasana 20s (96)

side whole body

Note: Aim at lowering the legs until they are held nearly parallel to the floor.

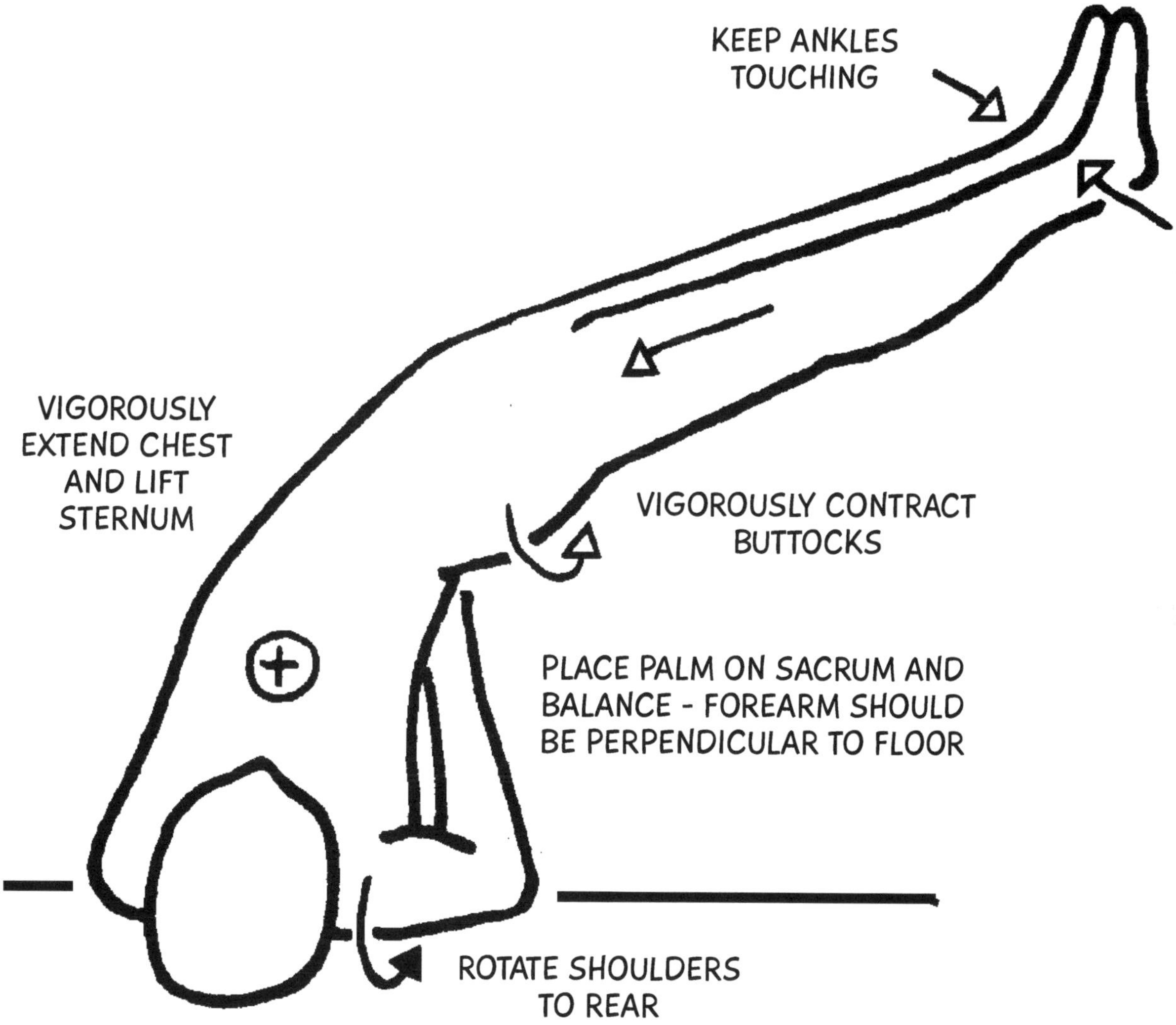
KEEP ANKLES
TOUCHING
VIGOROUSLY
EXTEND CHEST
AND LIFT
STERNUM
VIGOROUSLY CONTRACT
BUTTOCKS
PLACE PALM ON SACRUM AND
BALANCE - FOREARM SHOULD
BE PERPENDICULAR TO FLOOR
ROTATE SHOULDERS
TO REAR

Setu Bandha Sarvangasana 30s (97)

bridge, contracted whole body

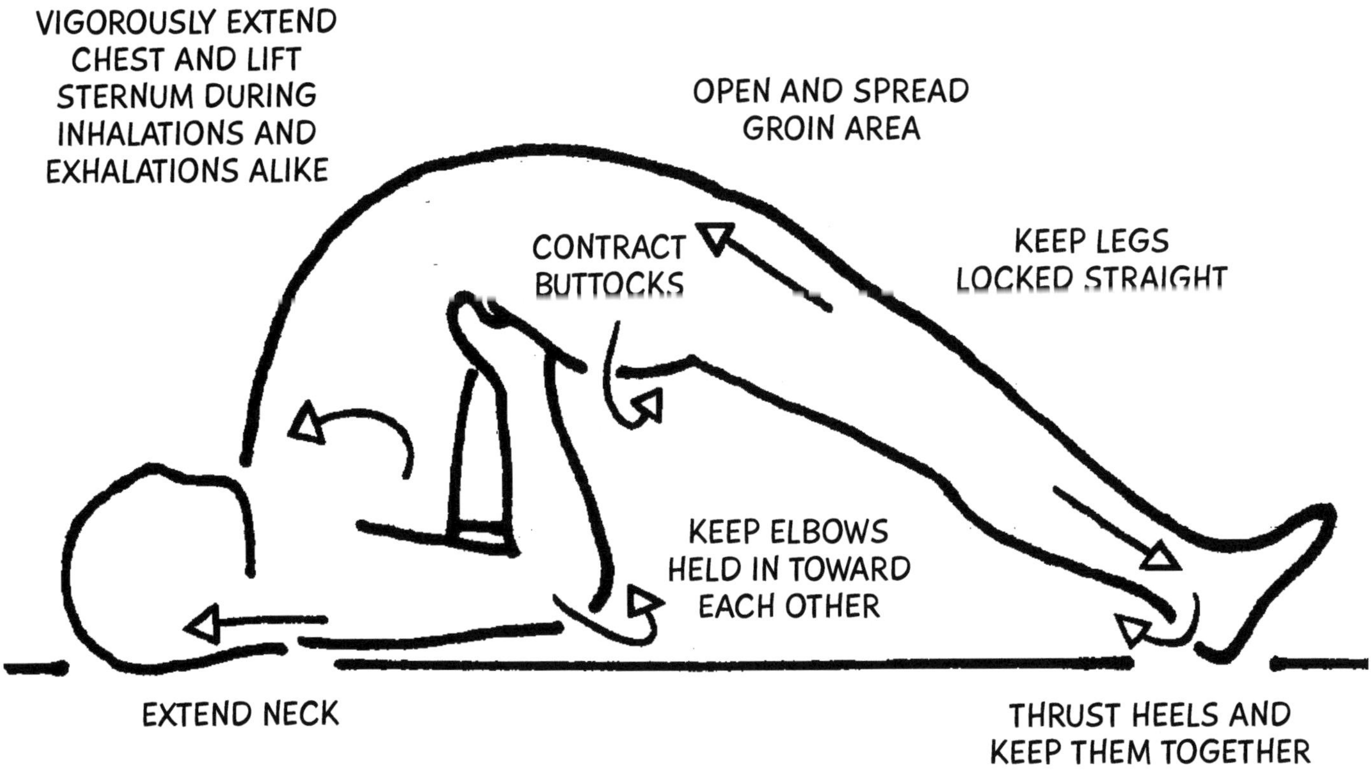
VIGOROUSLY EXTEND CHEST AND LIFT STERNUM DURING INHALATIONS AND EXHALATIONS ALIKE
OPEN AND SPREAD GROIN AREA
CONTRACT BUTTOCKS
KEEP LEGS LOCKED STRAIGHT
KEEP ELBOWS HELD IN TOWARD EACH OTHER
EXTEND NECK
THRUST HEELS AND KEEP THEM TOGETHER

Note: Later on you can do this posture with the palms supporting the hips (near the sacrum). Place the palms such that the fingers face outward.

Eka Pada Setu Bandha Sarvangasana 10s (98)

one leg bridge contracted

Note: How are those 'dead' little toes coming along? Here's another chance to wake them up.

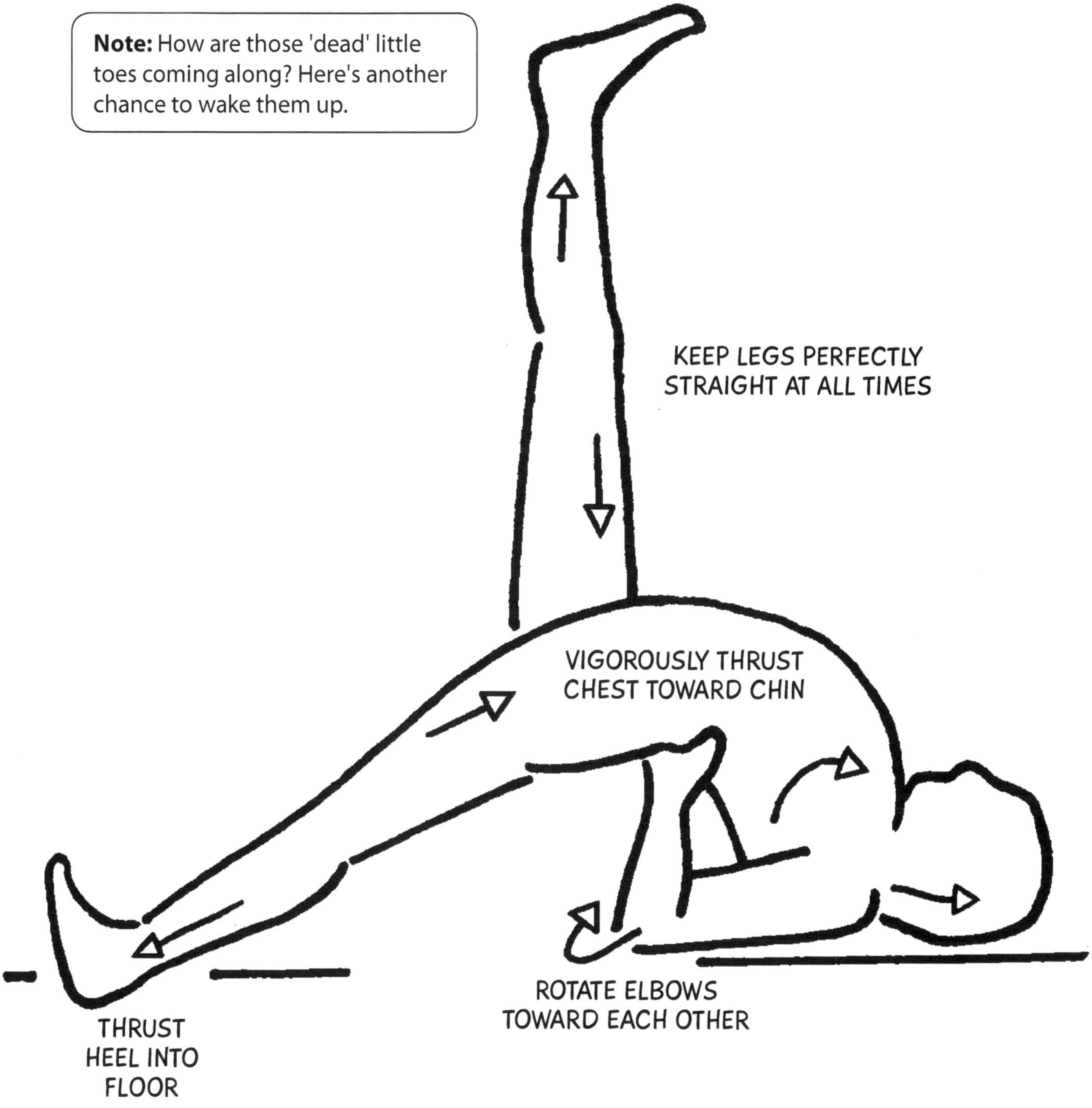
KEEP LEGS PERFECTLY
STRAIGHT AT ALL TIMES
VIGOROUSLY THRUST
CHEST TOWARD CHIN
THRUST
HEEL INTO
FLOOR
ROTATE ELBOWS
TOWARD EACH OTHER

Program 6

First Day: Begin with the **Headstand Cycle (page 103)**. Next do Sarvangasana and Halasana (below). Follow these with **Basic Arm Cycle (page 125)**. Again, half of these postures will be new to you. Skip any you don't feel up to now; return to them later when you are ready. Be patient, and do keep in mind that some you'll never do for various reasons. As always consistency of practice and watchfulness are the secrets to success , not which postures you do, or don't do.

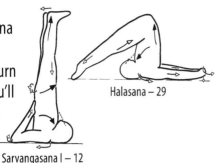

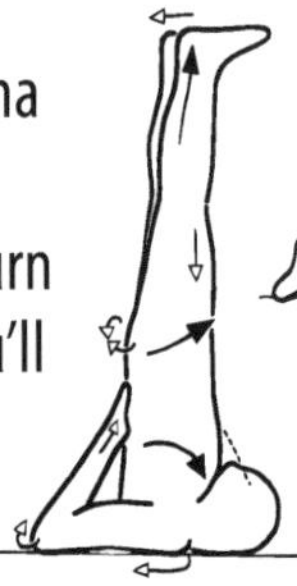
Sarvangasana I – 12

Halasana – 29

Next do the **Forward Cycle (page 73)**. Next do the leg-head postures below followed by the twist and backbends. By then you should be ready for a a few minutes of Savasana.

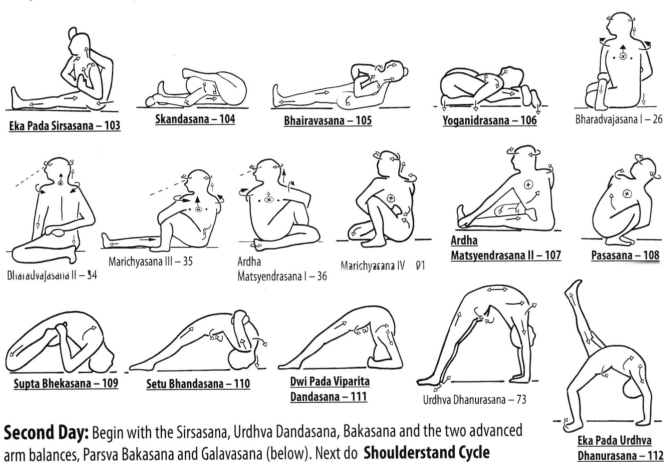

Eka Pada Sirsasana – 103

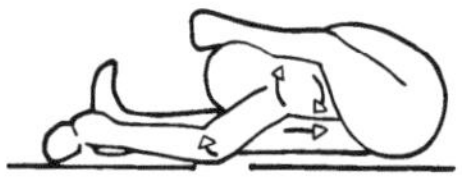
Skandasana – 104

Bhairavasana – 105

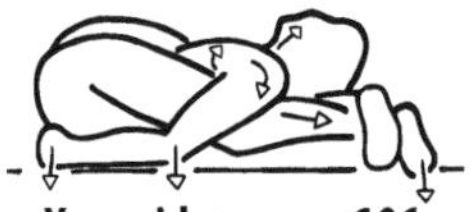
Yoganidrasana – 106

Bharadvajasana I – 26

Bharadvajasana II – 34

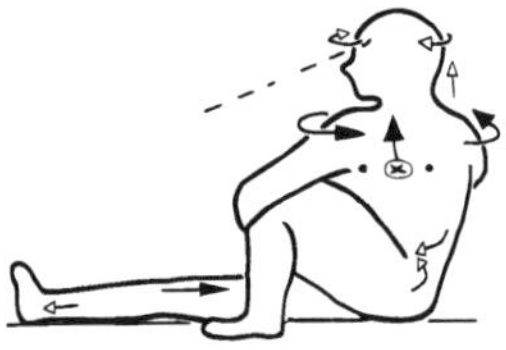
Marichyasana III – 35

Ardha Matsyendrasana I – 36

Marichyasana IV – 91

Ardha Matsyendrasana II – 107

Pasasana – 108

Supta Bhekasana – 109

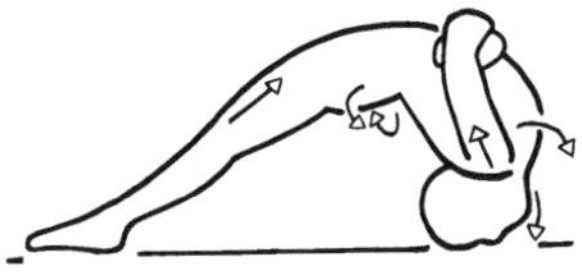
Setu Bhandasana – 110

Dwi Pada Viparita Dandasana – 111

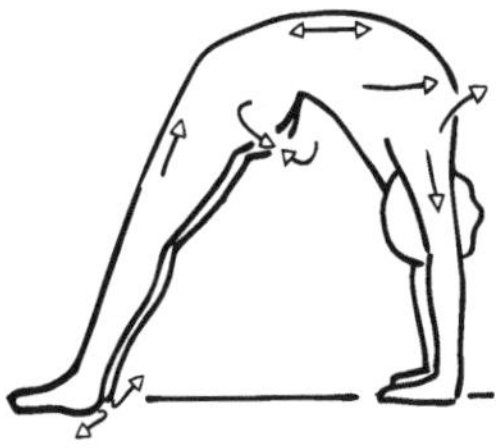
Urdhva Dhanurasana – 73

Eka Pada Urdhva Dhanurasana – 112

Second Day: Begin with the Sirsasana, Urdhva Dandasana, Bakasana and the two advanced arm balances, Parsva Bakasana and Galavasana (below). Next do **Shoulderstand Cycle (page 103)**.followed by the **Forward Cycle (page 73)**. Finally, repeat the leg-head, twists, and backbends shown above.

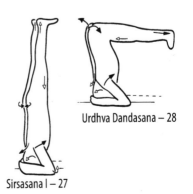

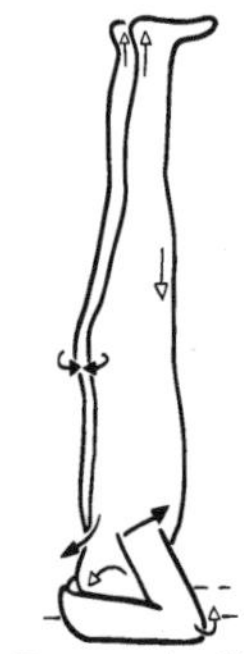
Sirsasana I – 27

Urdhva Dandasana – 28

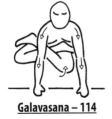

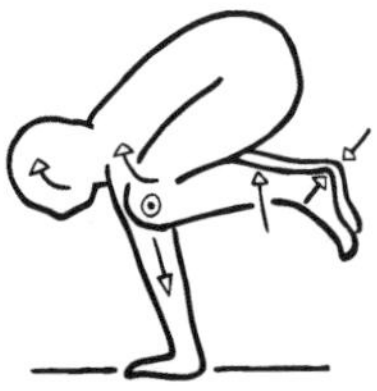
Bakasana – 74

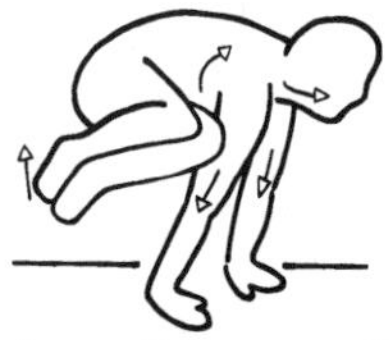
Parsva Bakasana – 113

Galavasana – 114

Review (or Third) Day: This is similar to Review day for Program 5. Begin with the Sirsasana, Urdhva Danadasana, Sarvangasana and Halasana below. Next do the **Standing Cycle (page 72)**, **Basic Cycle (page 73)** and **Lotus Cycle (page 73)**.

Basic Arm Cycle (About 13 minutes)

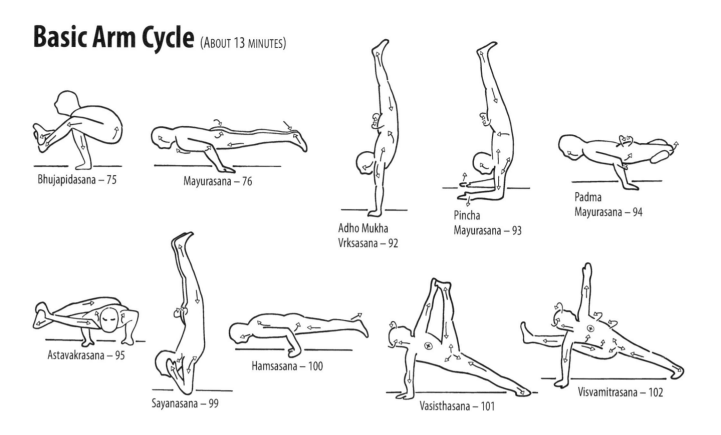

Bhujapidasana – 75

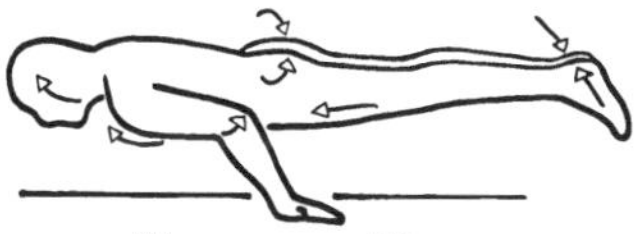
Mayurasana – 76

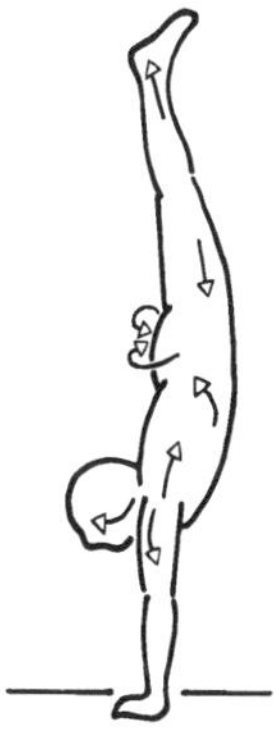
Adho Mukha Vrksasana – 92

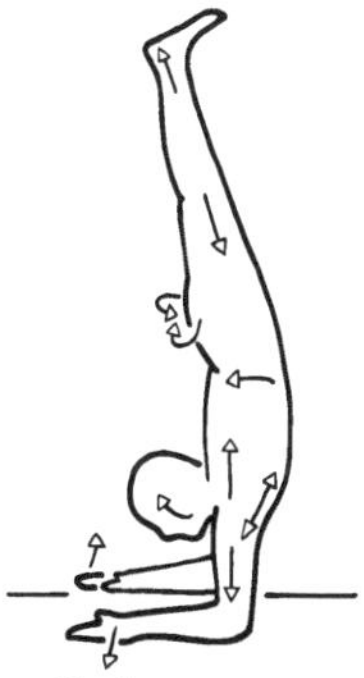
Pincha Mayurasana – 93

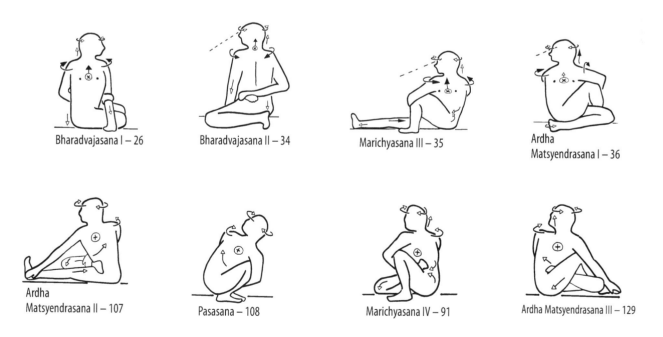
Padma Mayurasana – 94

Astavakrasana – 95

Sayanasana – 99

Hamsasana – 100

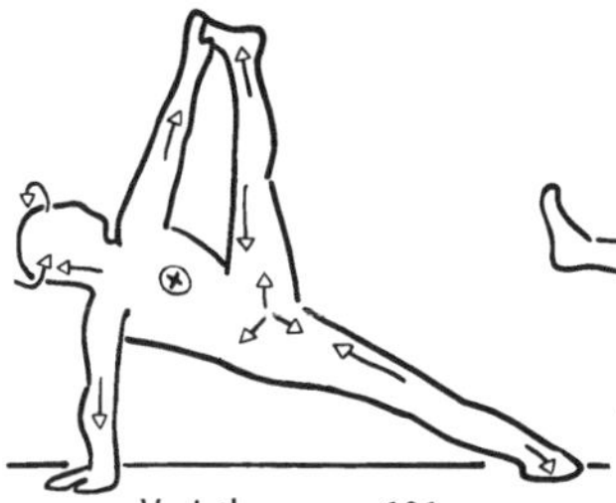
Vasisthasana – 101

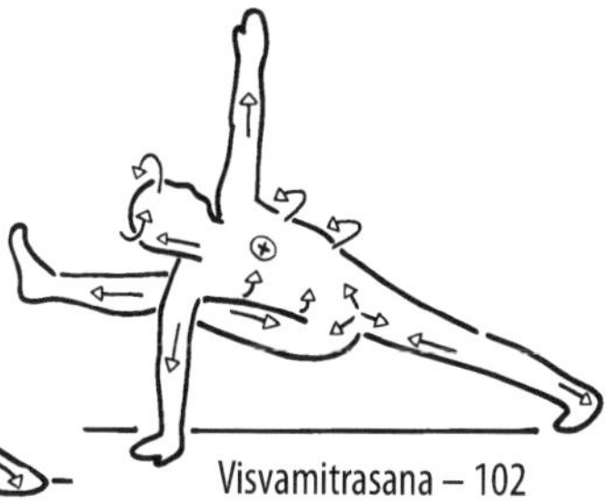
Visvamitrasana – 102

Twist Cycle (About 14 minutes)

Bharadvajasana I – 26

Bharadvajasana II – 34

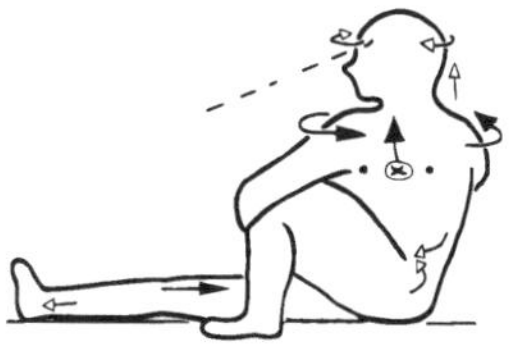
Marichyasana III – 35

Ardha Matsyendrasana I – 36

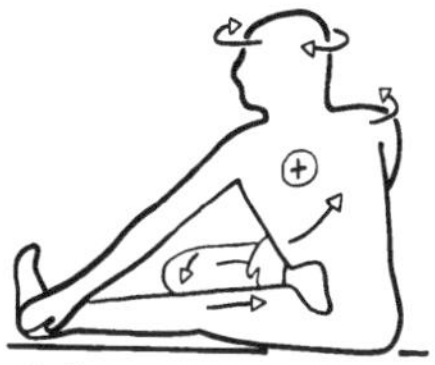
Ardha Matsyendrasana II – 107

Pasasana – 108

Marichyasana IV – 91

Ardha Matsyendrasana III – 129

Sayanasana a few sec (99)

couch

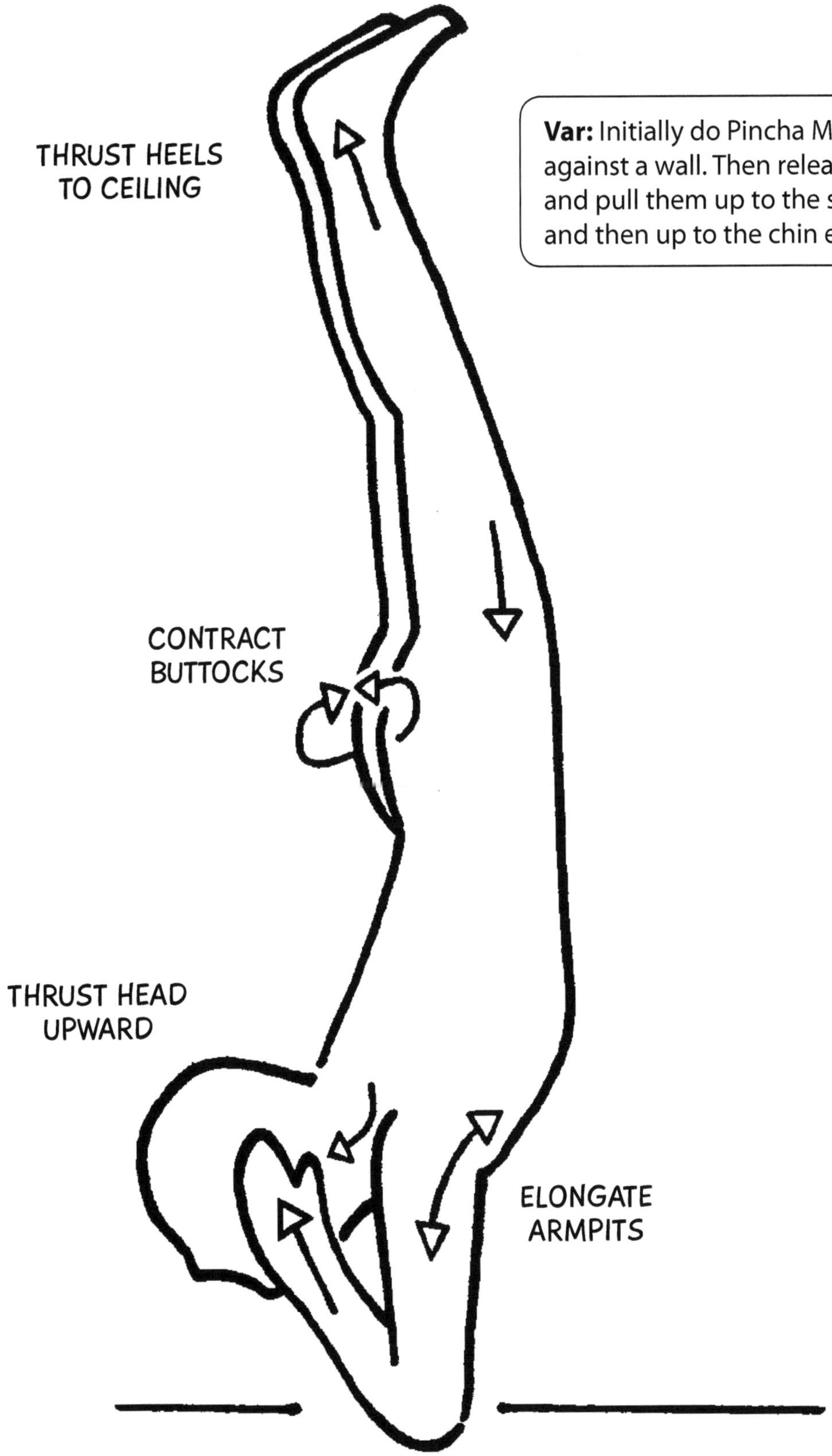
THRUST HEELS TO CEILING
CONTRACT BUTTOCKS
THRUST HEAD UPWARD
ELONGATE ARMPITS

Var: Initially do Pincha Mayurasana against a wall. Then release the hands and pull them up to the shoulders, and then up to the chin eventually.

Hamsasana 30-60s (100)

swan

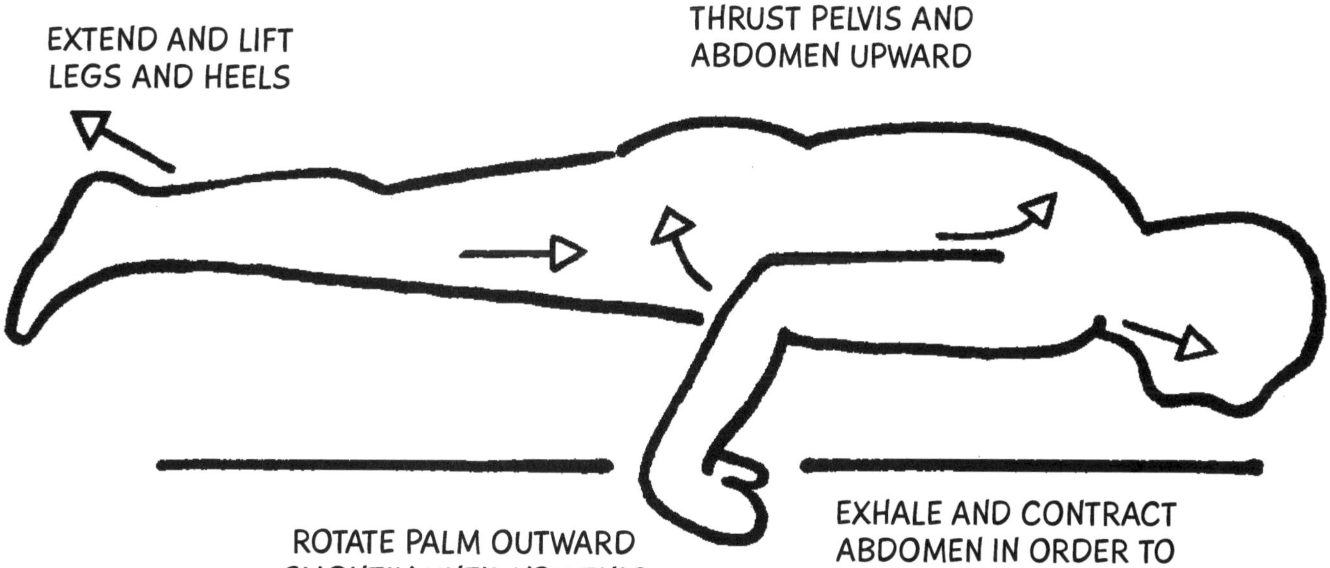
EXTEND AND LIFT
LEGS AND HEELS
THRUST PELVIS AND
ABDOMEN UPWARD
ROTATE PALM OUTWARD
SLIGHTLY UNTIL YOU THIS
POSTURE IS POSSIBLE
EXHALE AND CONTRACT
ABDOMEN IN ORDER TO
PLACE ELBOWS NEAR
MIDDLE OF ABDOMEN

Vasisthasana 20-30s (101)

an Indian sage

Var: Thrust lower foot firmly to the wall or prop trunk against a wall.

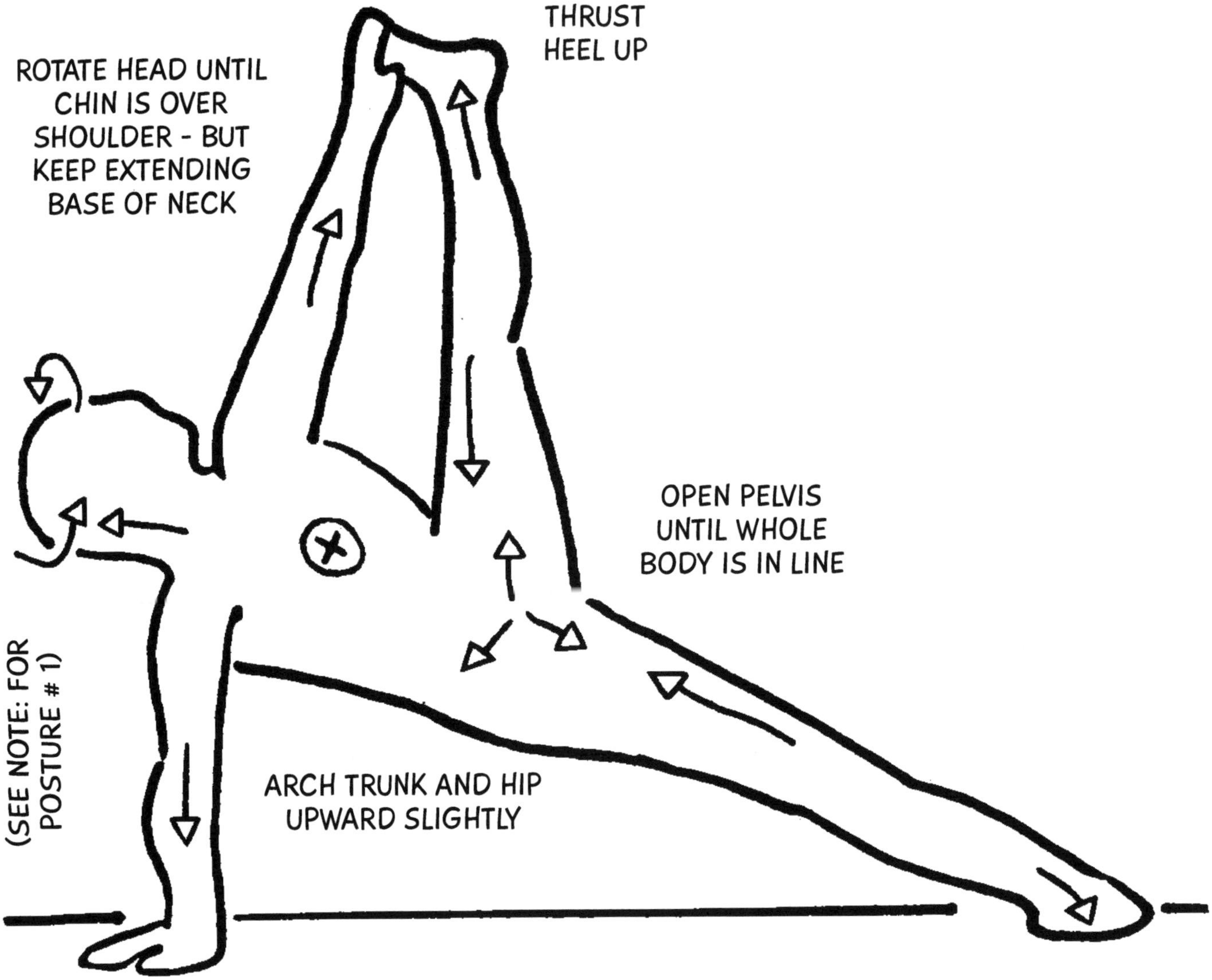

THRUST HEEL UP
ROTATE HEAD UNTIL CHIN IS OVER SHOULDER - BUT KEEP EXTENDING BASE OF NECK
OPEN PELVIS UNTIL WHOLE BODY IS IN LINE
(SEE NOTE: FOR POSTURE # 1)
ARCH TRUNK AND HIP UPWARD SLIGHTLY

Visvamitrasana 20-30s (102)

an Indian sage

Var: Begin this posture with the upper leg fully bent, kind of hanging on the arm. Once you have that, begin straightening the leg.

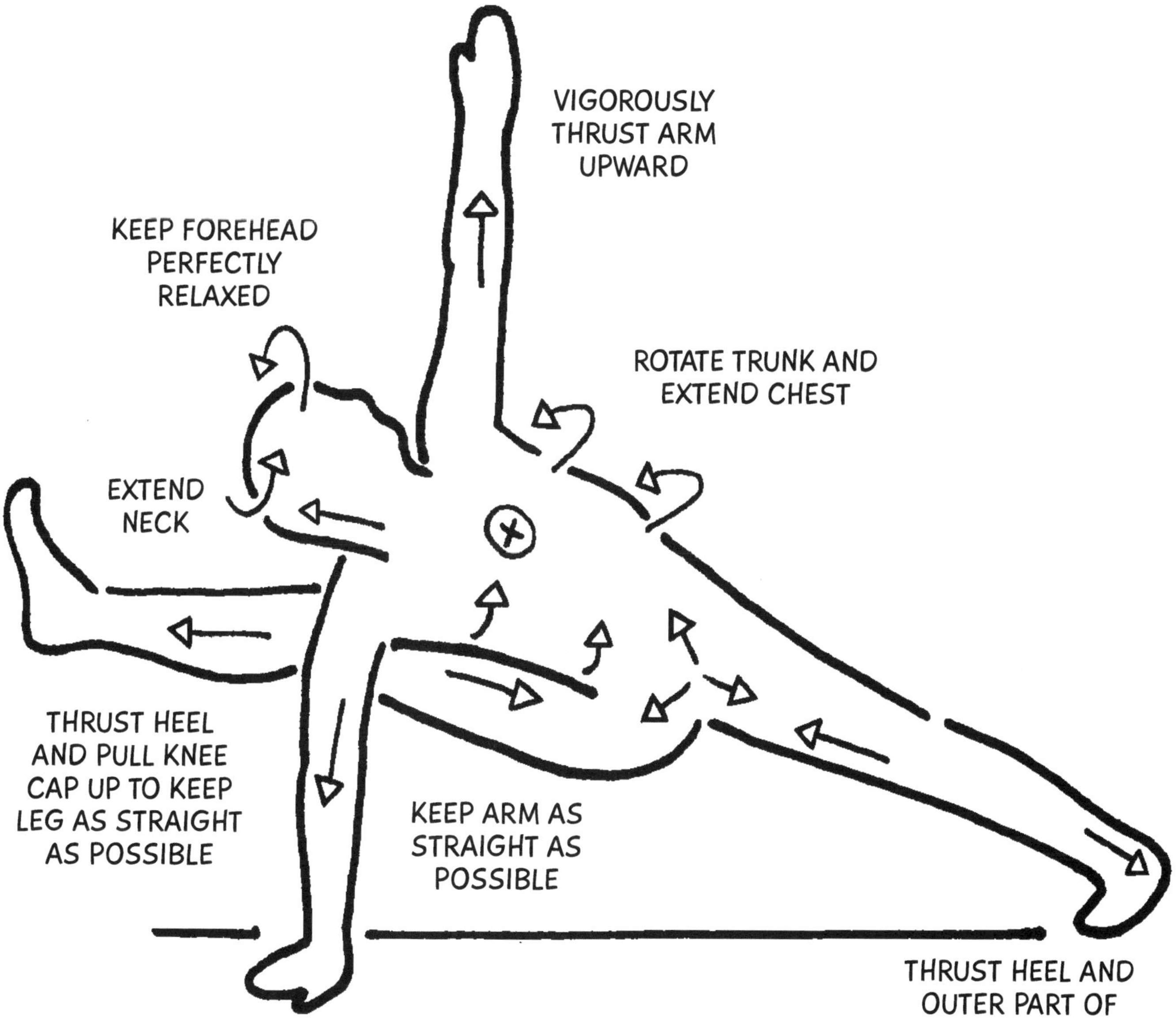

VIGOROUSLY THRUST ARM UPWARD
KEEP FOREHEAD PERFECTLY RELAXED
ROTATE TRUNK AND EXTEND CHEST
EXTEND NECK
THRUST HEEL AND PULL KNEE CAP UP TO KEEP LEG AS STRAIGHT AS POSSIBLE
KEEP ARM AS STRAIGHT AS POSSIBLE
THRUST HEEL AND OUTER PART OF FOOT INTO FLOOR

Enka Pada Sirsasana 15-60s (103)

one leg head

Note: In this and all other leg-head postures, you should bring as such of the trunk in front of the bent leg as possible. Strive to place as much of the foot beyond the neck as possible and extend the chest and lift the sternum vigorously. Vigorously extending the base of the neck up-ward and backward will help support this bent leg.

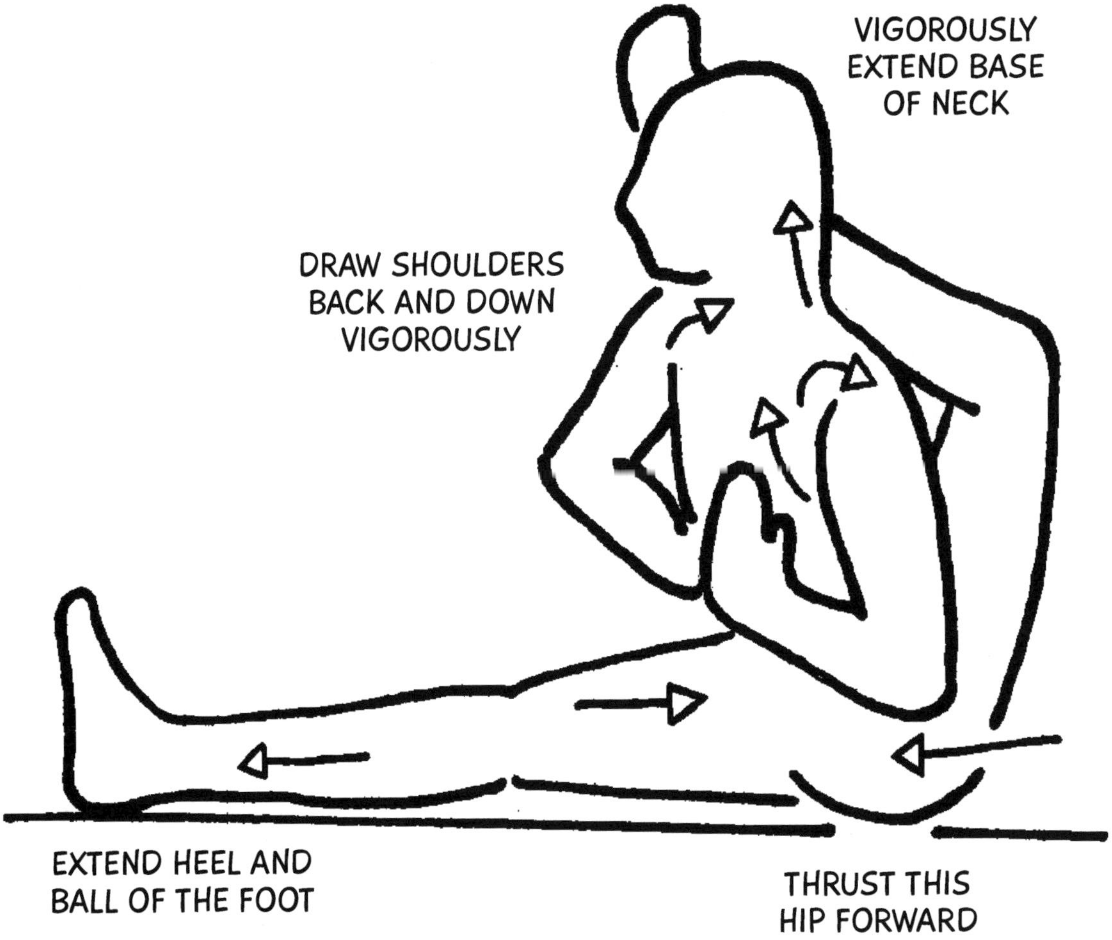

VIGOROUSLY EXTEND BASE OF NECK
DRAW SHOULDERS BACK AND DOWN VIGOROUSLY
EXTEND HEEL AND BALL OF THE FOOT
THRUST THIS HIP FORWARD

Skandasana 20-30s (104)

God of war

Note: In bending postures where the hands and wrists are grasped, use the hand running next to the instep on the inner side of the leg to grasp the wrist of the other arm.

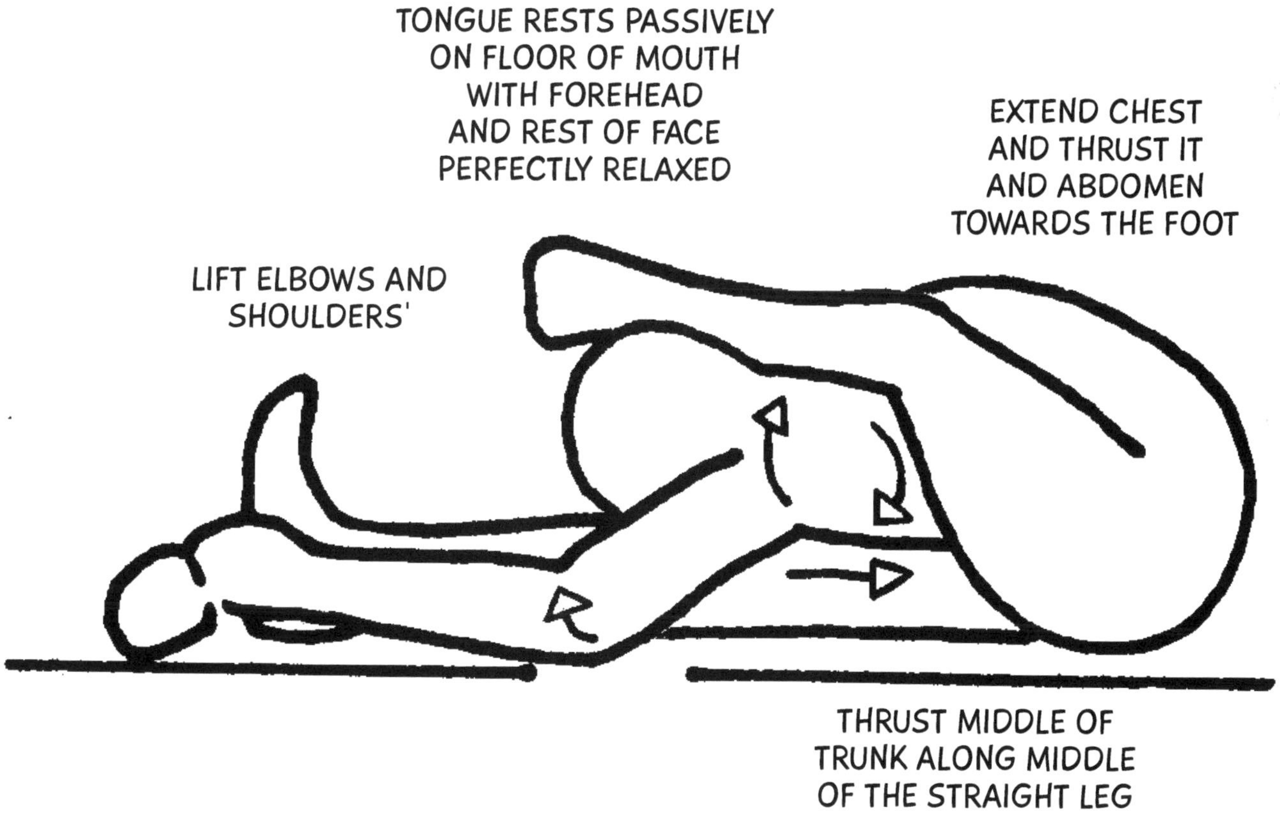
TONGUE RESTS PASSIVELY ON FLOOR OF MOUTH WITH FOREHEAD AND REST OF FACE PERFECTLY RELAXED
EXTEND CHEST AND THRUST IT AND ABDOMEN TOWARDS THE FOOT
LIFT ELBOWS AND SHOULDERS'
THRUST MIDDLE OF TRUNK ALONG MIDDLE OF THE STRAIGHT LEG

Bhairavasana 20-30s (105)

formidable

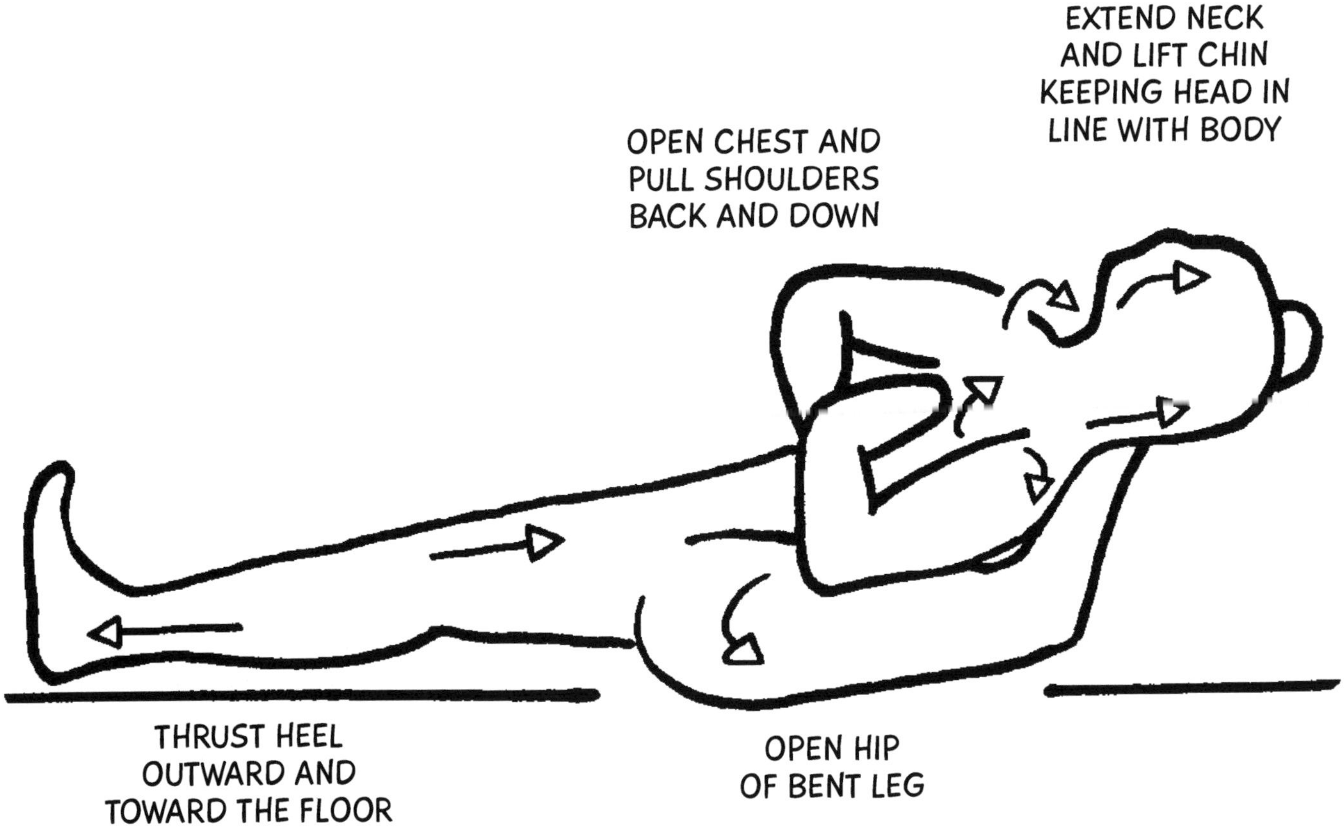
EXTEND NECK
AND LIFT CHIN
KEEPING HEAD IN
LINE WITH BODY
OPEN CHEST AND
PULL SHOULDERS
BACK AND DOWN
THRUST HEEL
OUTWARD AND
TOWARD THE FLOOR
OPEN HIP
OF BENT LEG

Yoganidrasana 30-60s (106)

Yoga sleep

Note: This posture is 'Yoga sleep', but I doubt it will be anything more than a short nap.

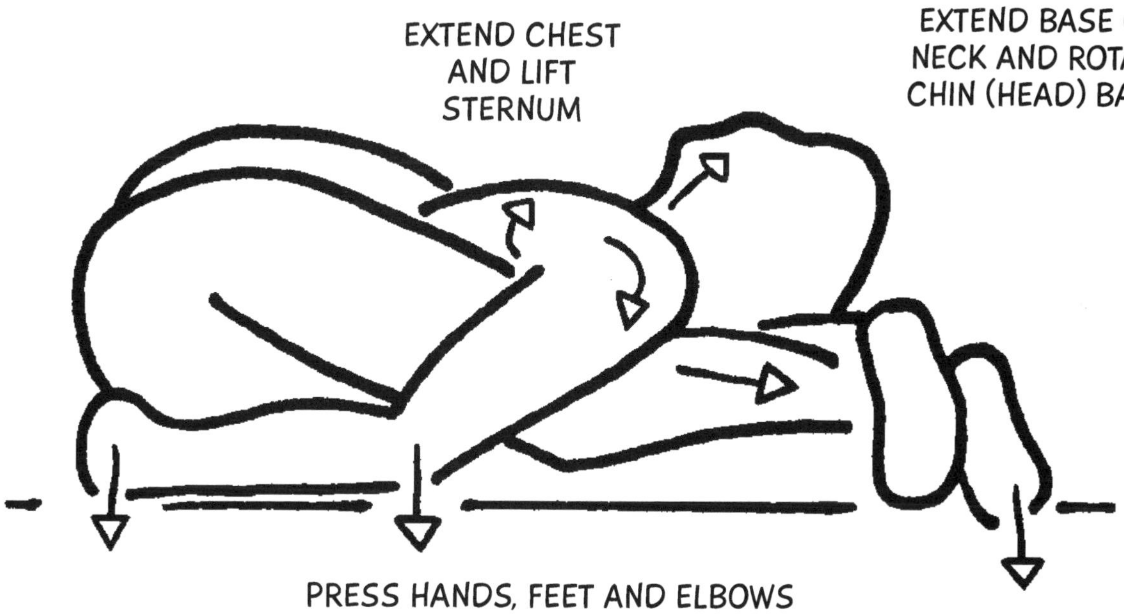

EXTEND CHEST
AND LIFT
STERNUM
EXTEND BASE OF
NECK AND ROTATE
CHIN (HEAD) BACK
PRESS HANDS, FEET AND ELBOWS
TO FLOOR AS MUCH AS POSSIBLE

Ardha Matsyendrasana II 30-60s (107)

a founder of Yoga

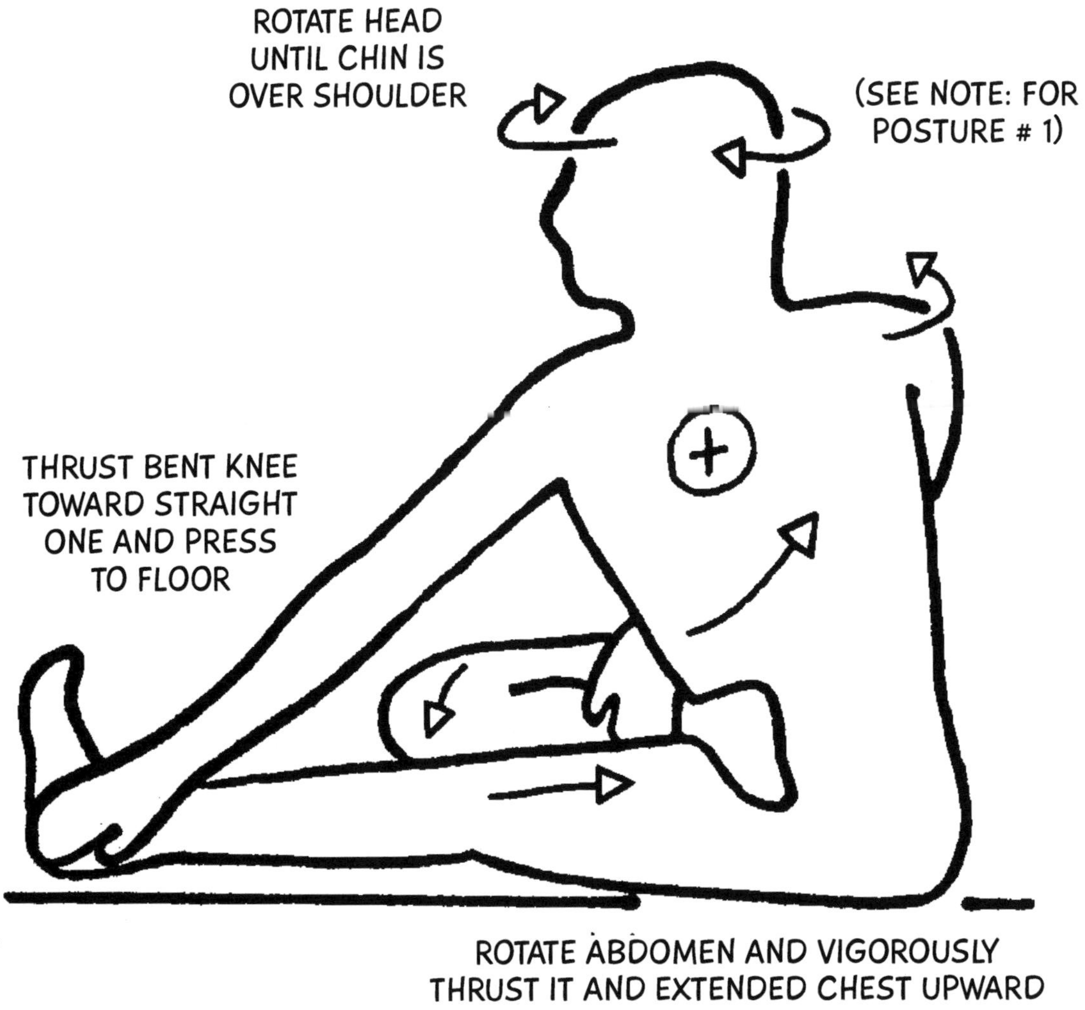
ROTATE HEAD
UNTIL CHIN IS
OVER SHOULDER
(SEE NOTE: FOR
POSTURE # 1)
THRUST BENT KNEE
TOWARD STRAIGHT
ONE AND PRESS
TO FLOOR
ROTATE ABDOMEN AND VIGOROUSLY
THRUST IT AND EXTENDED CHEST UPWARD

Var: Reach around and grasp the thigh of the bent leg instead of the ankle.

Pasasana 30-60s (108)

noose

Var: You can put a blanket under the back of the heels if ankle flexibility is too low. Also try propping the trunk up against the wall.

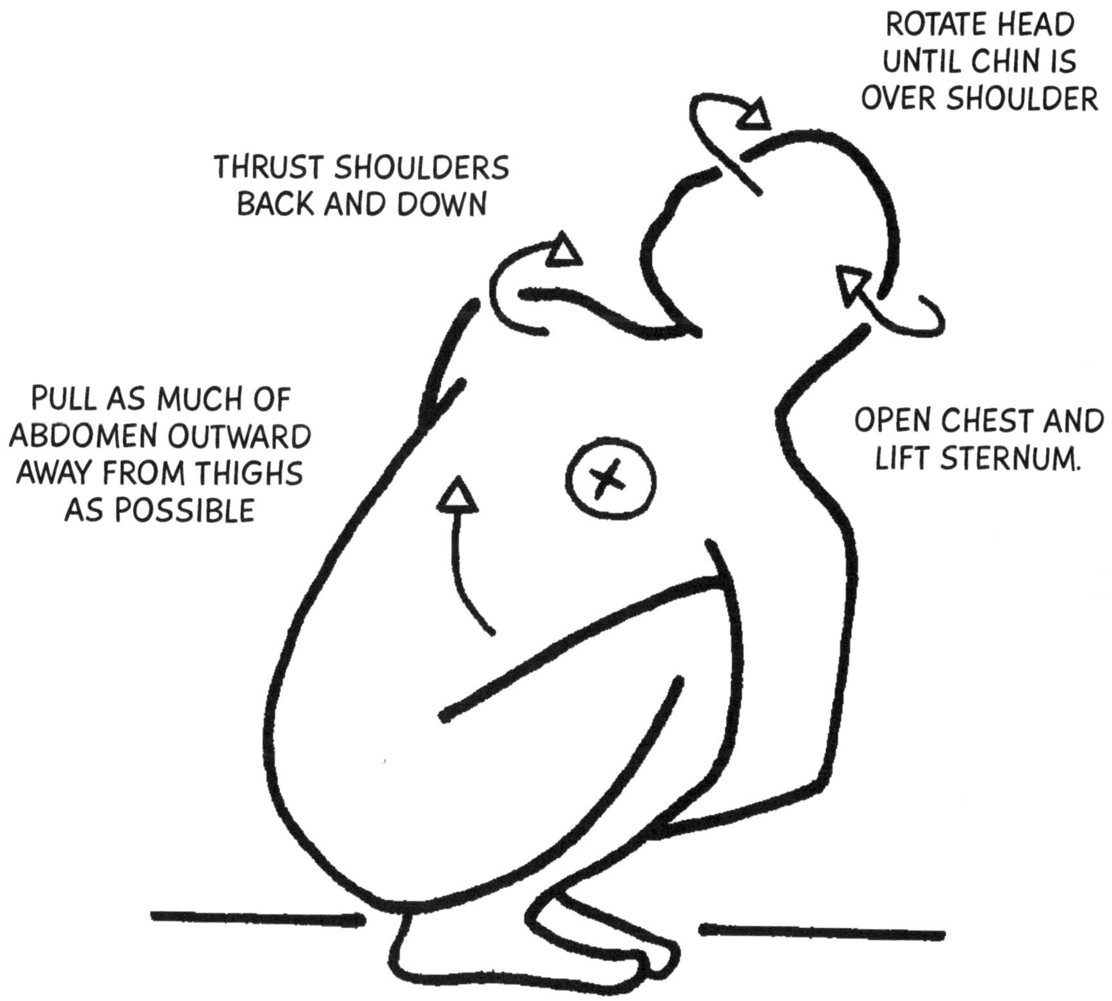
ROTATE HEAD
UNTIL CHIN IS
OVER SHOULDER
THRUST SHOULDERS
BACK AND DOWN
PULL AS MUCH OF
ABDOMEN OUTWARD
AWAY FROM THIGHS
AS POSSIBLE
OPEN CHEST AND
LIFT STERNUM.

Note: In this and most other twist postures, the arm passed behind the back is grasped by the hand of the bent arm, and is thrust downward.

Supta Bhekasana 20-30s (109)

reclining frog

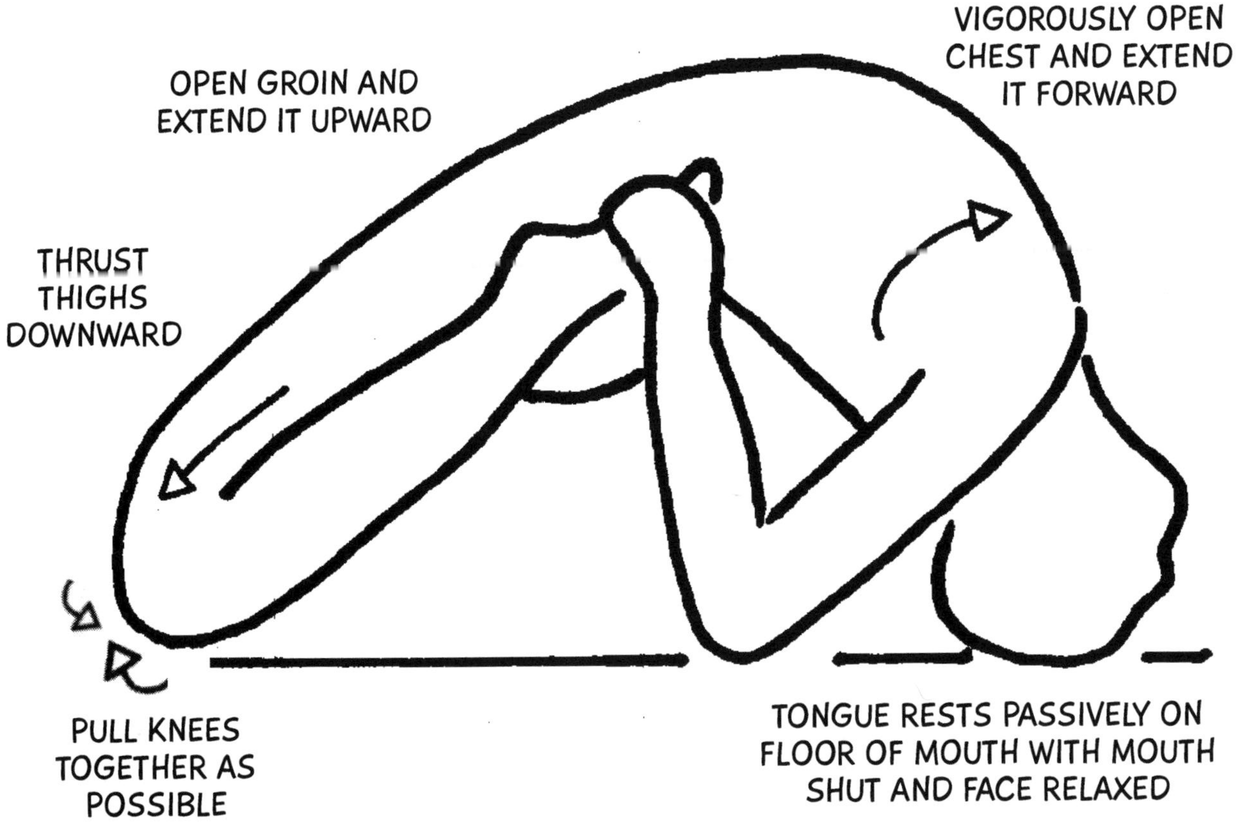

OPEN GROIN AND
EXTEND IT UPWARD
VIGOROUSLY OPEN
CHEST AND EXTEND
IT FORWARD
THRUST
THIGHS
DOWNWARD
PULL KNEES
TOGETHER AS
POSSIBLE
TONGUE RESTS PASSIVELY ON
FLOOR OF MOUTH WITH MOUTH
SHUT AND FACE RELAXED

Setu Bandhasana a few sec (110)

bridge contracted

Note: This posture feels like you're going to break your neck. It is an eerie feeling, but so far my neck is just fine (and stronger to boot). Obviously though, great care is necessary.

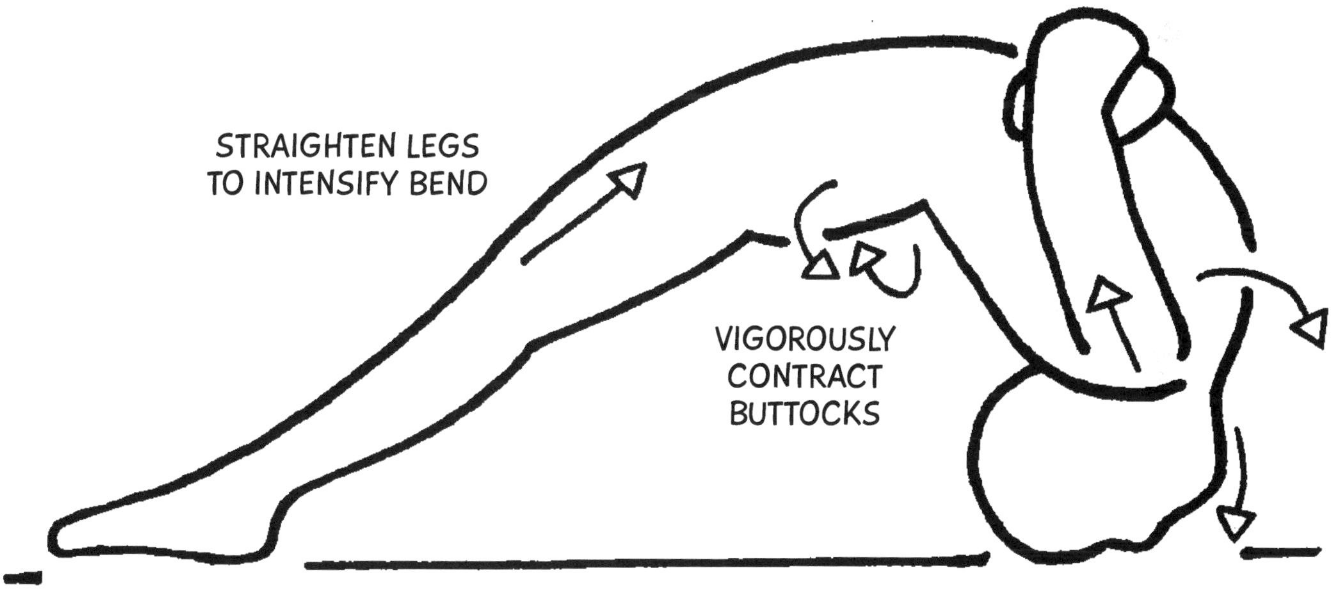
LIFT
SHOULDERS
UPWARD
STRAIGHTEN LEGS
TO INTENSIFY BEND
VIGOROUSLY
CONTRACT
BUTTOCKS
CAREFULLY ROTATE HEAD
TOWARD FLOOR UNTIL
NOSE TOUCHES FLOOR

Dwi Pada Viparita Dandasana 1-2min (111)

two leg inverted staff

Var: Prop the elbows up firmly against a wall and thrust the chest towards the wall.

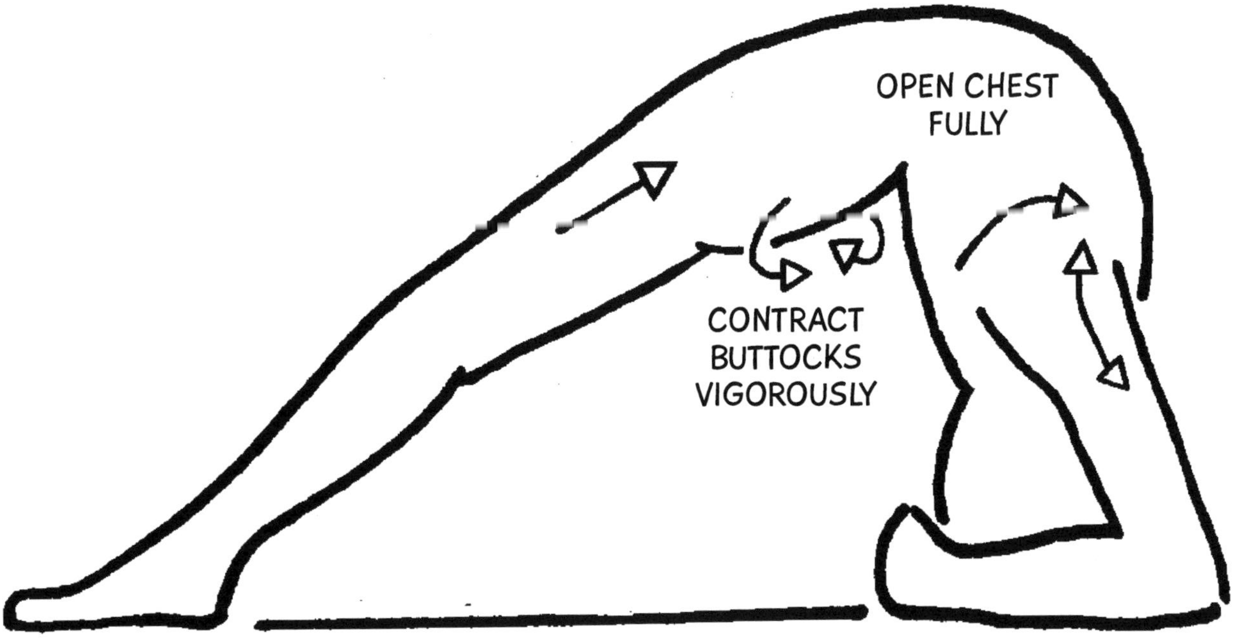
OPEN CHEST
FULLY
CONTRACT
BUTTOCKS
VIGOROUSLY
KEEP FEET
PARALLEL
OPEN ARM-PITS AND THRUST
ELBOWS TO FLOOR

Note: In this and some of the other back bending postures, you can keep the legs bent and move them closer toward the head until your back bending flexibility allows you to keep them straight.

Eka Pada Urdhva Dhanurasana 15s (112)

one leg up bow

Var: In order to help you balance, initially do this posture in a doorway - prop the upper leg next to the door opening.

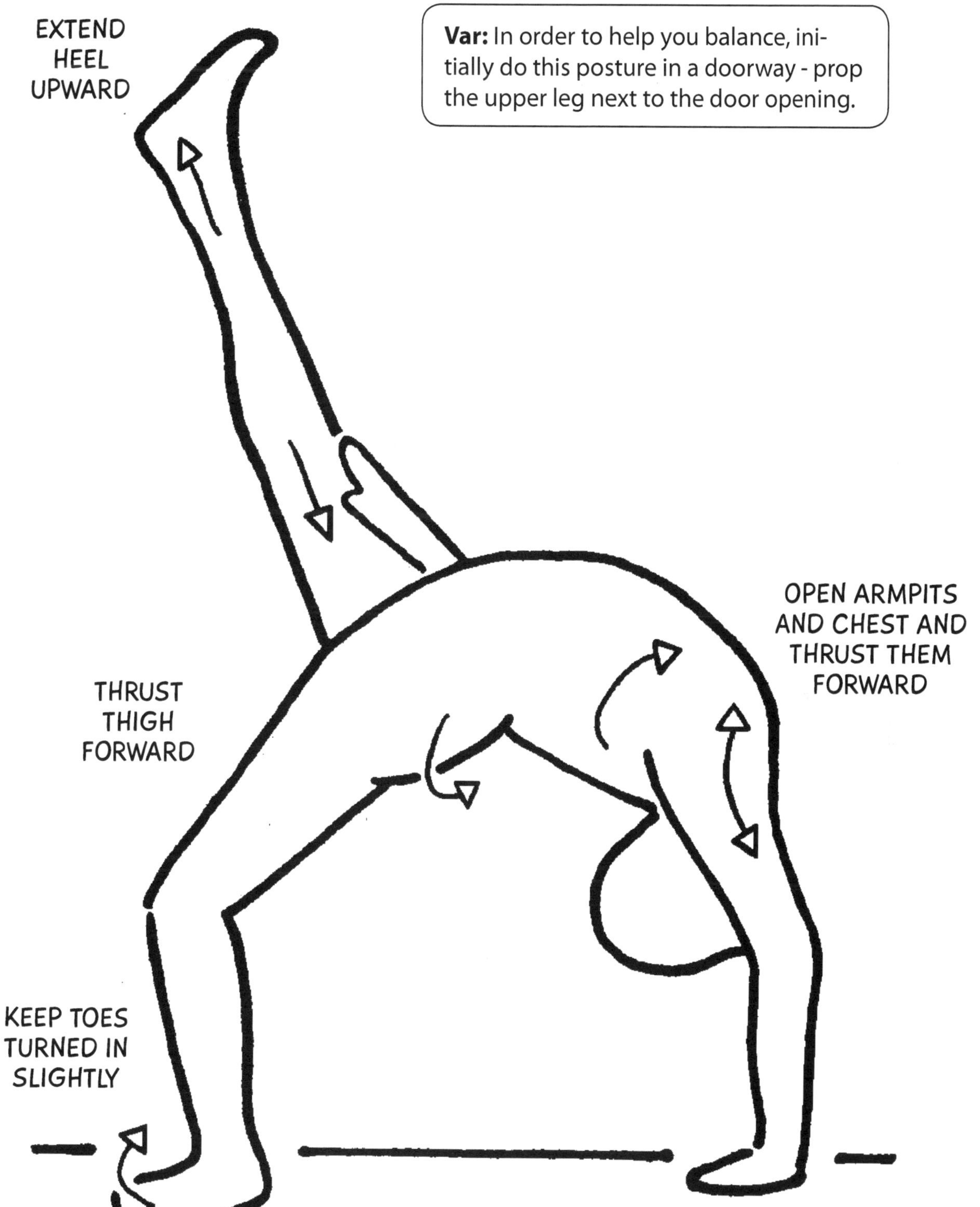

EXTEND HEEL UPWARD
THRUST THIGH FORWARD
OPEN ARMPITS AND CHEST AND THRUST THEM FORWARD
KEEP TOES TURNED IN SLIGHTLY

Parsva Bakasana 20s (113)

side crane

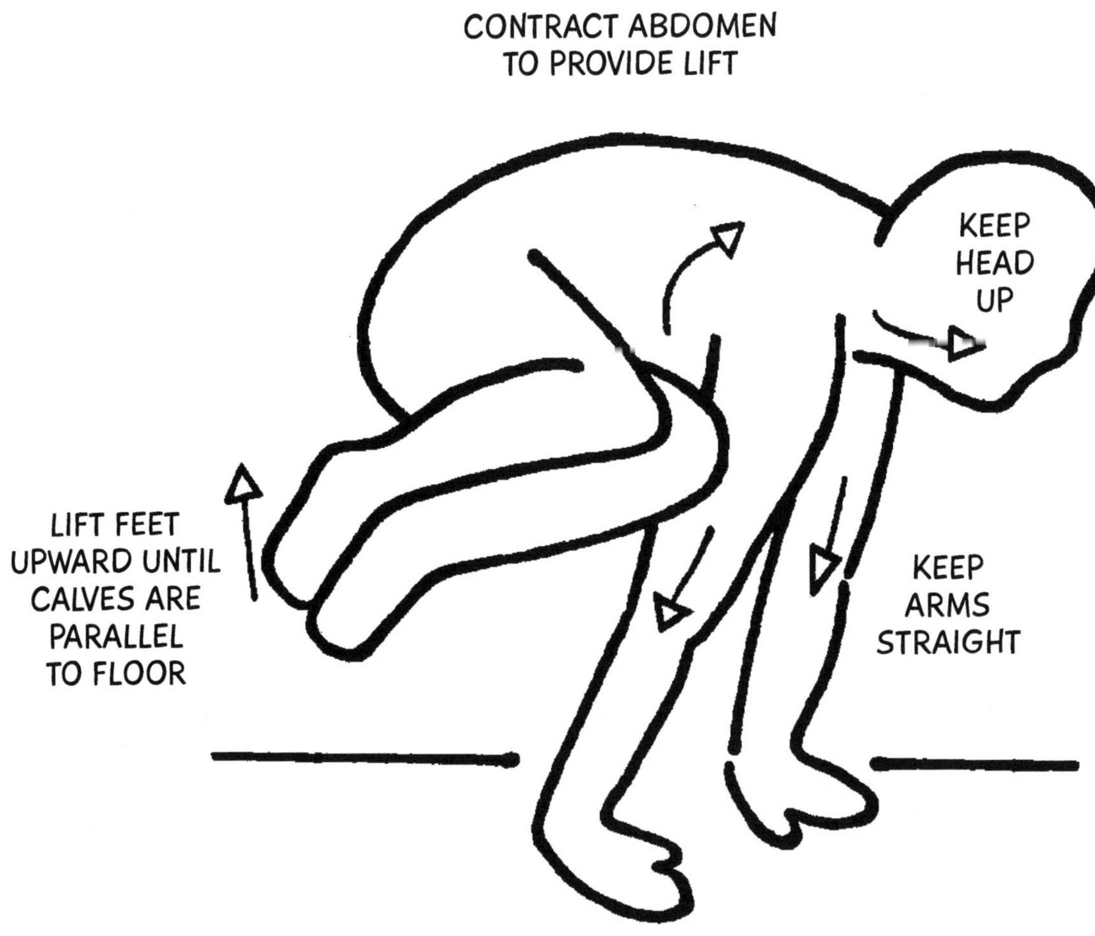

CONTRACT ABDOMEN
TO PROVIDE LIFT
KEEP
HEAD
UP
LIFT FEET
UPWARD UNTIL
CALVES ARE
PARALLEL
TO FLOOR
KEEP
ARMS
STRAIGHT

Note: Rest the knee just above the elbow and use the elbow for leverage in rotating as much of the abdomen toward the bent knees as possible. For added challenge, lift the upper knee, separating it a few inches from the lower one.

Galavasana 20s (114)

an Indian sage

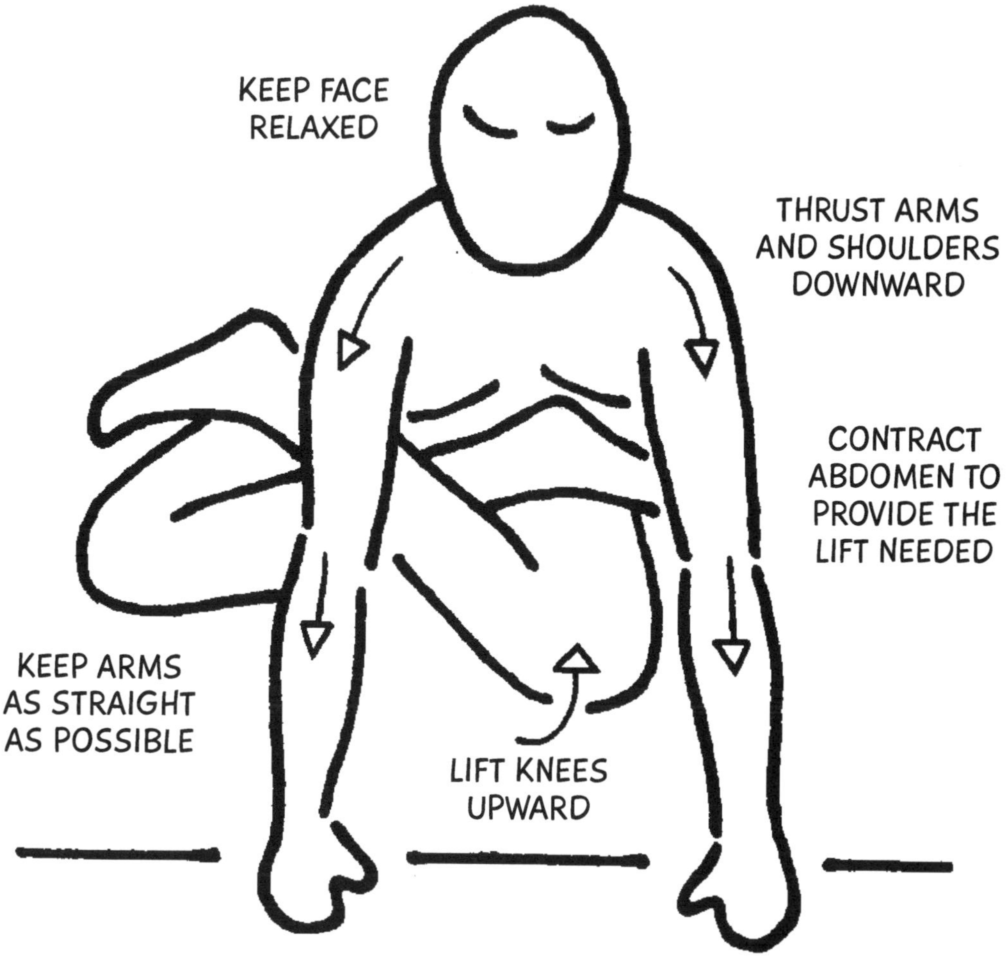
KEEP FACE
RELAXED
THRUST ARMS
AND SHOULDERS
DOWNWARD
CONTRACT
ABDOMEN TO
PROVIDE THE
LIFT NEEDED
KEEP ARMS
AS STRAIGHT
AS POSSIBLE
LIFT KNEES
UPWARD

Note: In this and all advanced arm balance postures, keep the wrist firm and feel them rooted to the floor. This should help stabilize your balance.

Program 7

First Day: Begin with the **Headstand Cycle (page 103)**. Next do the advanced arm balances, of which three are new, then Sarvangasana and Halasana.

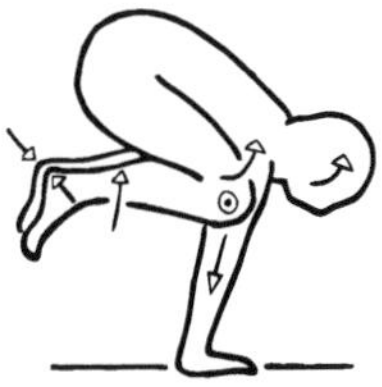
Bakasana – 74

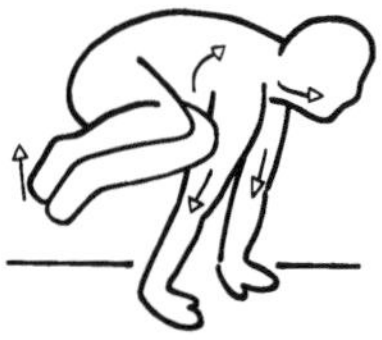
Parsva Bakasana – 113

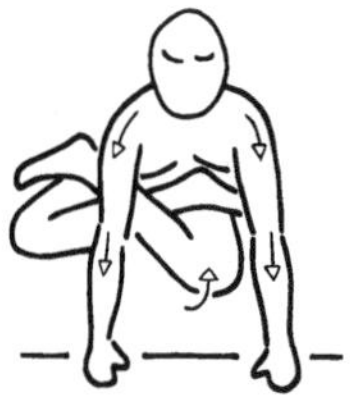
Galavasana – 114

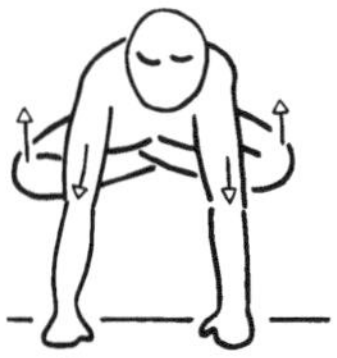
Urdhva Kukkutasana – 115

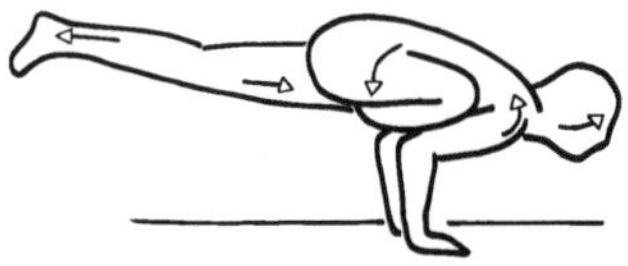
Eka Pada Galavasana – 116

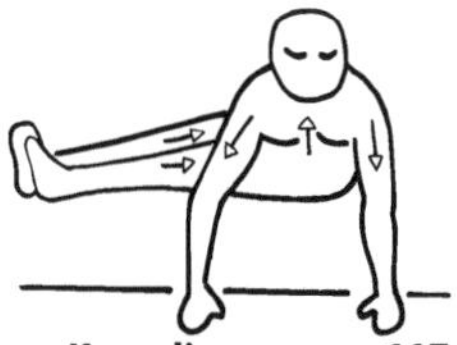
Koundinyasana – 117

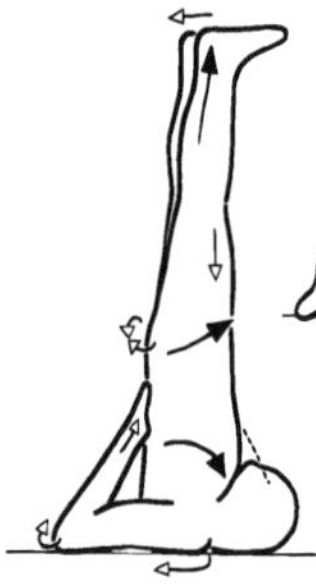
Sarvangasana I – 12

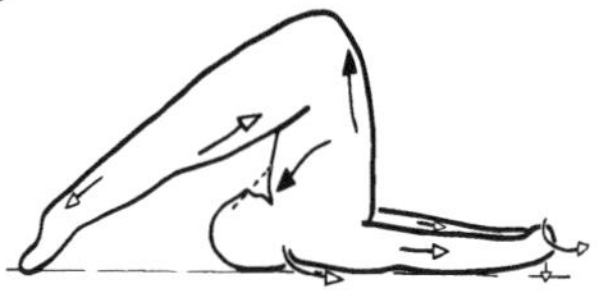
Halasana – 29

After Halasana, do the **Forward Cycle (page 73)**, continue on with the leg-head, twists, and back bends (right and below). Gradually add the new ones to your practice.

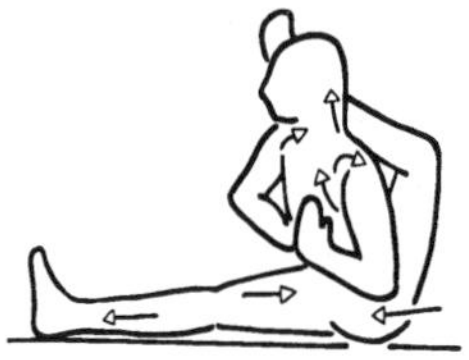
Eka Pada Sirsasana – 103

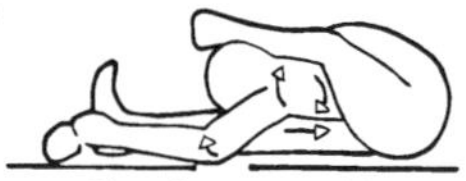
Skandasana – 104

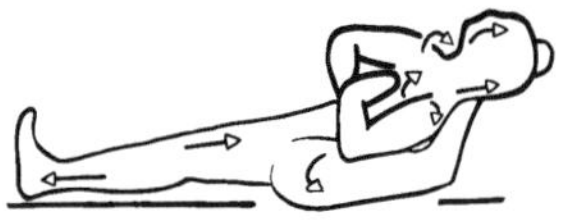
Bhairavasana – 105

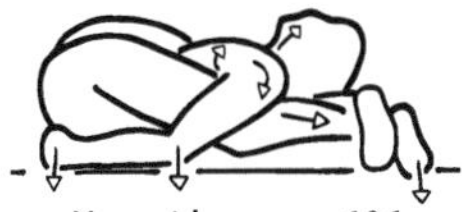
Yoganidrasana – 106

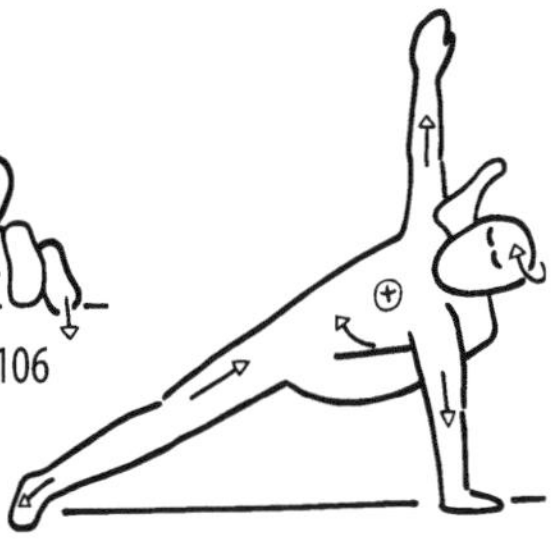
Kalabhairavasana – 118

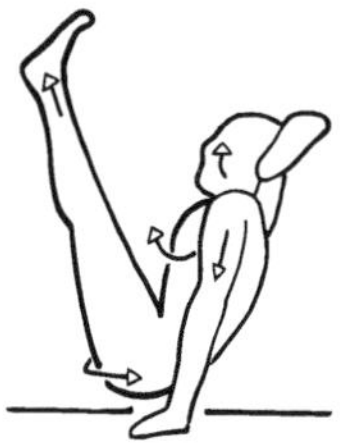
Chakorasana – 119

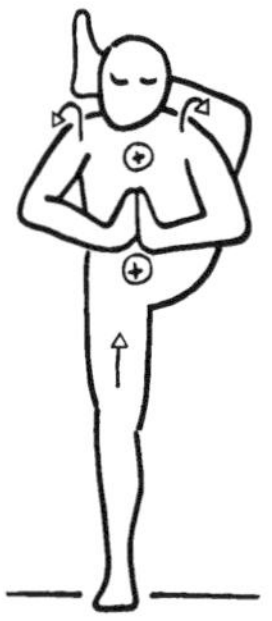
Durvasana – 120

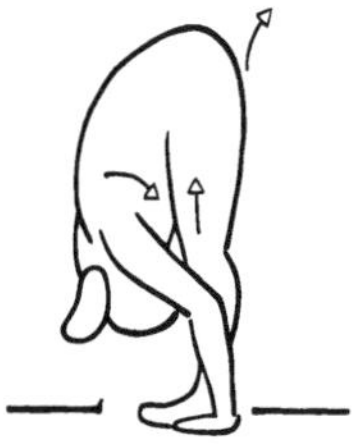
Ruchikasana – 121

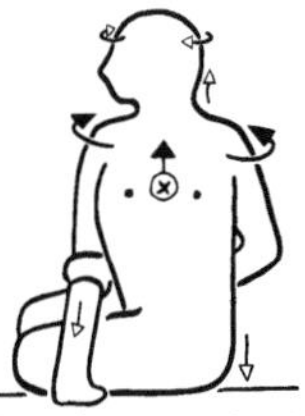
Bharadvajasana I – 26

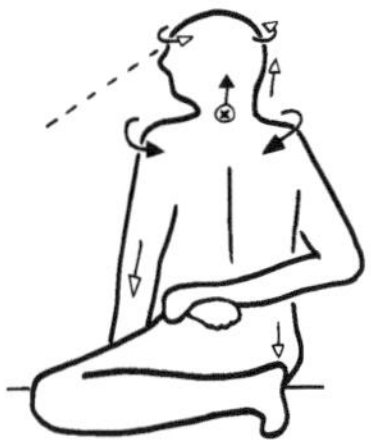
Bharadvajasana II – 34

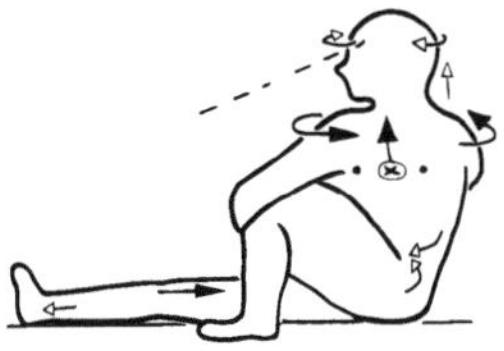
Marichyasana III – 35

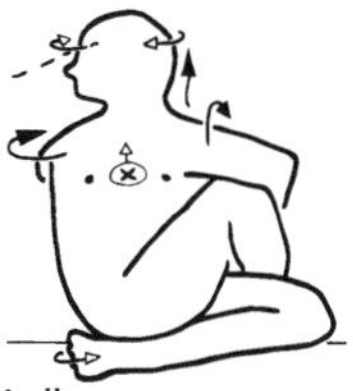
Ardha Matsyendrasana I – 36

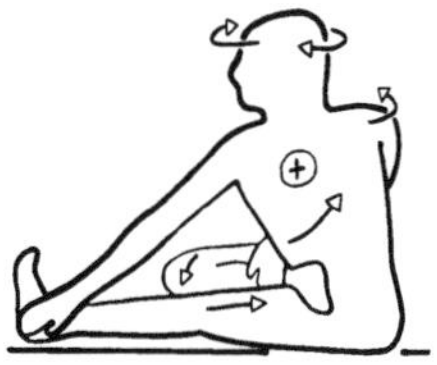
Ardha Matsyendrasana II – 107

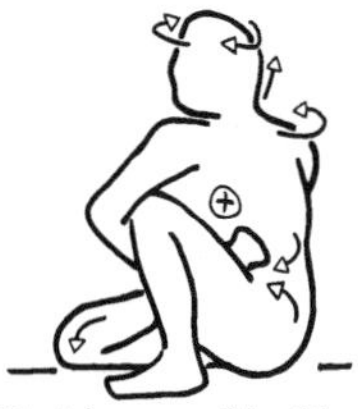
Marichyasana IV – 91

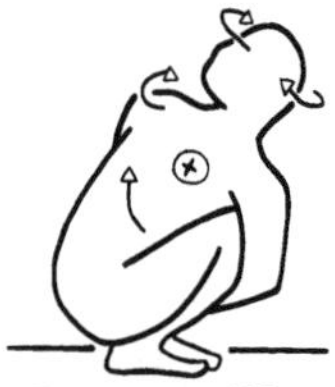
Pasasana – 108

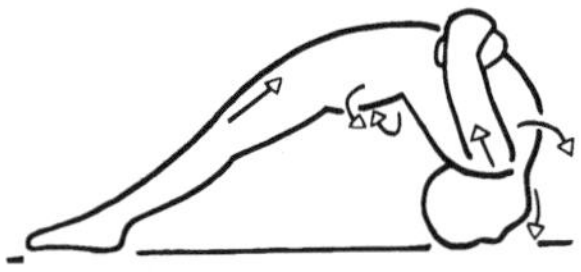
Setu Bhandasana – 110

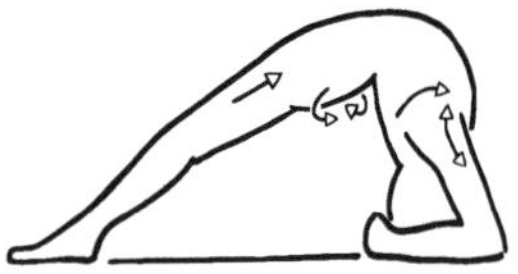
Dwi Pada Viparita Dandasana – 111

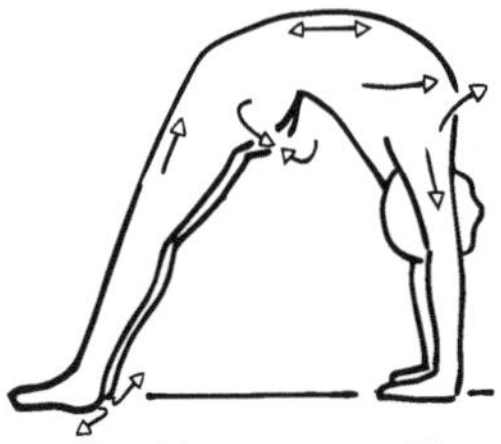
Urdhva Dhanurasana – 73

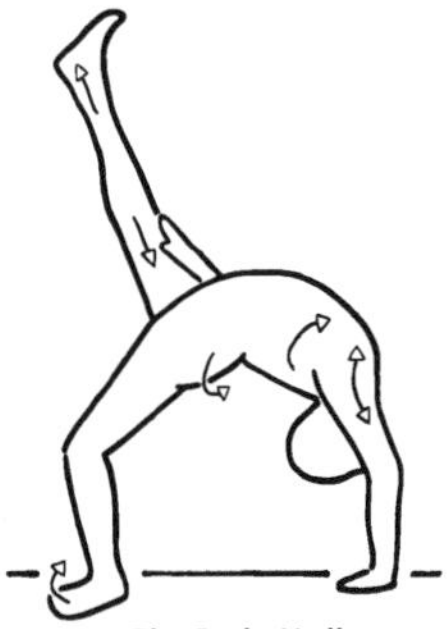
Eka Pada Urdhva Dhanurasana – 112

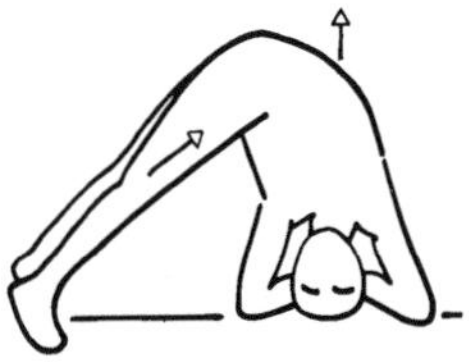
Mandalasana – 122

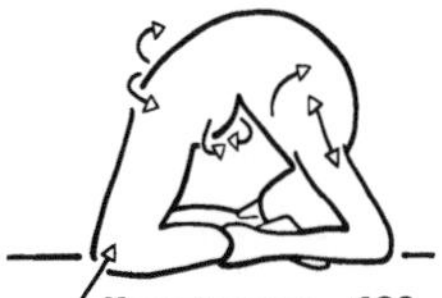
Kapotasana – 123

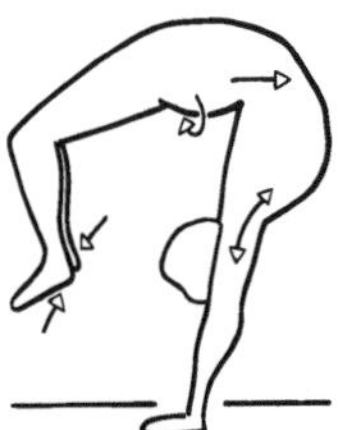
Viparita Chakrasana – 124

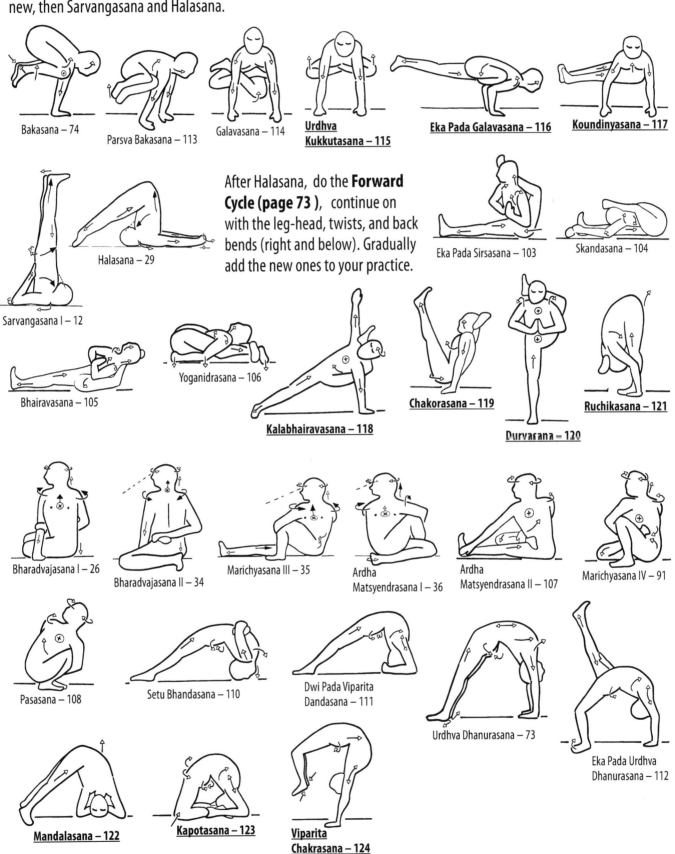

(Program 7: Continued)

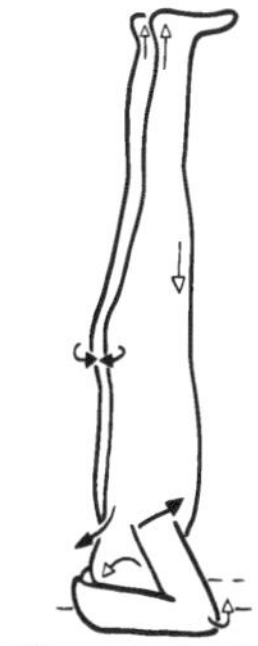

Sirsasana I – 27

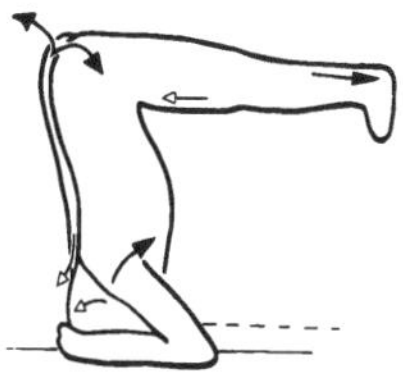

Urdhva Dandasana – 28

Second Day: Begin with the Sirsasana and Urdhva Dandasana (left). Next do three cycles: **Basic Arm Cycle (page 125)**, **Shoulderstand Cycle (page 103)**, and the **Forward Cycle (page 73)**. Continue on with these postures below.

Review (or Third) Day: The same as Program 6's Review Day.

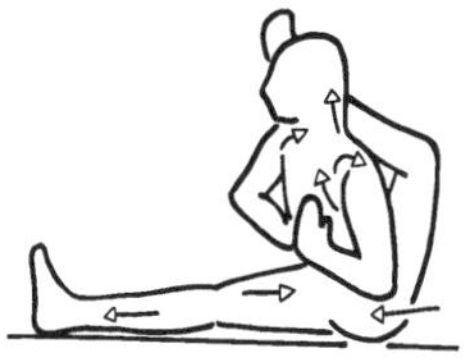

Eka Pada Sirsasana – 103

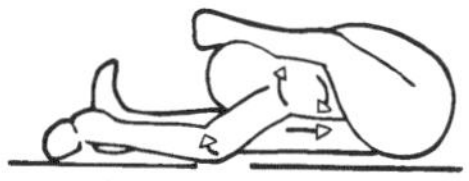

Skandasana – 104

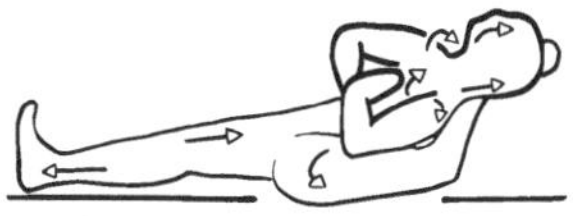

Bhairavasana – 105

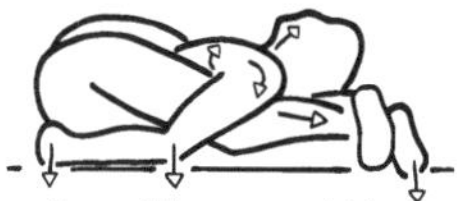

Yoganidrasana – 106

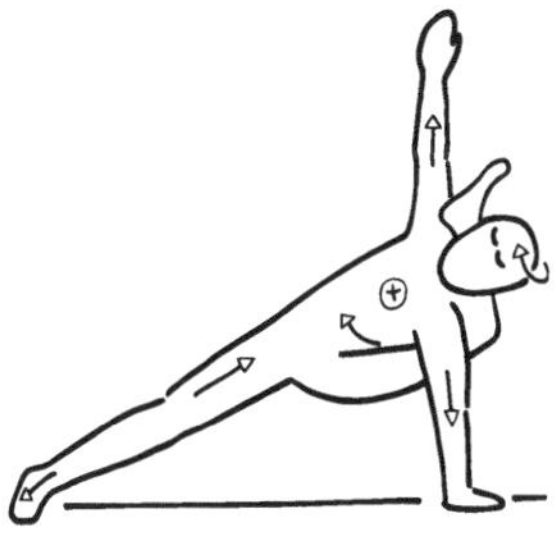

Kalabhairavasana – 118

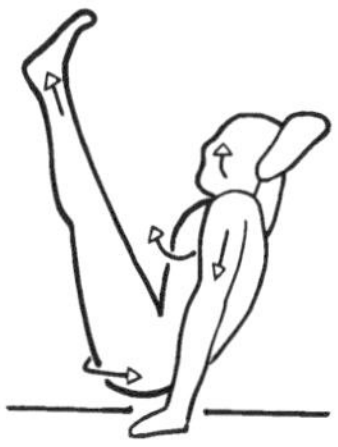

Chakorasana – 119

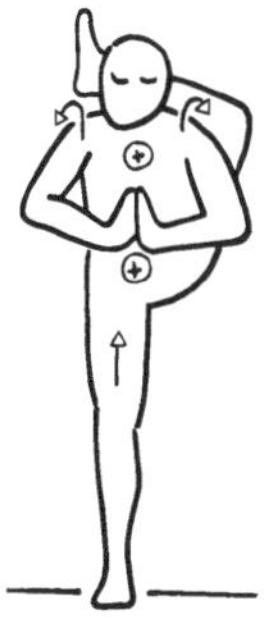

Durvasana – 120

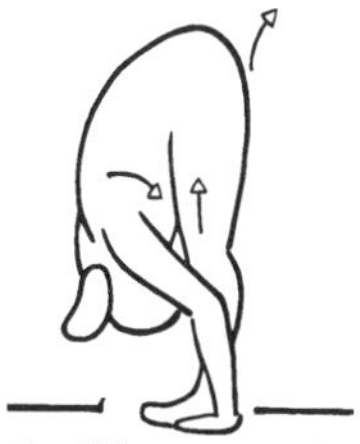

Ruchikasana – 121

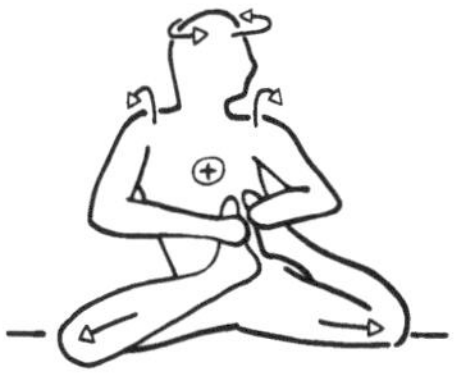

Vamedevasana – 125

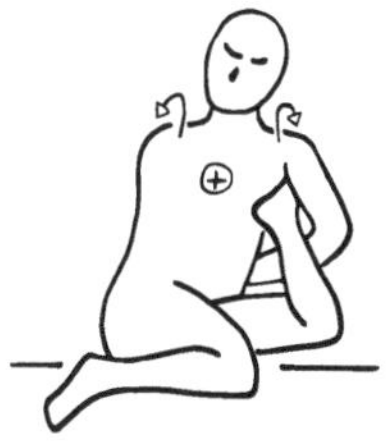

Yoga Dandasana – 126

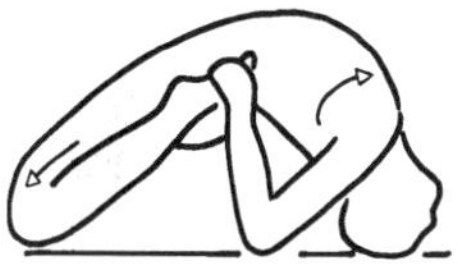

Supta Bhekasana – 109

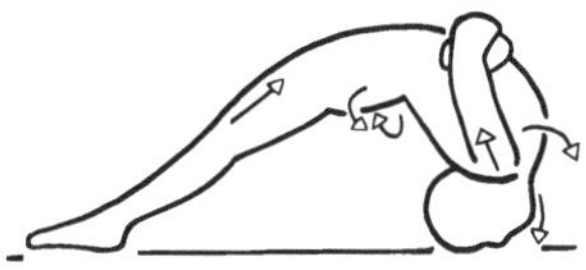

Setu Bhandasana – 110

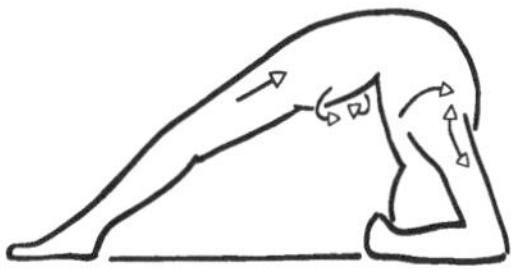

Dwi Pada Viparita Dandasana – 111

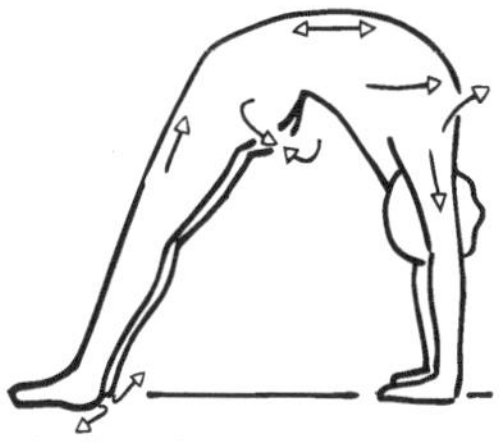

Urdhva Dhanurasana – 73

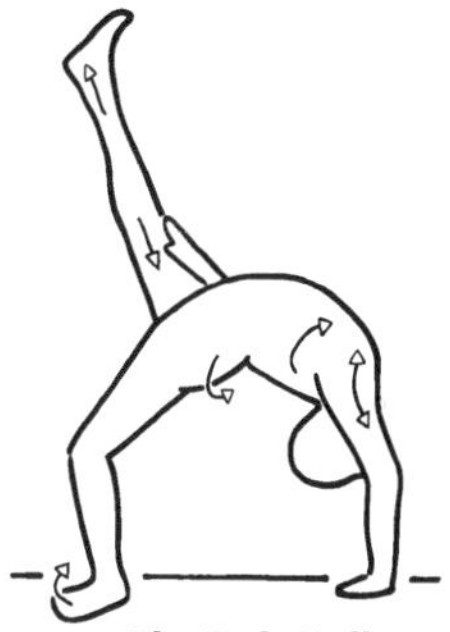

Eka Pada Urdhva Dhanurasana – 112

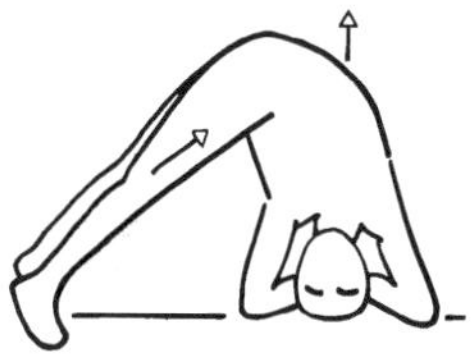

Mandalasana – 122

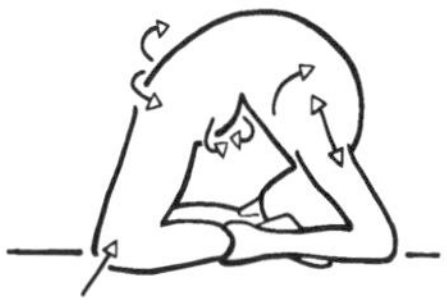

Kapotasana – 123

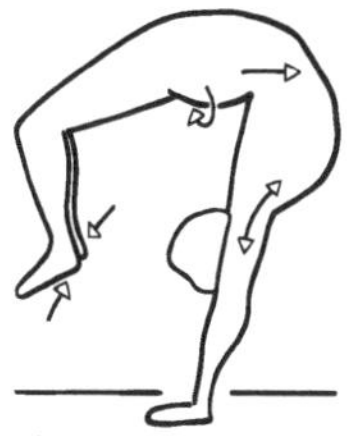

Viparita Chakrasana – 124

Note: Even though you are able to do certain advanced postures, wait until you reach them in due course by working up through the programs. Resist the temptation to work pursue advanced postures that come naturally easy and neglect the more basic (or advanced) ones in your actual program level which you dislike, i.e. can't do well. After all, working in your weakest areas grows determination, patience and self honesty. A balanced approach means applying more effort to areas in which you are reluctance to work, and decrease the intensity of effort in areas you habitually and/or unconsciously work hardest in.

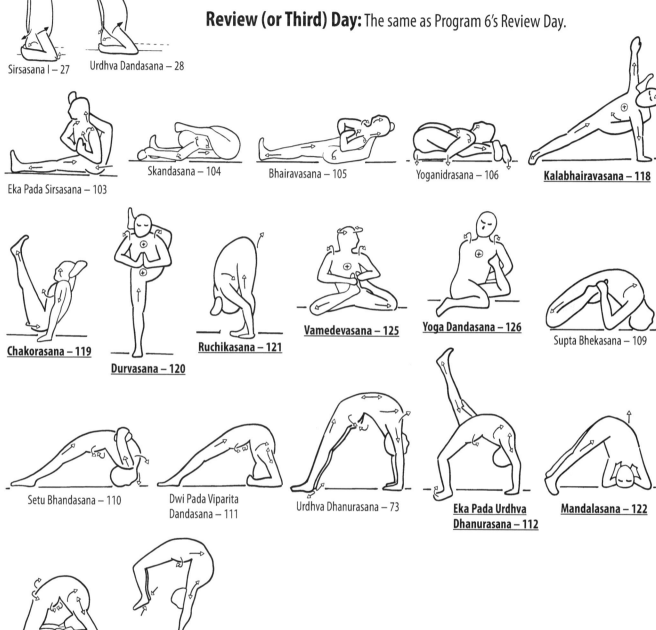

Urdhva Kukkutasana 20s (115)

up rooster

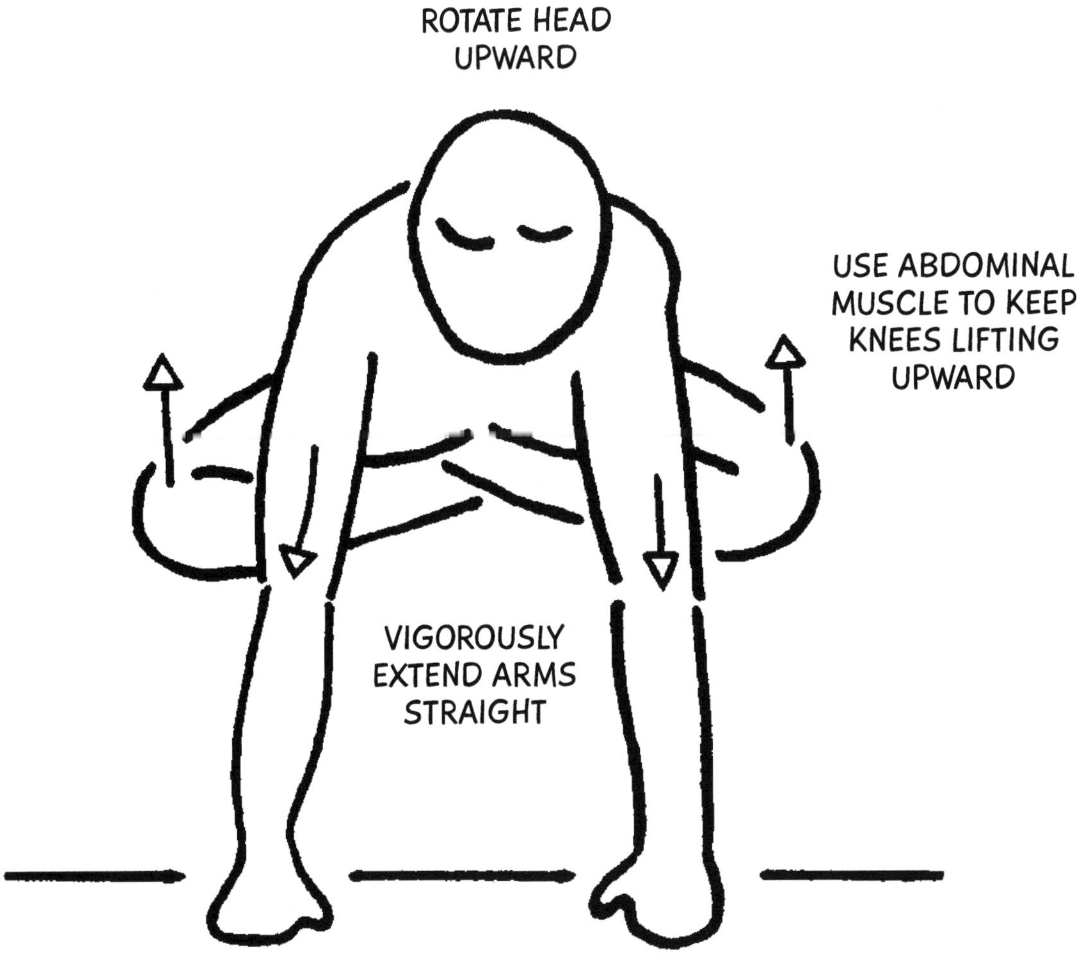
ROTATE HEAD UPWARD
USE ABDOMINAL MUSCLE TO KEEP KNEES LIFTING UPWARD
VIGOROUSLY EXTEND ARMS STRAIGHT

Eka Pada Galavasana 20s (116)

one leg sage

Note: the arrow (in both basic and advanced postures) which indicates thrusting of the heel away from the body. When you thrust the heel away from the body this pulls the knee caps up, which is correct, but this can also lead to unnecessary tightness in the ankle. Strive to thrust the ball of the foot and the heel simultaneously with just enough effort to bring "life" to this area, without tension in the ankle. In some postures, however, the heel is still vigorously thrust outward with the toes and ball of the foot curled in towards the body. This principle of vigorous effort without tension applies to the other postures as well.

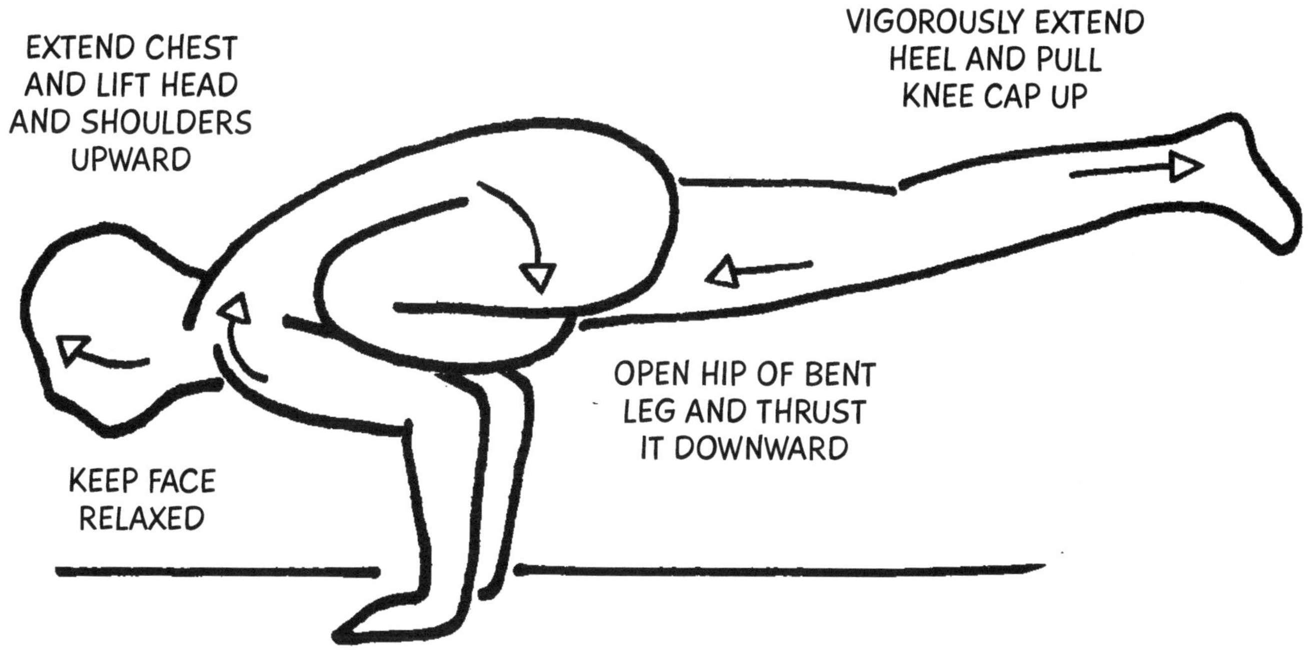
EXTEND CHEST AND LIFT HEAD AND SHOULDERS UPWARD
VIGOROUSLY EXTEND HEEL AND PULL KNEE CAP UP
OPEN HIP OF BENT LEG AND THRUST IT DOWNWARD
KEEP FACE RELAXED

Koundinyasana 20s (117)

an Indian sage

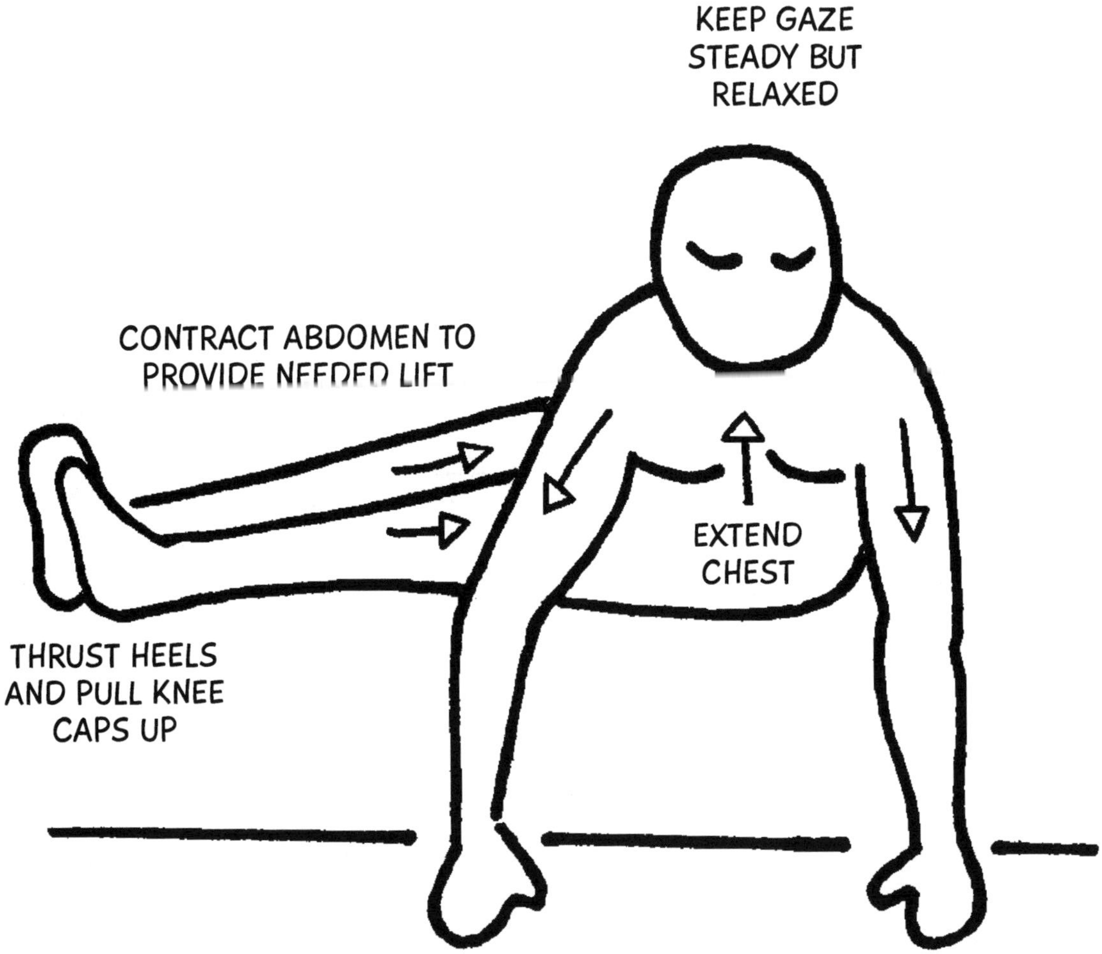
KEEP GAZE
STEADY BUT
RELAXED
CONTRACT ABDOMEN TO
PROVIDE NEEDED LIFT
EXTEND
CHEST
THRUST HEELS
AND PULL KNEE
CAPS UP

Note: For added challenge, lift one leg a few inches to separate and raise it above the other one. Keep both straight.

Kala Bhairavasana 20s (118)

destroyer of the universe

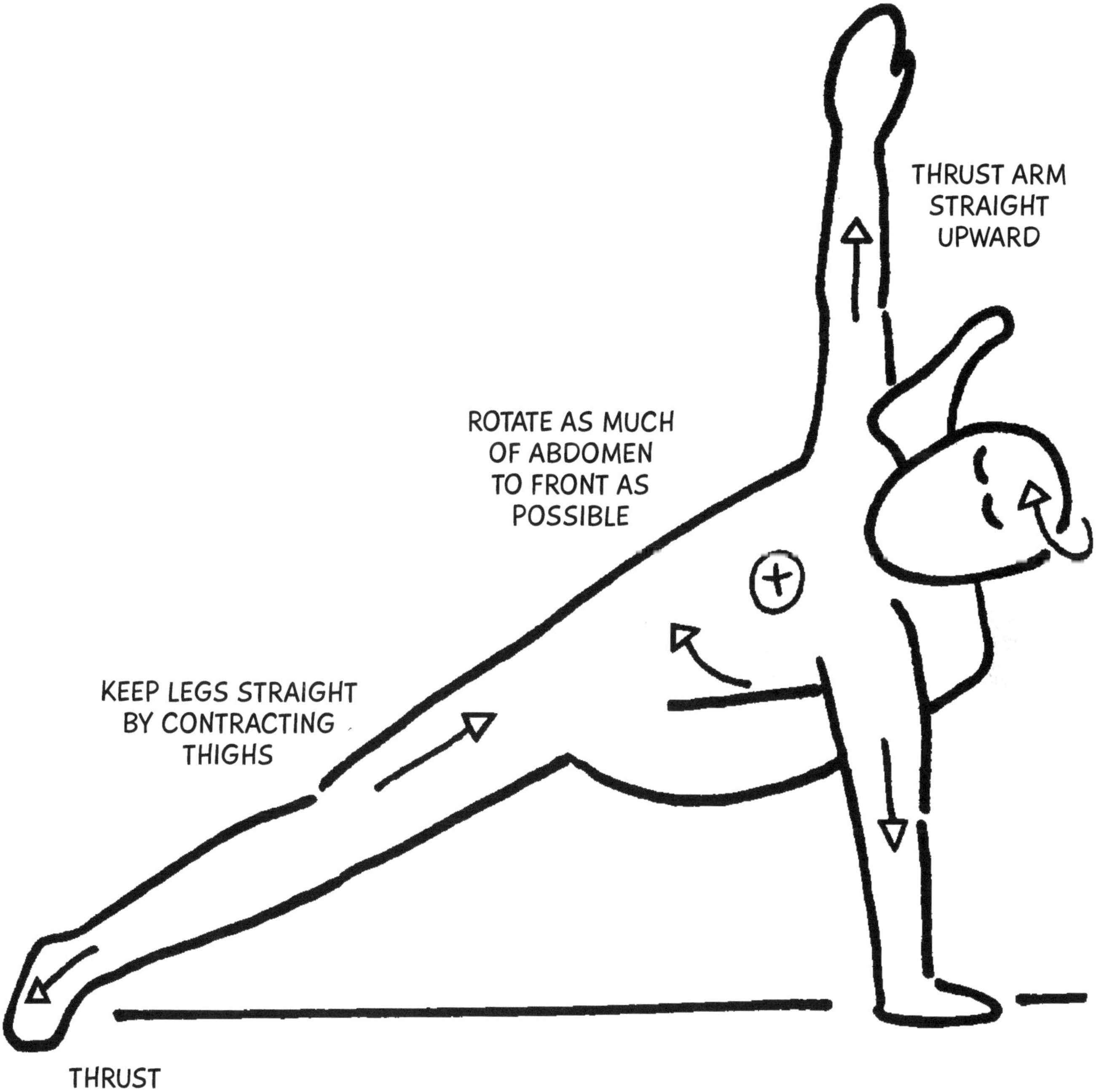

THRUST ARM STRAIGHT UPWARD
ROTATE AS MUCH OF ABDOMEN TO FRONT AS POSSIBLE
KEEP LEGS STRAIGHT BY CONTRACTING THIGHS
THRUST HEEL INTO FLOOR

Chakorasana 20s

a moon beam eating partridge

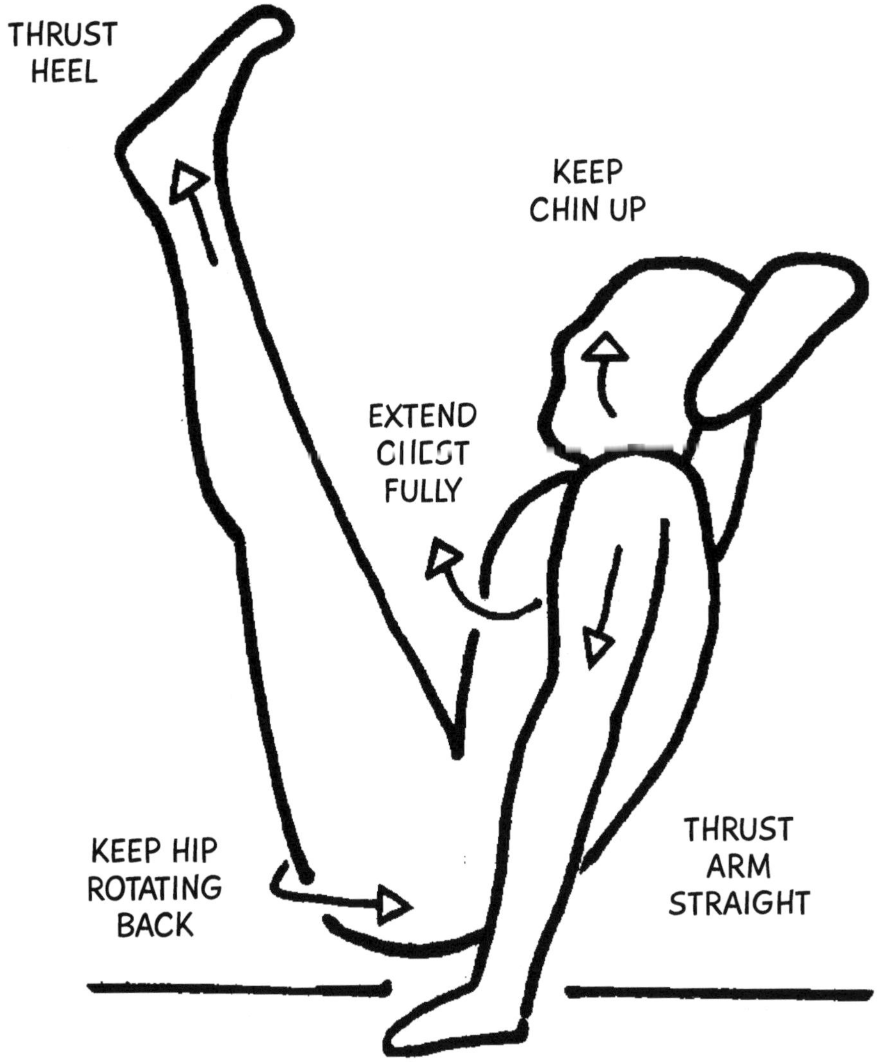
THRUST
HEEL
KEEP
CHIN UP
EXTEND
CHEST
FULLY
KEEP HIP
ROTATING
BACK
THRUST
ARM
STRAIGHT

Note: In this and other postures, never use strained exhalations.

Durvasana 20s (120)

an irascible sage

Note: Balance can be precarious. Leave space around you in case you fall.

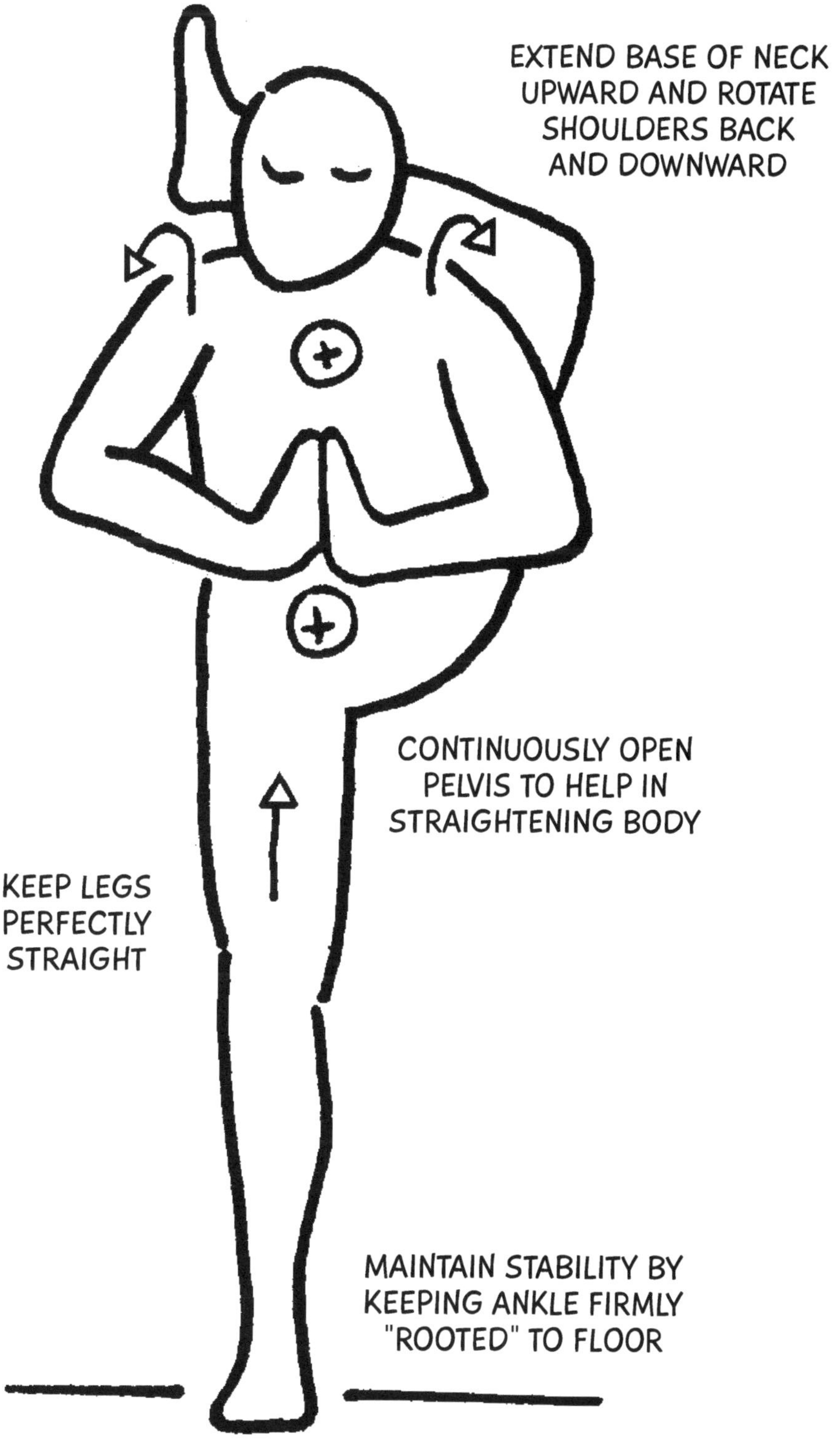

EXTEND BASE OF NECK UPWARD AND ROTATE SHOULDERS BACK AND DOWNWARD
CONTINUOUSLY OPEN PELVIS TO HELP IN STRAIGHTENING BODY
KEEP LEGS PERFECTLY STRAIGHT
MAINTAIN STABILITY BY KEEPING ANKLE FIRMLY "ROOTED" TO FLOOR

Ruchikasana 20s

an Indian sage

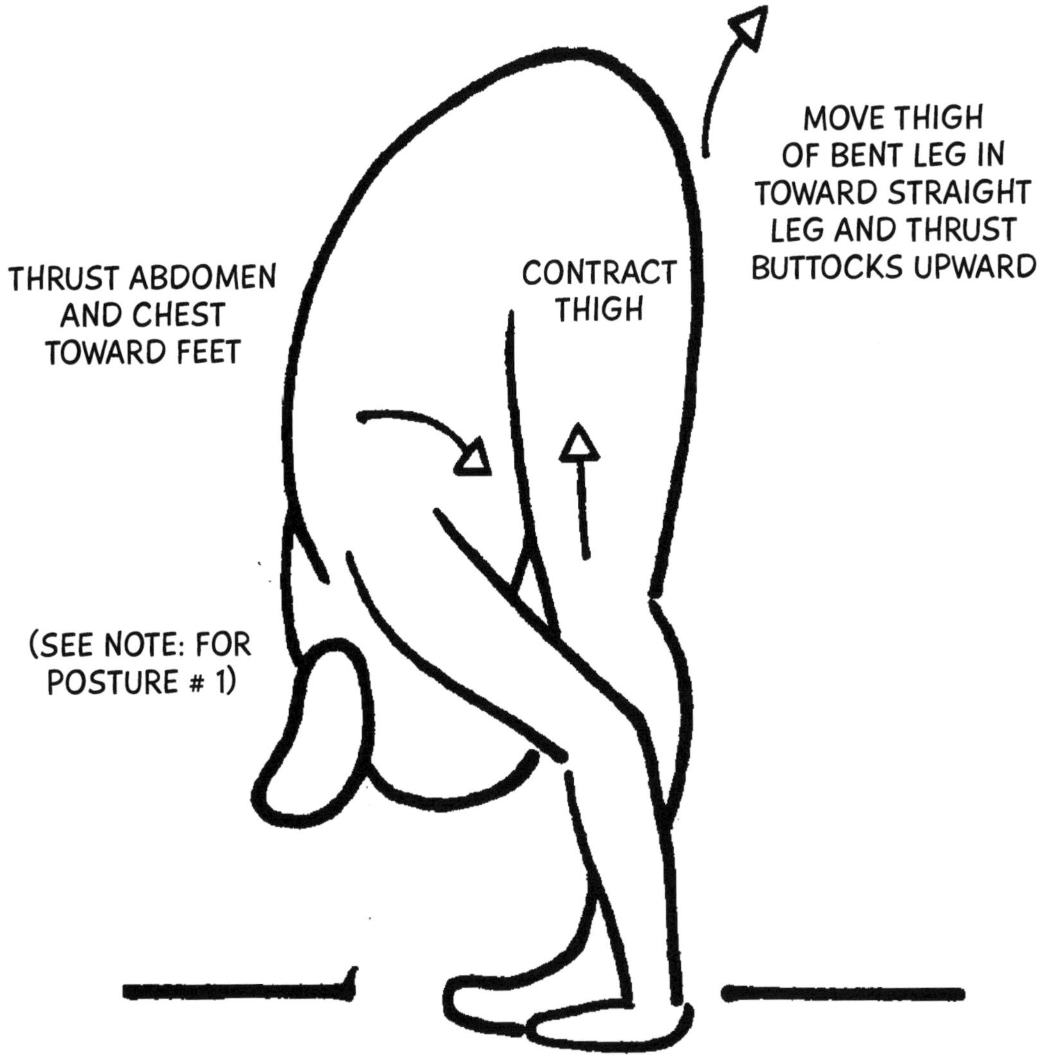
MOVE THIGH
OF BENT LEG IN
TOWARD STRAIGHT
LEG AND THRUST
BUTTOCKS UPWARD
THRUST ABDOMEN
AND CHEST
TOWARD FEET
CONTRACT
THIGH
(SEE NOTE: FOR
POSTURE # 1)

Mandalasana 3-6 revolutions (122)

wheel or ring

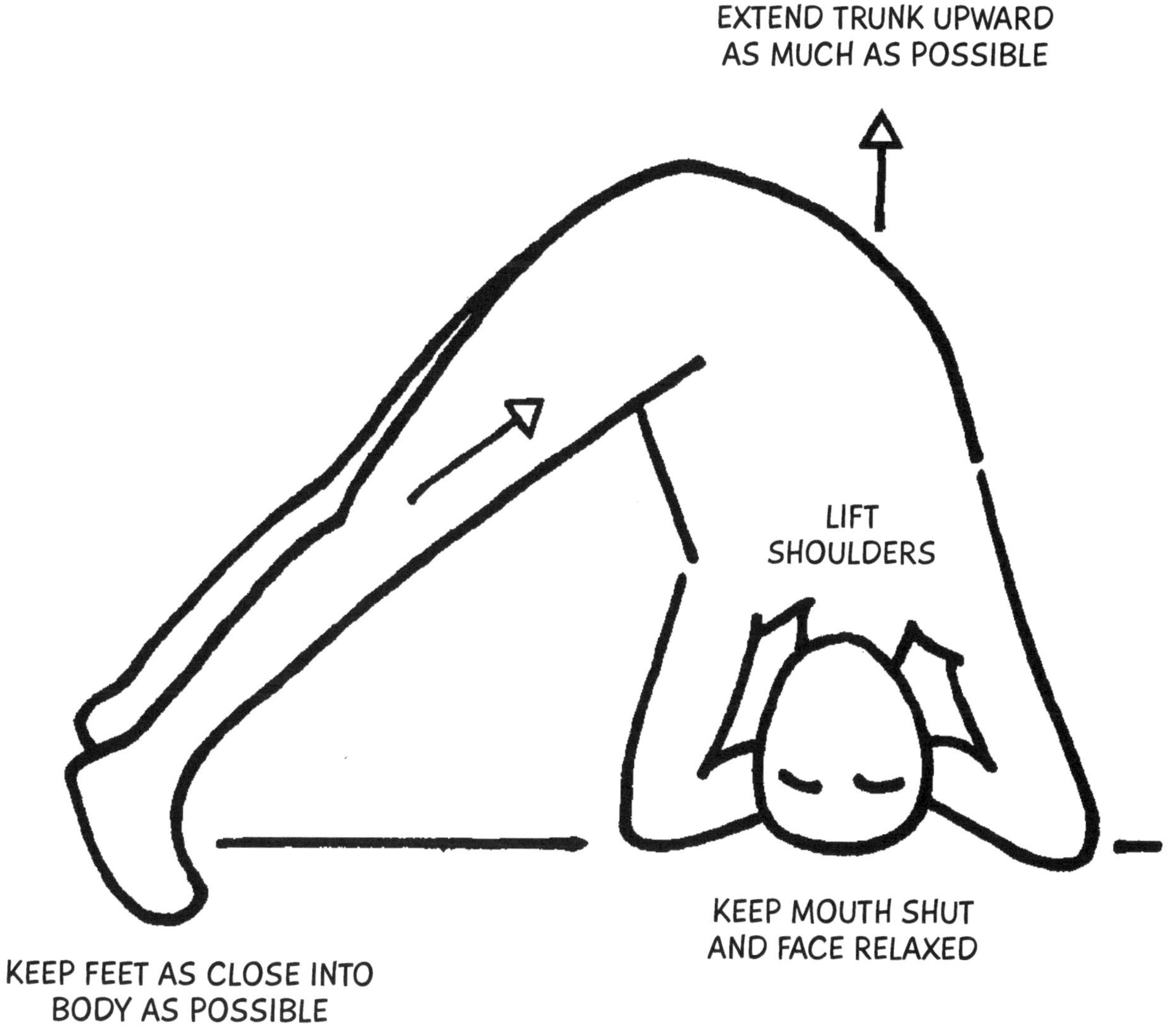
EXTEND TRUNK UPWARD
AS MUCH AS POSSIBLE
LIFT
SHOULDERS
KEEP MOUTH SHUT
AND FACE RELAXED
KEEP FEET AS CLOSE INTO
BODY AS POSSIBLE

Kapotasana 10-60s

pigeon or dove

(123)

Var: Use a rope looped around the ankles to grasp on to. Later grasp the toes and gradually work the hands (grasp) toward the ankles. Also start the posture with the knees spread 18" or so apart.

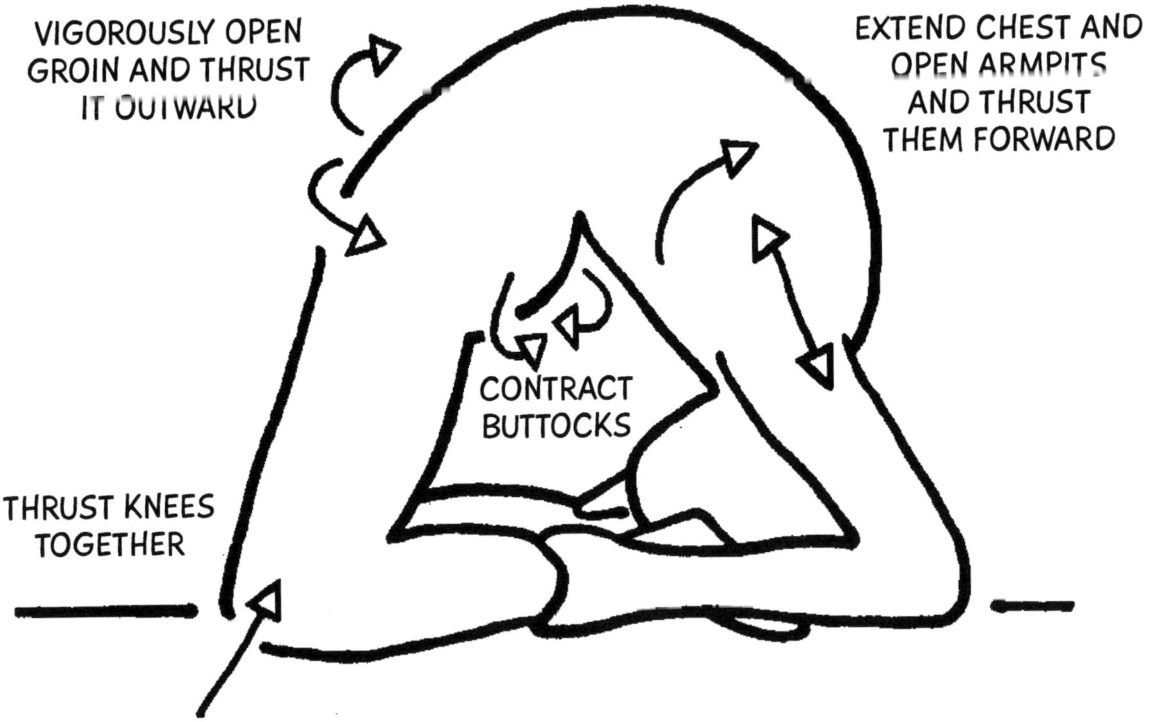
VIGOROUSLY OPEN
GROIN AND THRUST
IT OUTWARD
EXTEND CHEST AND
OPEN ARMPITS
AND THRUST
THEM FORWARD
CONTRACT
BUTTOCKS
THRUST KNEES
TOGETHER

Note: Move into this and other back bends slowly. First thrust thumbs into lower lumbar area of the spine. Extend the spine to make space between these lower vertebrae.

Viparita Chakrasana repeat 3-9 times (124)

inverted wheel

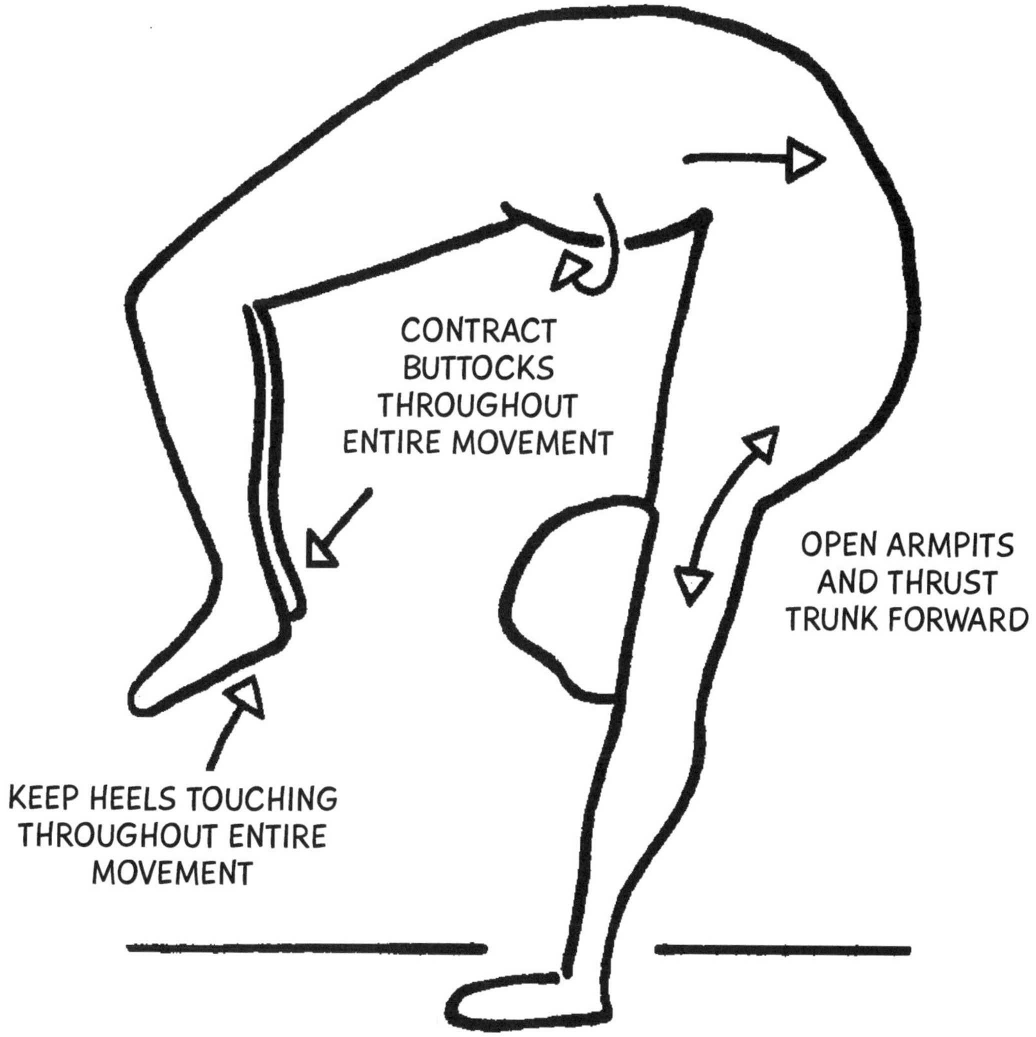
CONTRACT BUTTOCKS THROUGHOUT ENTIRE MOVEMENT
OPEN ARMPITS AND THRUST TRUNK FORWARD
KEEP HEELS TOUCHING THROUGHOUT ENTIRE MOVEMENT

Var: Initially you can do this posture from Urdhva Dhanurasana with the feet next to a wall. Walk feet up the wall and use them to push against the wall to propel you upward and over.

Vamadevasana 30s (125)

knot

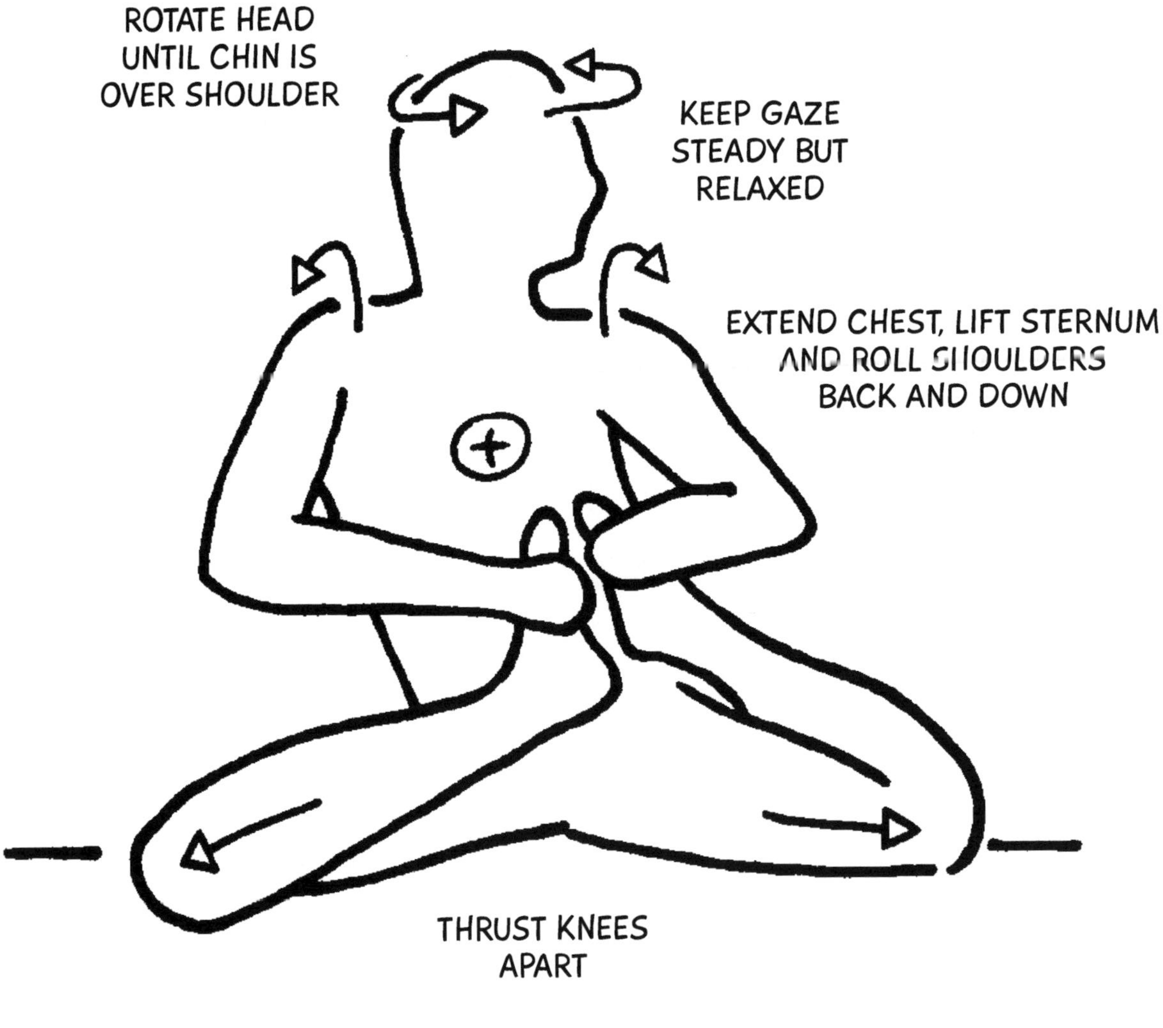
ROTATE HEAD
UNTIL CHIN IS
OVER SHOULDER
KEEP GAZE
STEADY BUT
RELAXED
EXTEND CHEST, LIFT STERNUM
AND ROLL SHOULDERS
BACK AND DOWN
THRUST KNEES
APART

Yogadandasana 30s (126)

Yogi's staff

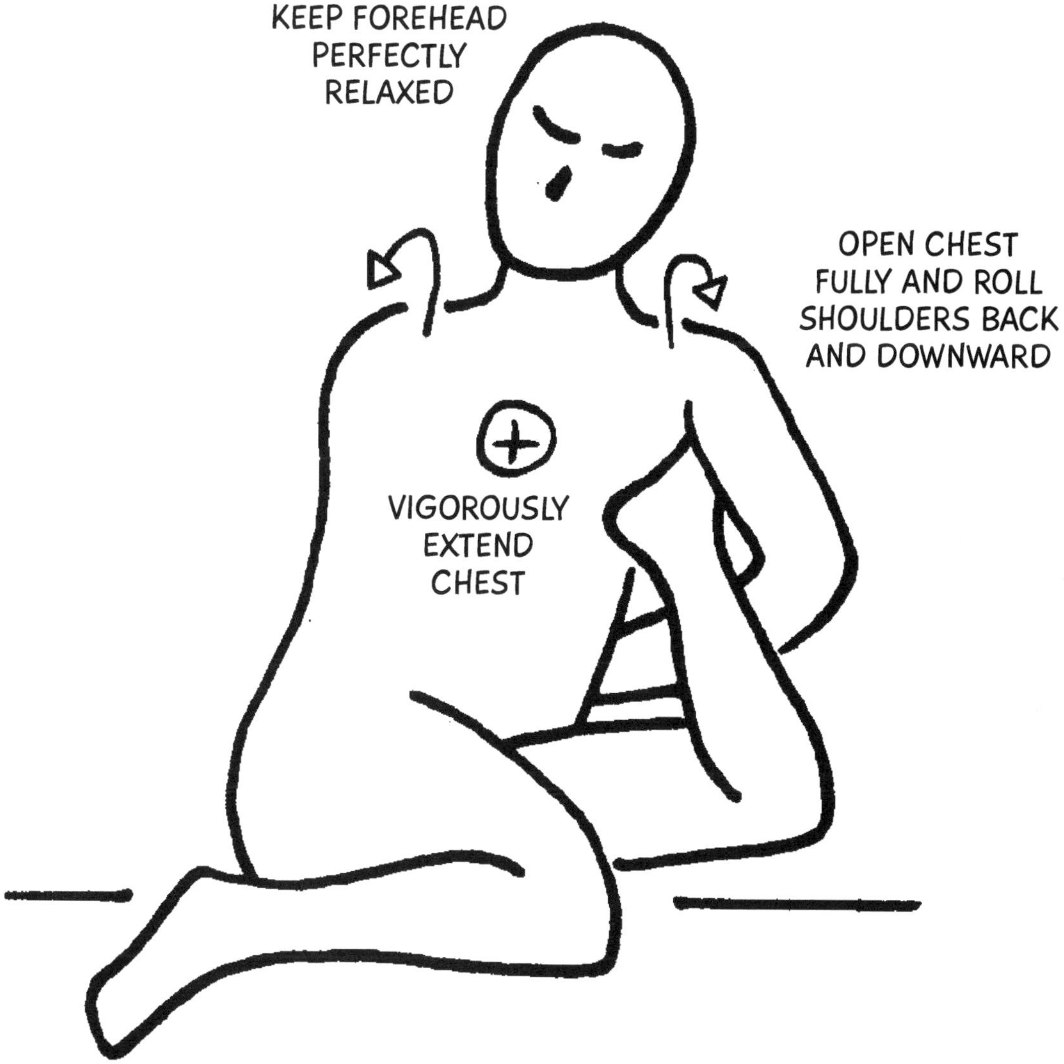
KEEP FOREHEAD PERFECTLY RELAXED
OPEN CHEST FULLY AND ROLL SHOULDERS BACK AND DOWNWARD
VIGOROUSLY EXTEND CHEST

Var: Start by bringing this foot up to the chest. Next bring it to the elbow, then the middle of the arm. Work the foot higher and higher up on the arm until you can place it in the armpit.

Program 8

First Day: Begin with the **Headstand Cycle (page 103)**. Next do Sarvangasana and Halasana. Follow these with **Basic Arm Cycle (page 125)**, and the **Forward Cycle (page 73)** Next do the **Leg Head Cycle (page 157)** followed by the **Twist Cycle (page 125)**. As always, skip any you are not ready for now. You may wait years, if ever, before feeling you are ready to take them on. Yoga is one of the few things one can do, day in and day out, over a lifetime, and with each passing year discover more your true ('original') nature. Other activities, like brushing one's teeth don't, by their nature, generally offer this opportunity for profound insight through their practice.

Second Day: Begin with Sirsasana and Urdhva Danadasana. Next do the **Shoulderstand Cycle (page 103)**, the **Advanced Arm Cycle (page 158)**, and the **Backward Cycle (page 157)**. End with the short **Knee-Hip Cycle (page 158)**.

> **Note:** When you complete each advanced arm balance, you can return to Sirsasana before doing the next one. Even better: After the some of the arm balances, (Parsva Bakasana, Parsva Kukkutasana, Eka Pada Galavasana, Eka Pada Bakasana II, and both Eka Pada Koundinyanasana I and II) return to headstand as usual. From here, arch backward and drop down into Dwi Pada Viparita Dandasana. Next, move into Urdhva Dhanurasana, and then into Viparita Chakrasana. After Viparita Chakrasana go briefly to Uttanasana. Finally, go back into a head stand and from there do the next arm balance posture in the program.

Review (or Third) Day: Begin with the Sirsasana I (5-15 minutes), Urdhva Danadasana, Sarvangasana (5 - 15 minutes) and Halasana. Next do the **Standing Cycle (page 72)** followed by the **Basic Cycle (page 73)**, and the **Lotus Cycle (page 73)**. Finish up with a few minute of Savasana, Pranayama in Savasana, and Meditation (to suit).

After Program 8, Then What?

What do you do now? That's easy, Consolidate! The beauty of doing yoga over decades is the opportunity to consolidate what you think and do. Yoga is well suited for this type of self discovery...there is no economic reward, no show business or national acclaim, no chance to win a gold medal or other measures of competitive competence, and certainly no instant gratification. It is just you an inward journey.

What do I do now? From the mid 90's I've been doing these cycles in a weekly program. The order works well for me. You may find an order that suits you better. Arthritis has forced me to ease up on a few postures from the Backward, Lotus, and Knee-Hip Cycles, otherwise all is going well, if not better than ever. In fact, had it not been for Yoga I'd probably would have had to have knee and hip replacements by now.

Mon: Head & Shoulder Stand <> Standing<> Advanced Arm Balance
Tue: Head & Shoulder Stand <> Basic <> Backward
Wed: Head & Shoulder Stand <> Forward <> Leg-Head
Thurs: Head & Shoulder Stand <> Twists <> Knee-Hip <> Lotus
Fri: Head & Shoulder Stand <> Standing <> Basic Arm Balance
Sat & Sun: (Sometimes) Head & Shoulder Stand

My kids began doing these with me around age five. They did what they could, as earnestly as possible for kids unpressured by an adult. Interestingly, they did it voluntarily. I imagine they couldn't resist joining in when they saw us (parents) doing yoga daily, after all, that is nature's way. In fact, I found children follow naturally if you don't bear down on them. Now, in their twenties, they are more earnest and so more on the way of self discovery, I assume.

Leg Head Cycle (About 11 minutes)

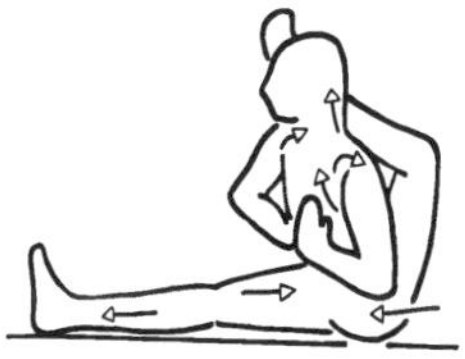

Eka Pada Sirsasana – 103

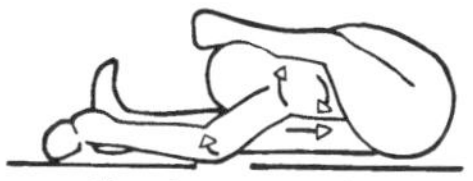

Skandasana – 104

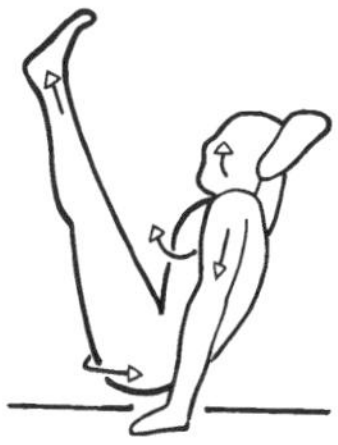

Chakorasana – 119

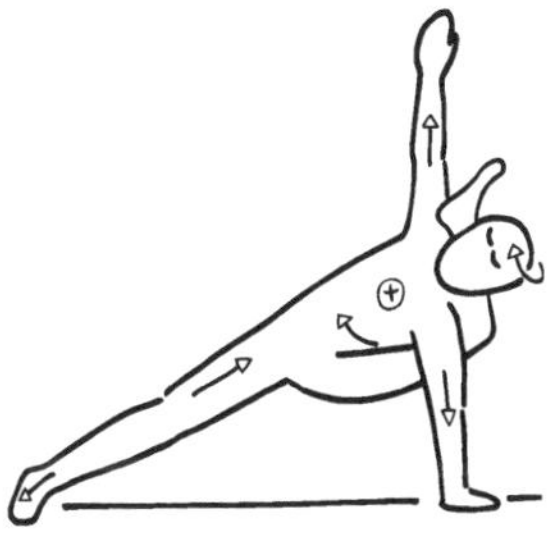

Kalabhairavasana – 118

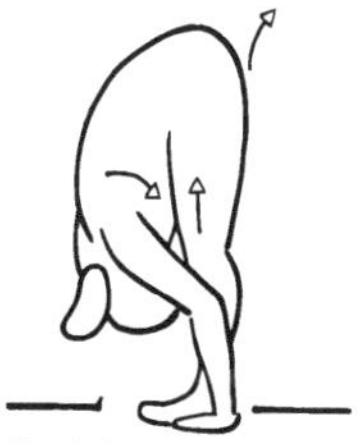

Ruchikasana – 121

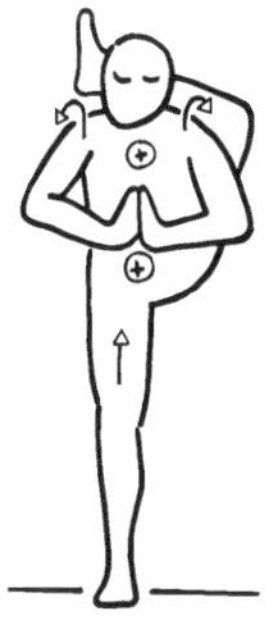

Durvasana – 120

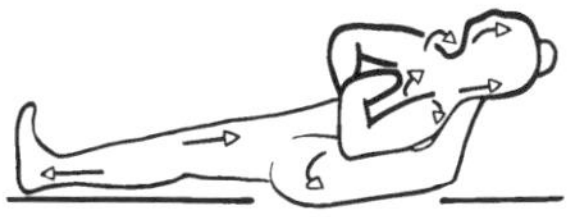

Bhairavasana – 105

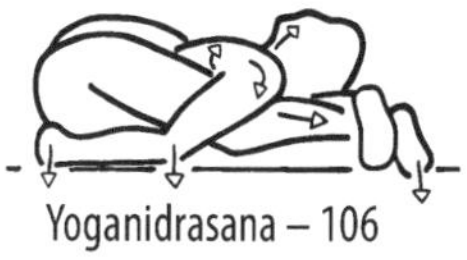

Yoganidrasana – 106

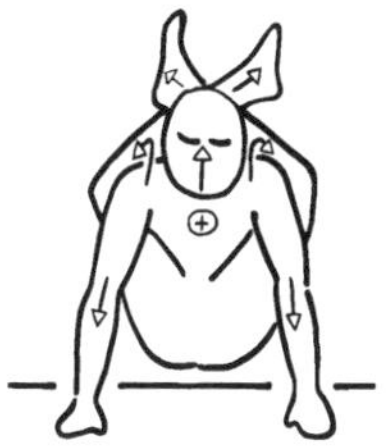

Dwi Pada Sirsasana – 127

Backward Cycle (About 15 minutes)

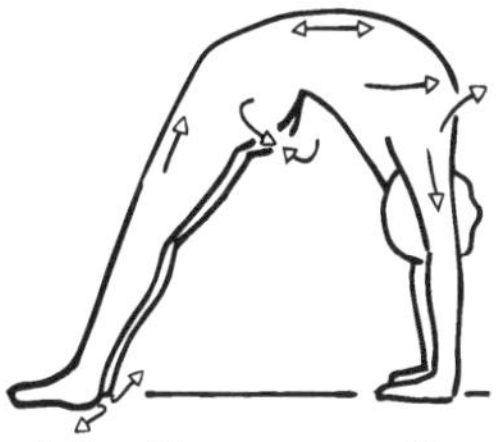

Urdhva Dhanurasana – 73

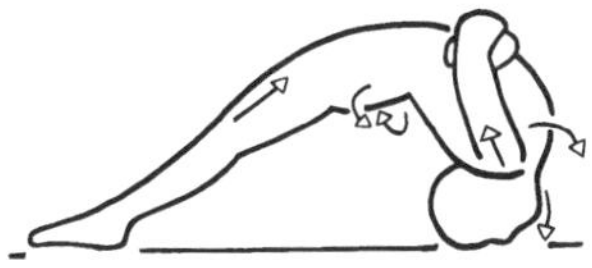

Setu Bhandasana – 110

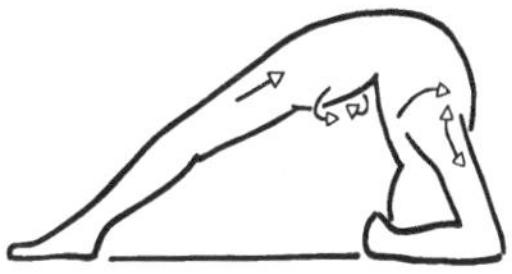

Dwi Pada Viparita Dandasana – 111

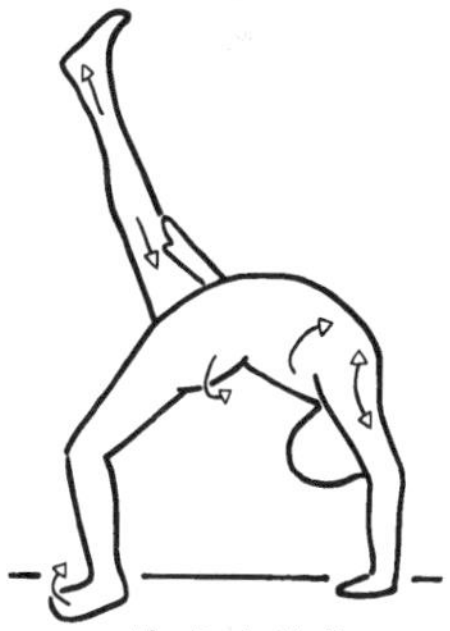

Eka Pada Urdhva Dhanurasana – 112

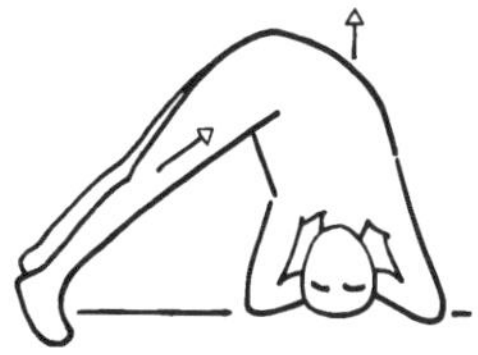

Mandalasana – 122

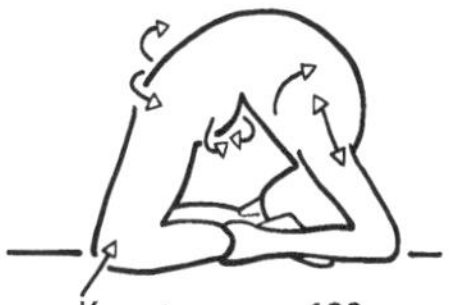

Kapotasana – 123

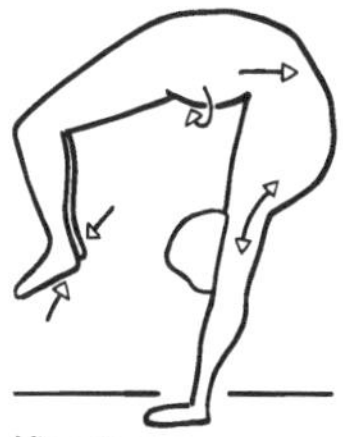

Viparita Chakrasana – 124

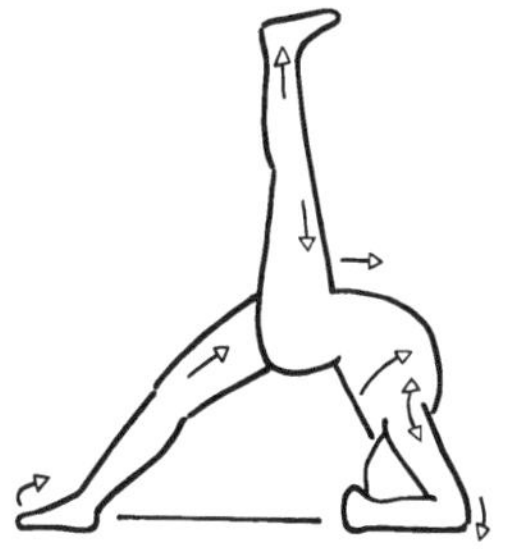

Eka Pada Viparita Dandasana I – 135

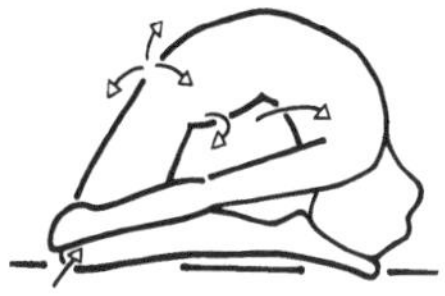

Lagu Vajrasana – 136

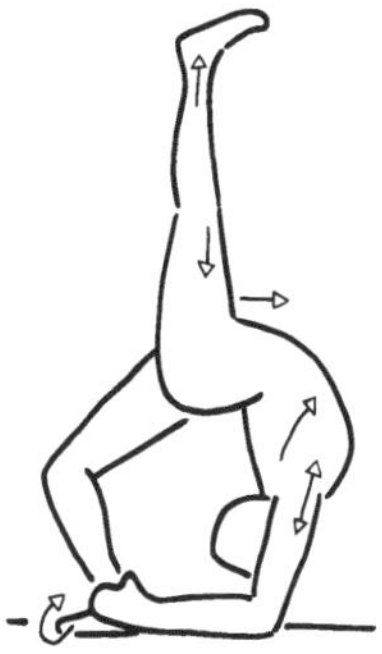

Eka Pada Viparita Dandasana II – 137

Advanced Arm Cycle (About 15 minutes)

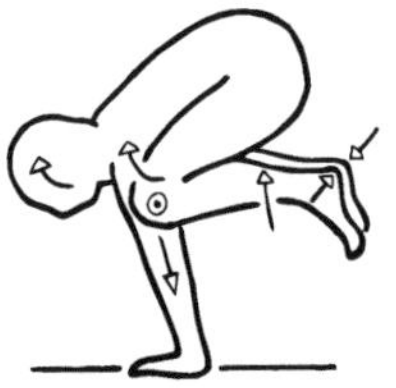

Bakasana – 74

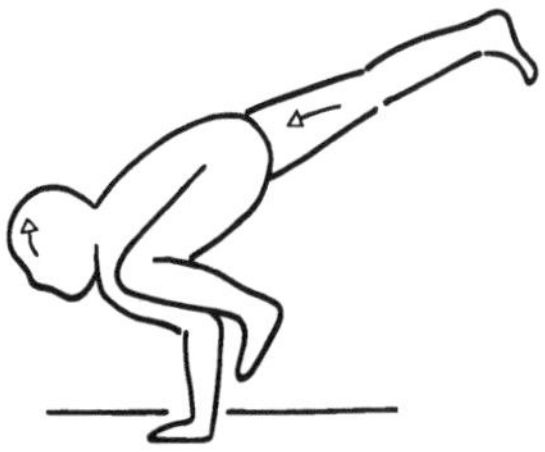

Eka Pada Bakasana II – 132

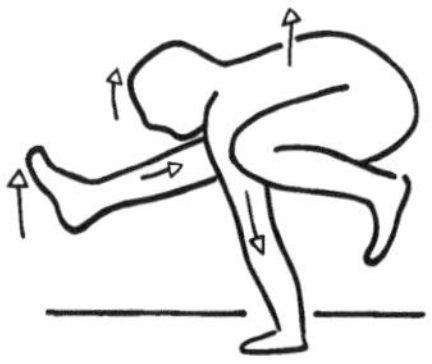

Eka Pada Bakasana I – 131

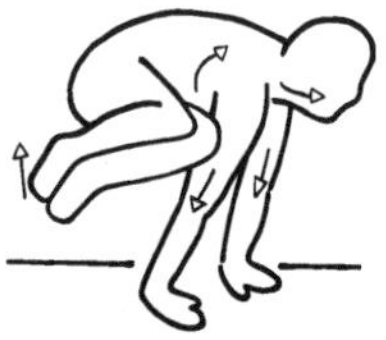

Parsva Bakasana – 113

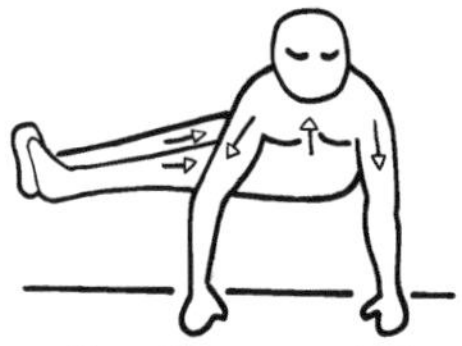

Koundinyasana – 117

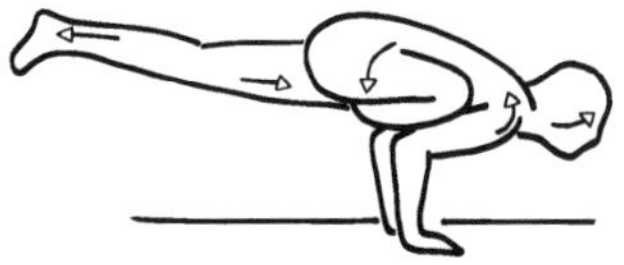

Eka Pada Galavasana – 116

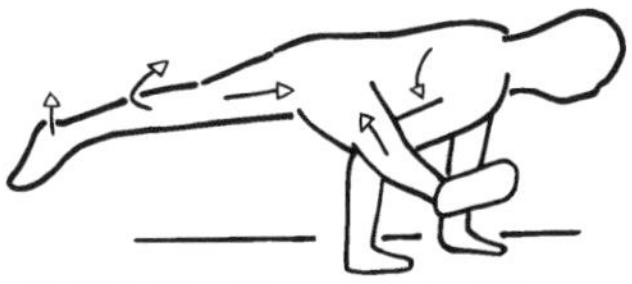

Eka Pada Koundinyanasana I – 133

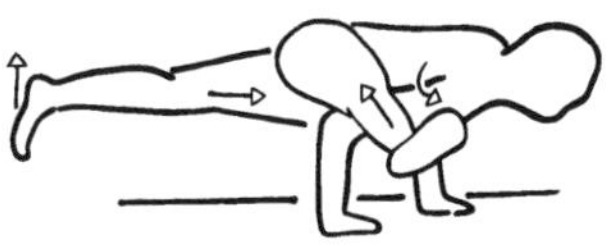

Eka Pada Koundinyanasana II – 134

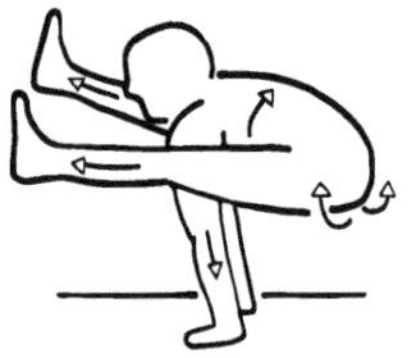

Tittibhasana – 128

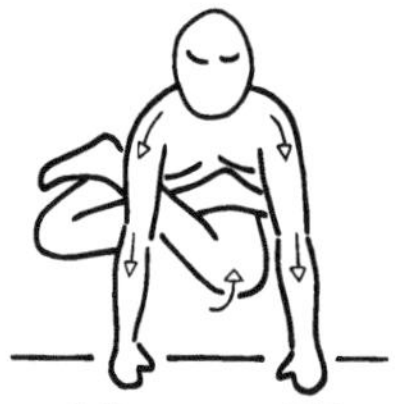

Galavasana – 114

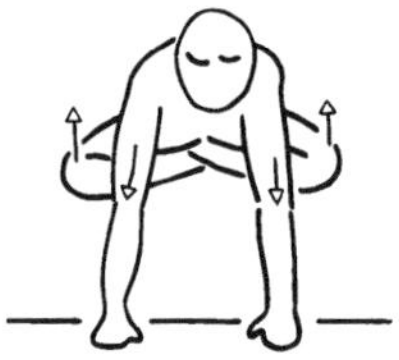

Urdhva
Kukkutasana – 115

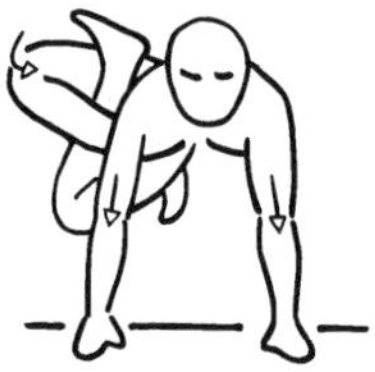

Parsva
Kukkutasana – 130

Knee-Hip Cycle (About 6 minutes)

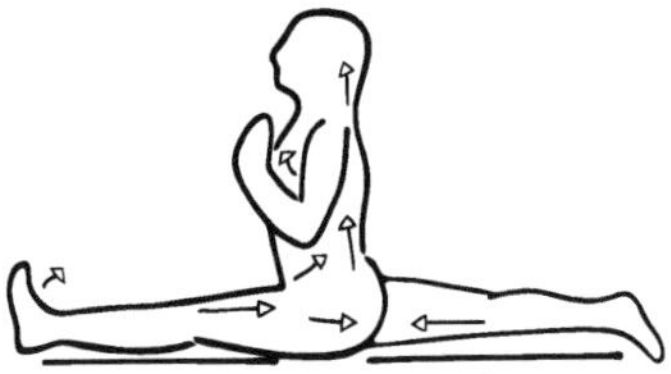

Hanumanasana – 138

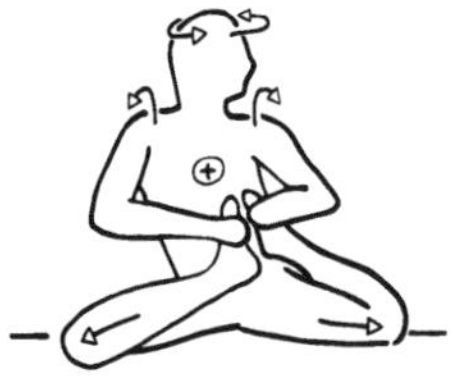

Vamedevasana – 125

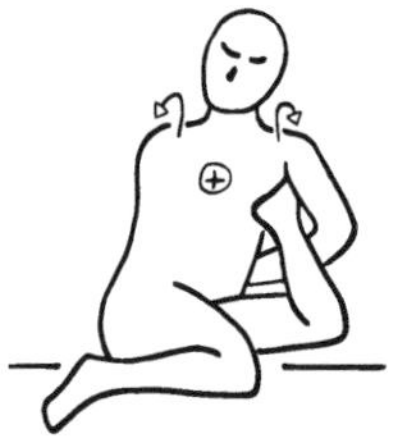

Yoga Dandasana – 126

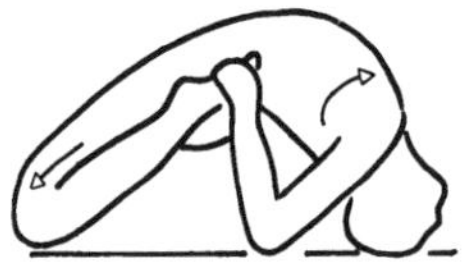

Supta Bhekasana – 109

Dwi Panda Sirsasana 10-30s (127)

both legs head

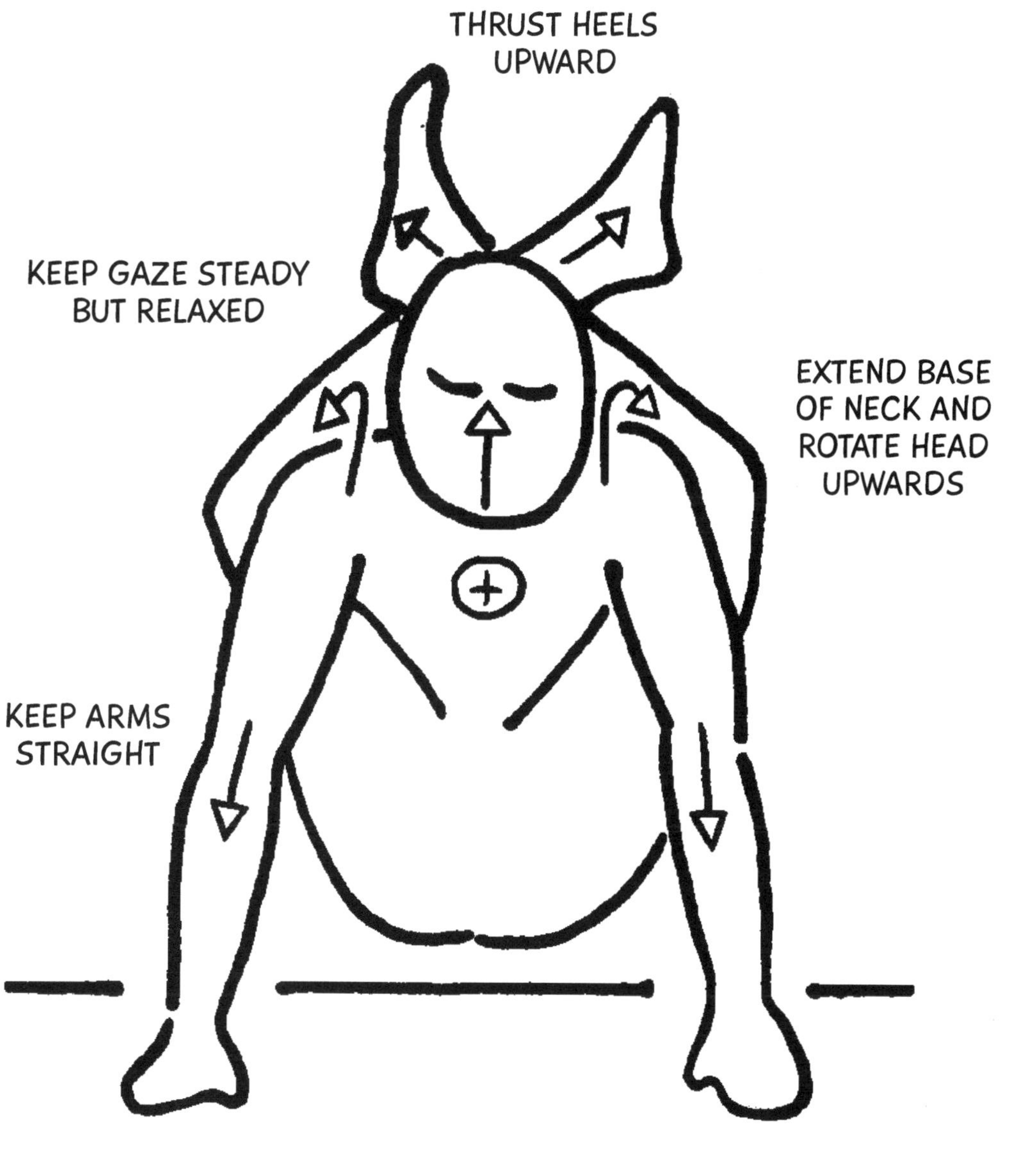
THRUST HEELS
UPWARD
KEEP GAZE STEADY
BUT RELAXED
EXTEND BASE
OF NECK AND
ROTATE HEAD
UPWARDS
KEEP ARMS
STRAIGHT

Tittibhasana   10-20s   (128)

firefly

Note: Pull trunk between legs to bring underside of knee as much up on the shoulder as possible before lifting feet off the ground. Going from Bakasana [72] straight into this posture works well.

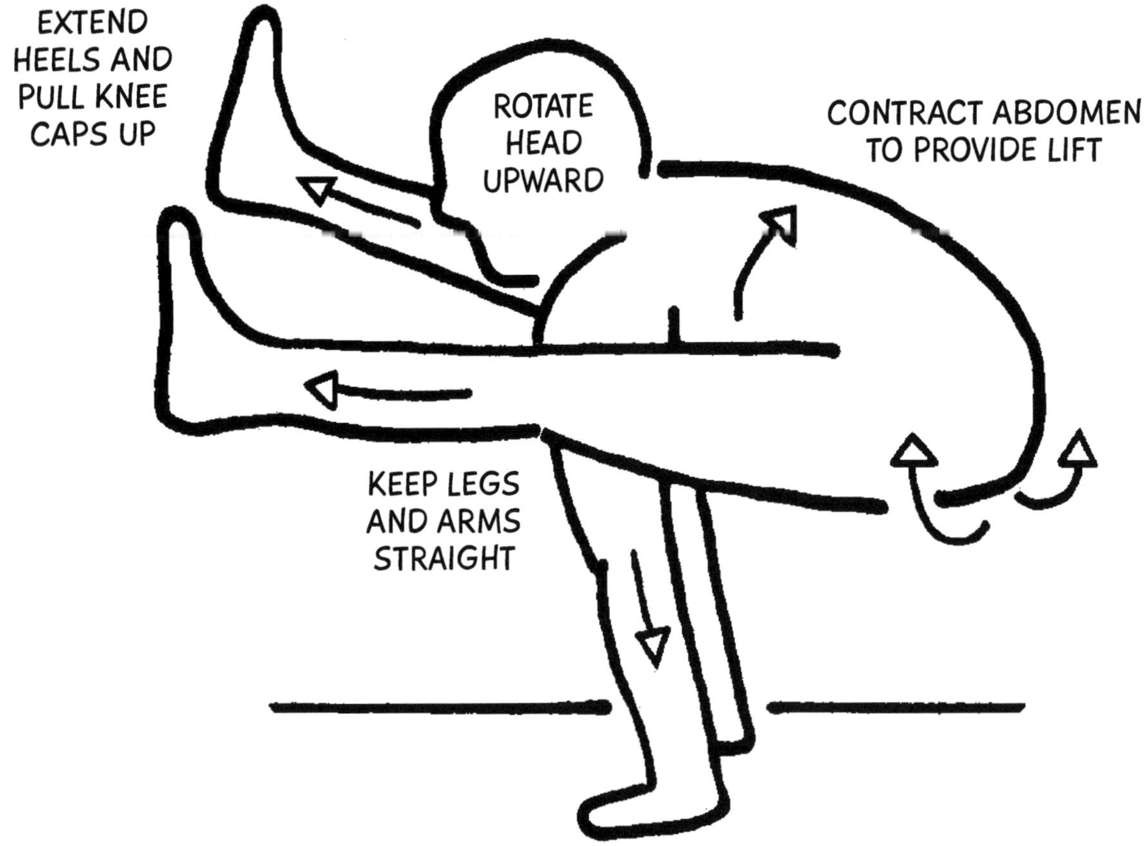
EXTEND HEELS AND PULL KNEE CAPS UP
ROTATE HEAD UPWARD
CONTRACT ABDOMEN TO PROVIDE LIFT
KEEP LEGS AND ARMS STRAIGHT

Ardha Matsyendrasana III 30-60s (129)

half founder of Yoga

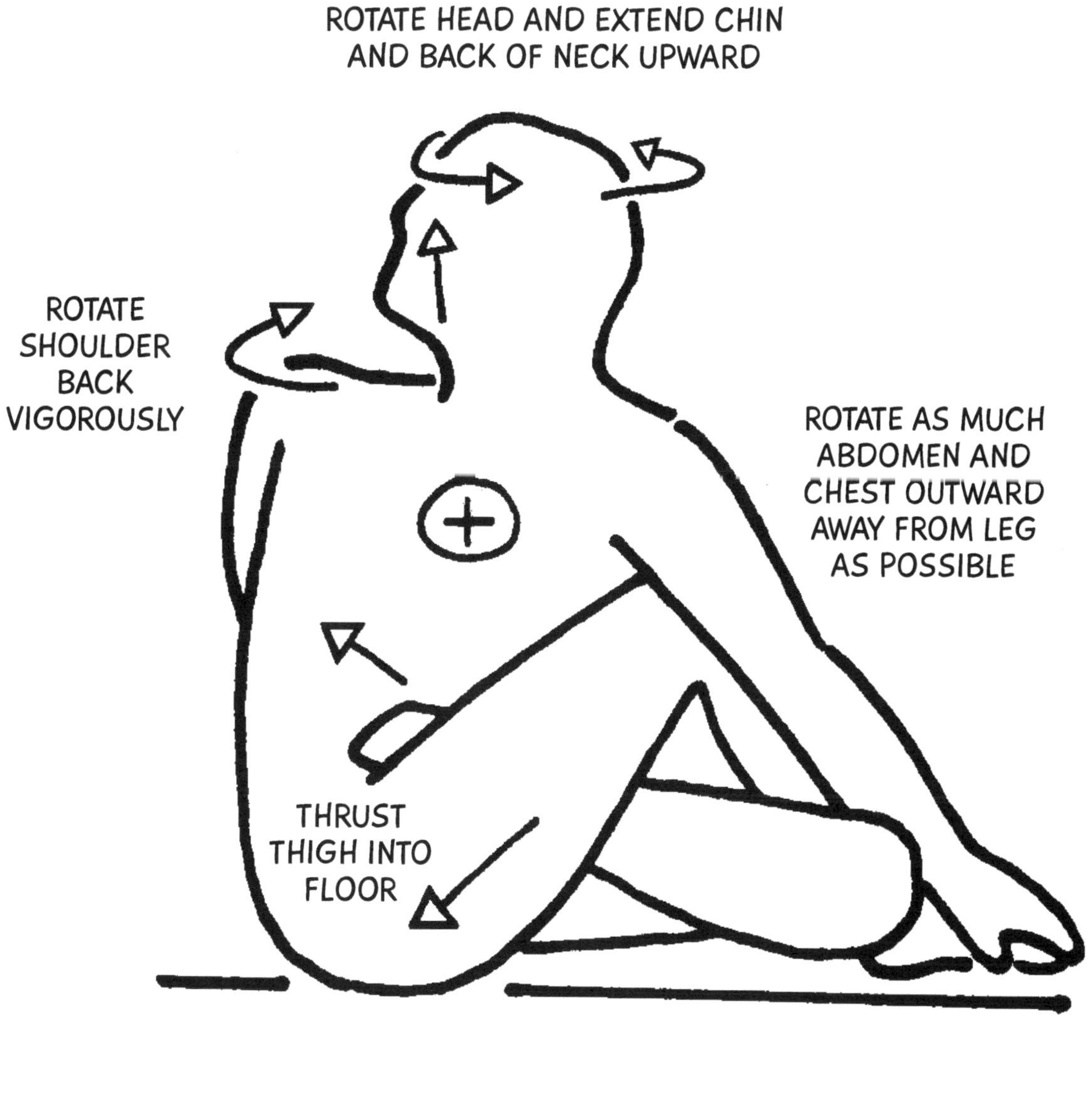
ROTATE HEAD AND EXTEND CHIN AND BACK OF NECK UPWARD
ROTATE SHOULDER BACK VIGOROUSLY
ROTATE AS MUCH ABDOMEN AND CHEST OUTWARD AWAY FROM LEG AS POSSIBLE
THRUST THIGH INTO FLOOR

Parsva Kukkutasana 20s (130)

side cock

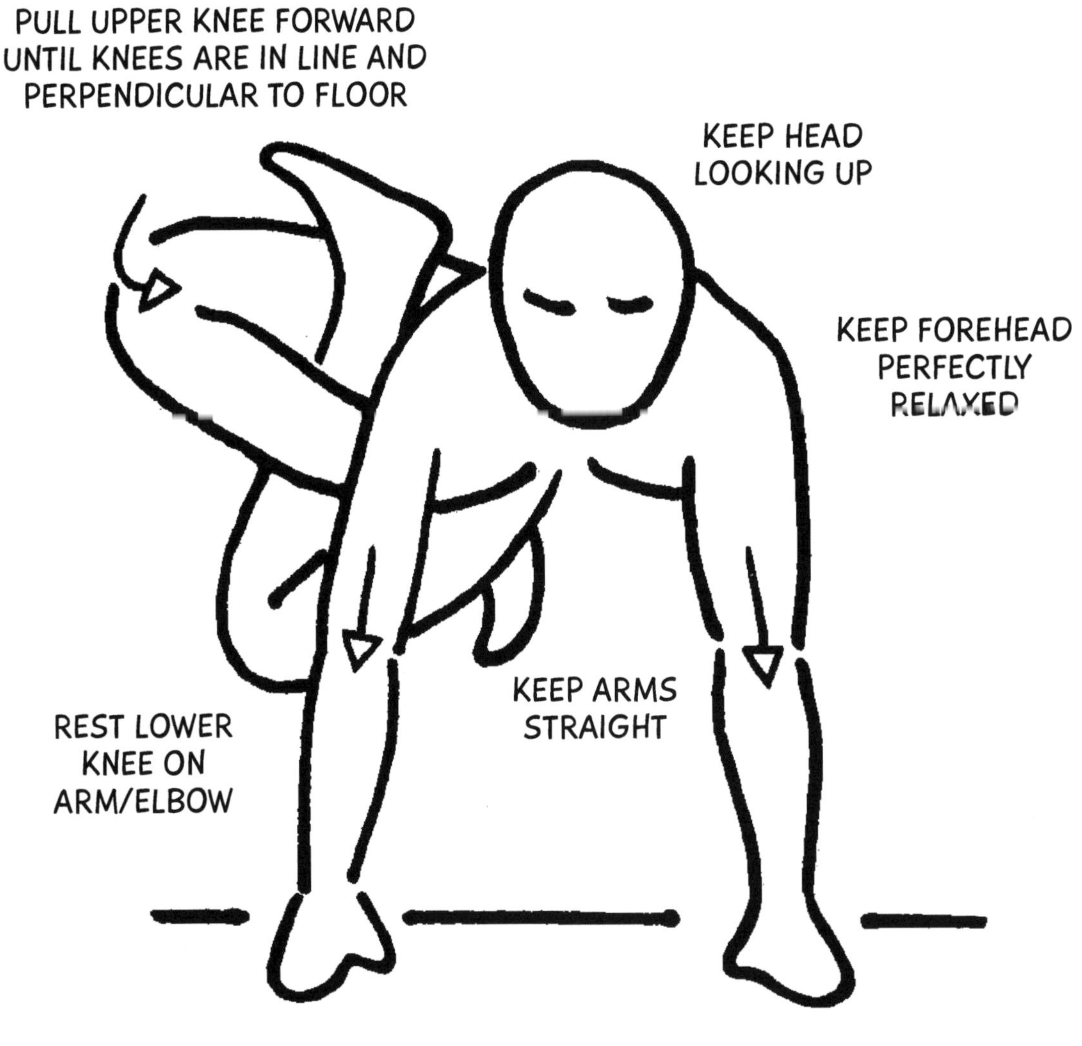
PULL UPPER KNEE FORWARD
UNTIL KNEES ARE IN LINE AND
PERPENDICULAR TO FLOOR
KEEP HEAD
LOOKING UP
KEEP FOREHEAD
PERFECTLY
RELAXED
KEEP ARMS
STRAIGHT
REST LOWER
KNEE ON
ARM/ELBOW

Eka Pada Bakasana I 20s (131)

one leg crane

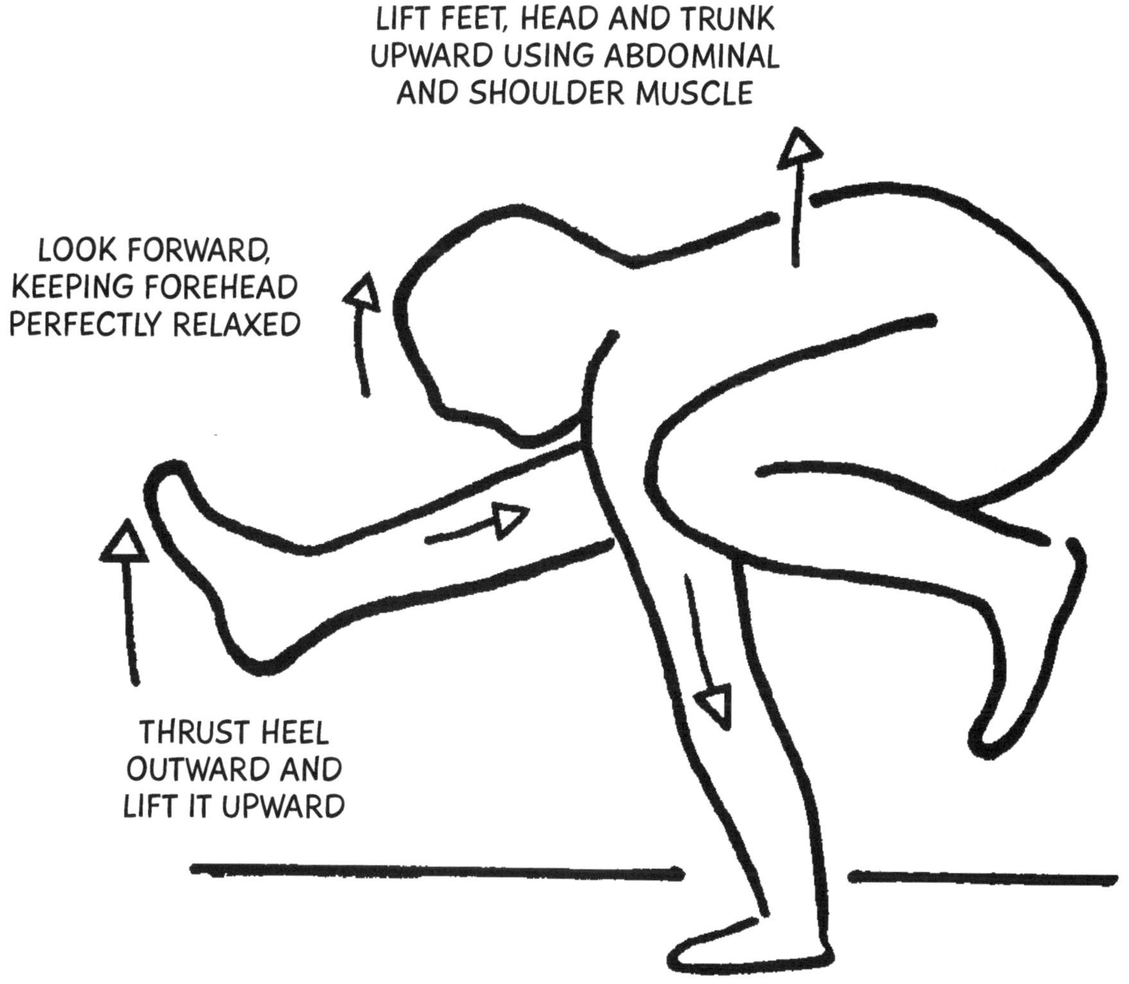
LIFT FEET, HEAD AND TRUNK UPWARD USING ABDOMINAL AND SHOULDER MUSCLE
LOOK FORWARD, KEEPING FOREHEAD PERFECTLY RELAXED
THRUST HEEL OUTWARD AND LIFT IT UPWARD

Eka Pada Bakasana II 20s (132)

one leg crane

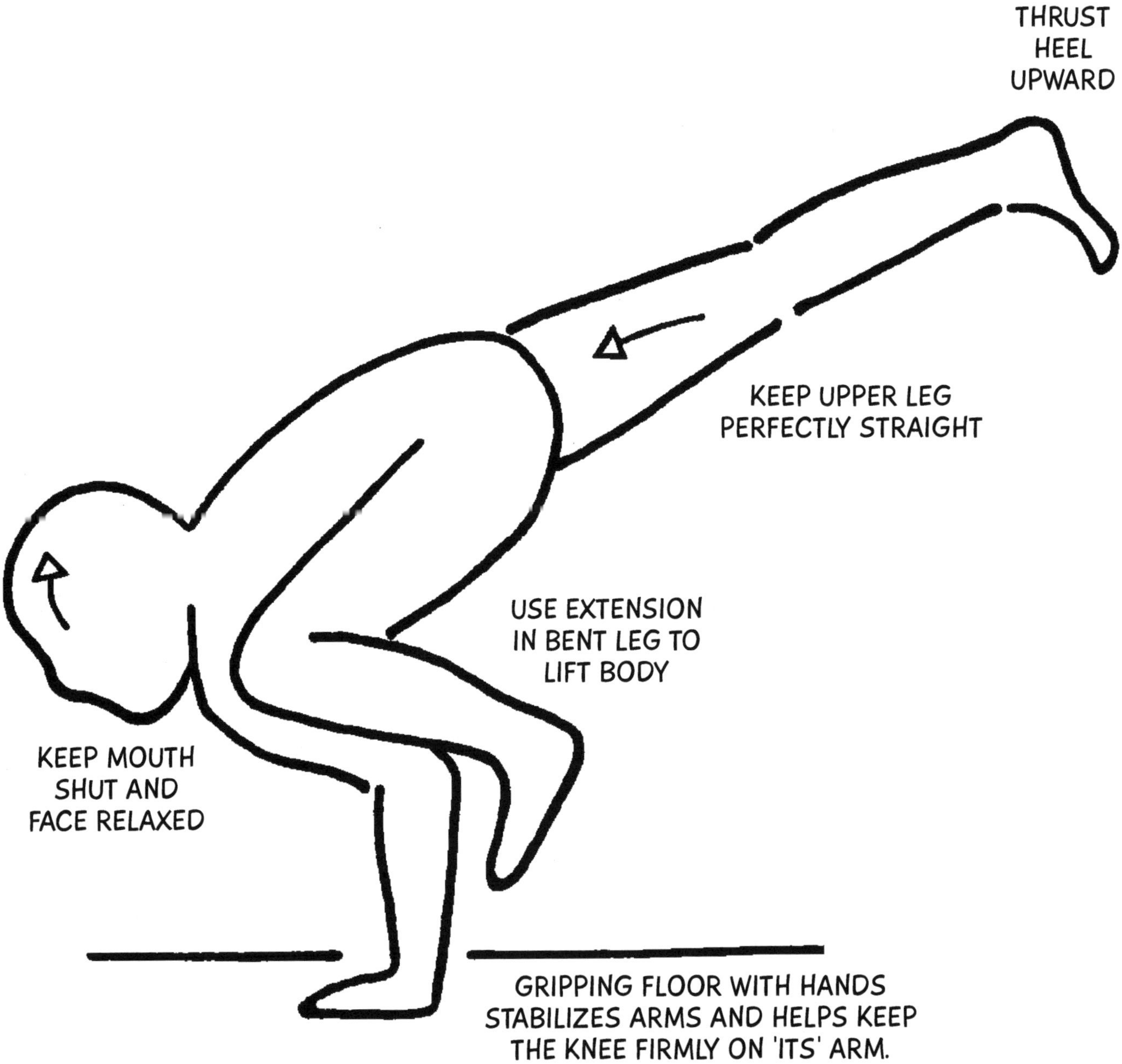

THRUST
HEEL
UPWARD
KEEP UPPER LEG
PERFECTLY STRAIGHT
USE EXTENSION
IN BENT LEG TO
LIFT BODY
KEEP MOUTH
SHUT AND
FACE RELAXED
GRIPPING FLOOR WITH HANDS
STABILIZES ARMS AND HELPS KEEP
THE KNEE FIRMLY ON 'ITS' ARM.

Eka Pada Koundinyasana I 20s (133)

one leg sage

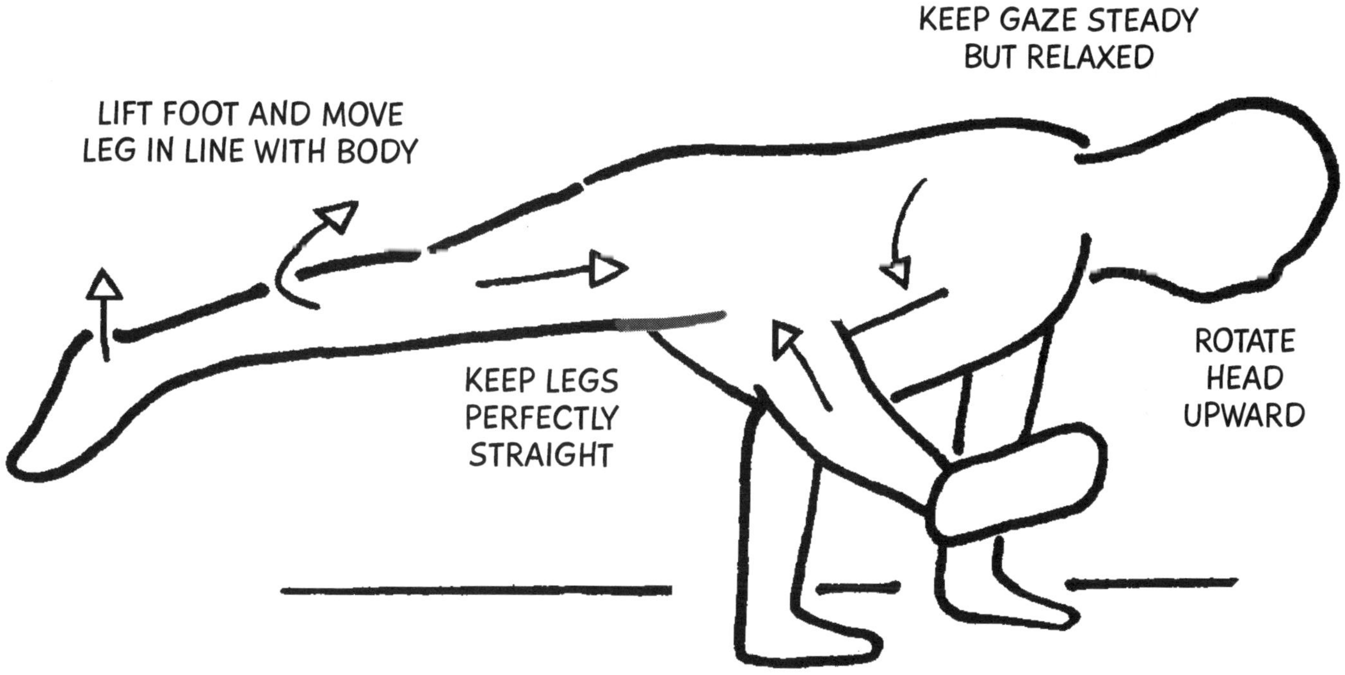
KEEP GAZE STEADY
BUT RELAXED
LIFT FOOT AND MOVE
LEG IN LINE WITH BODY
KEEP LEGS
PERFECTLY
STRAIGHT
ROTATE
HEAD
UPWARD

Eka Pada Koundinyasana II 20s (134)

one leg sage

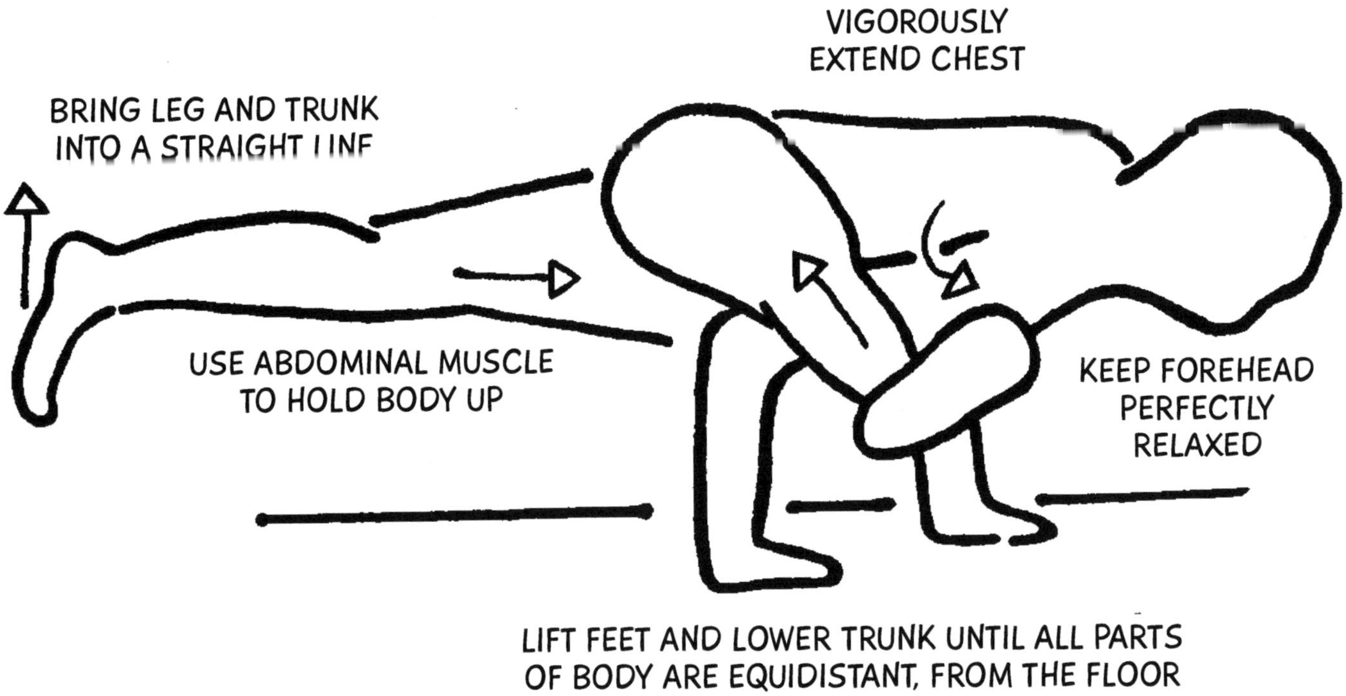
VIGOROUSLY
EXTEND CHEST
BRING LEG AND TRUNK
INTO A STRAIGHT LINE
USE ABDOMINAL MUSCLE
TO HOLD BODY UP
KEEP FOREHEAD
PERFECTLY
RELAXED
LIFT FEET AND LOWER TRUNK UNTIL ALL PARTS
OF BODY ARE EQUIDISTANT, FROM THE FLOOR

Eka Pada Viparita Dandasana I 15s (135)

one leg inverted staff

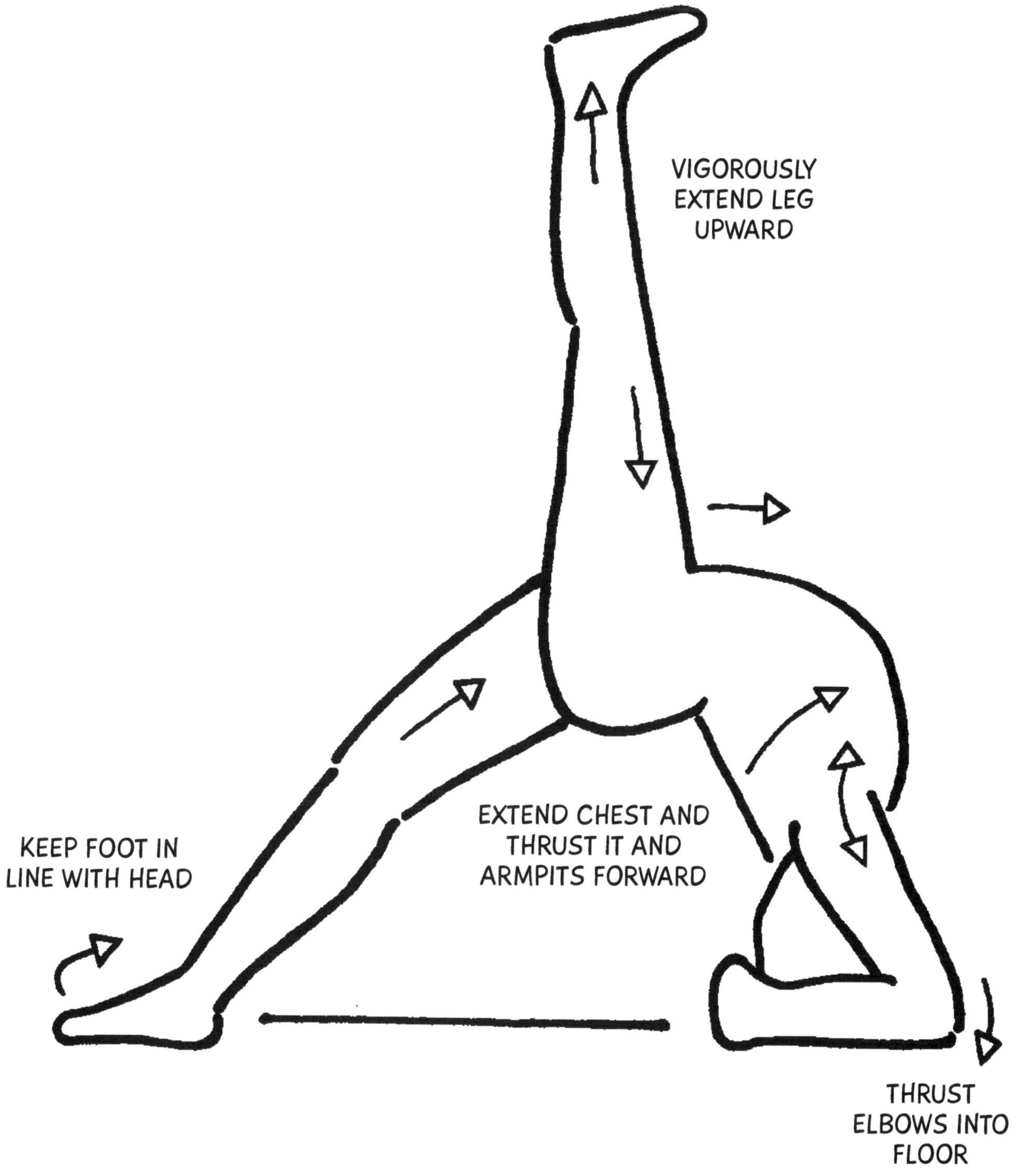
VIGOROUSLY
EXTEND LEG
UPWARD
KEEP FOOT IN
LINE WITH HEAD
EXTEND CHEST AND
THRUST IT AND
ARMPITS FORWARD
THRUST
ELBOWS INTO
FLOOR

Laghu Vajrasana 10-15s (136)

small thunderbolt

Note: Initially grasp the thighs and do a warm up bend - contracting the buttocks, opening the groin, and extending the lower spine to make space between the lower vertebrae. Then slide the hands down the thighs further and further, bending at each stage until you can grasp the knees.

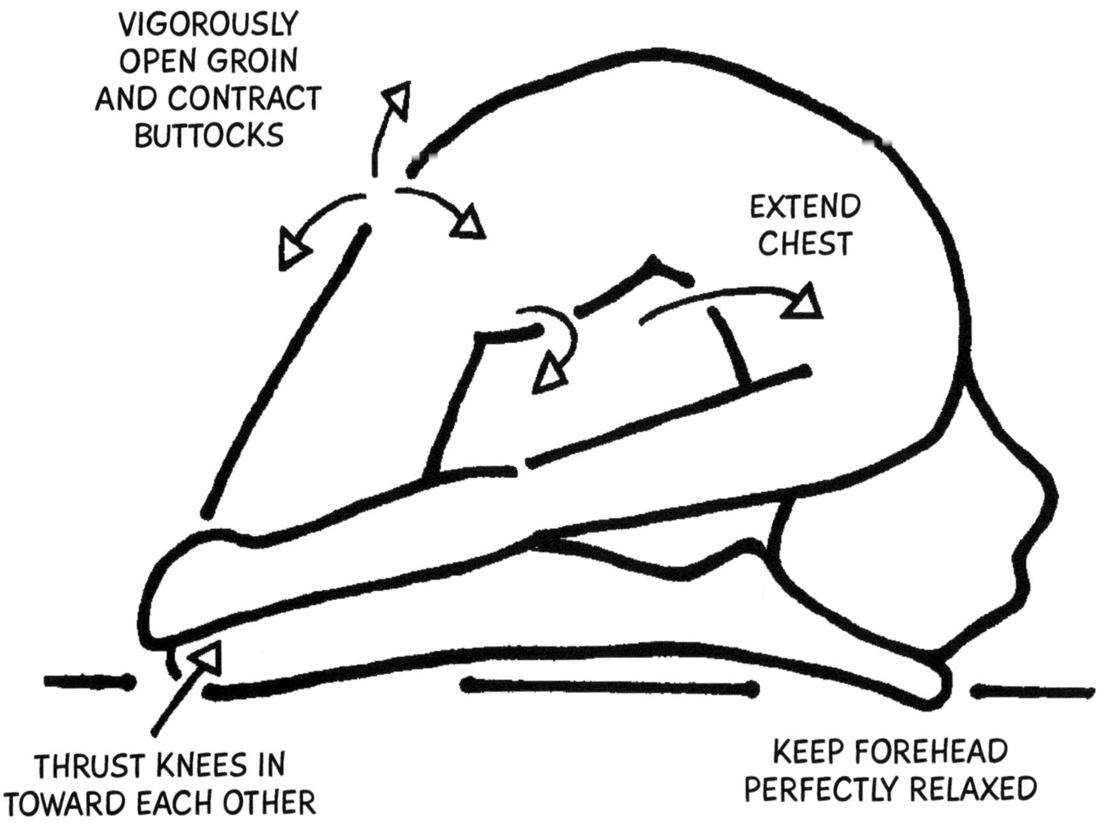
VIGOROUSLY OPEN GROIN AND CONTRACT BUTTOCKS
EXTEND CHEST
THRUST KNEES IN TOWARD EACH OTHER
KEEP FOREHEAD PERFECTLY RELAXED

Eka Pada Viparita Dandasana II 15s (137)

one leg inverted staff

Var.: Loop a rope around the ankle and grasp it with both hands.

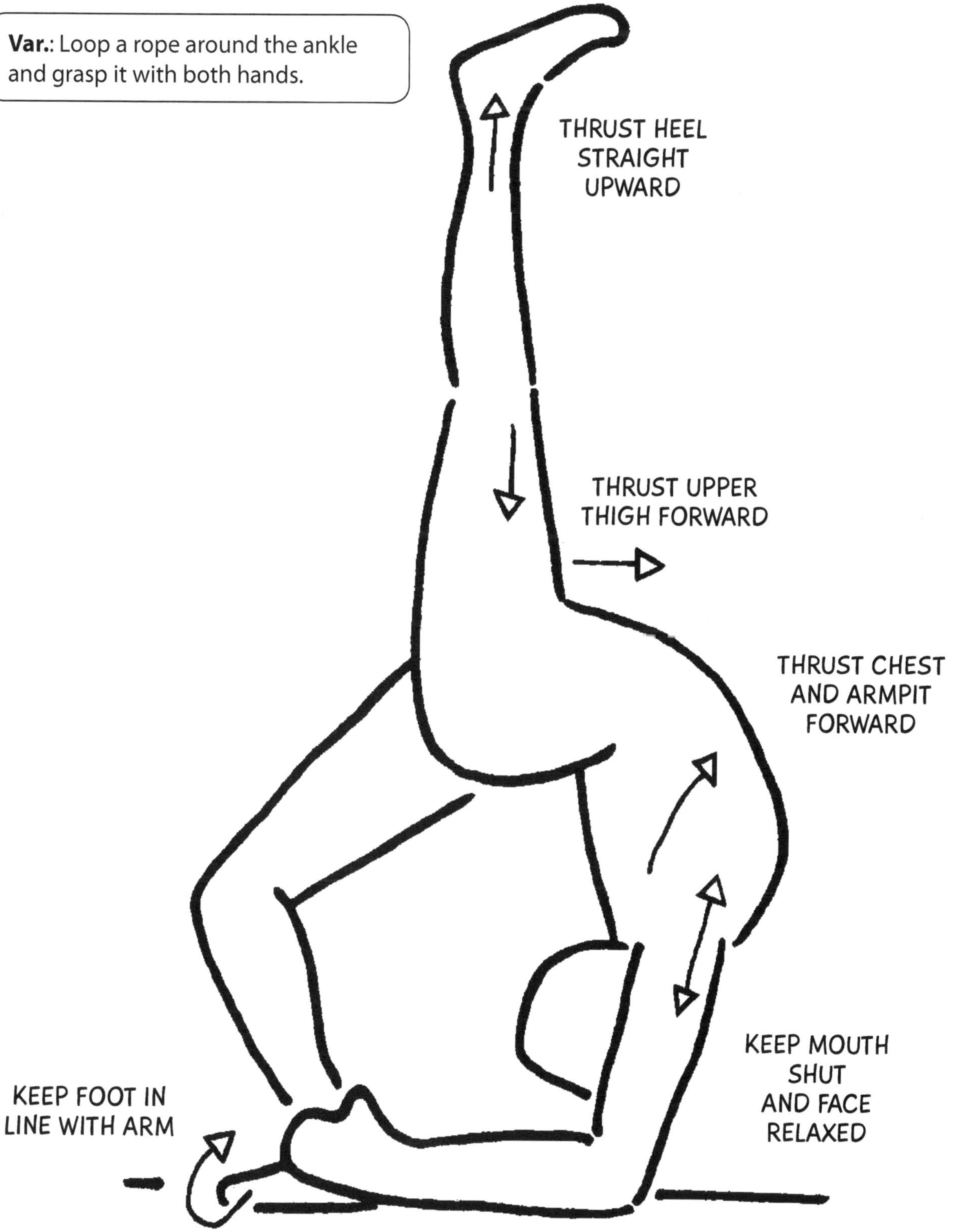
THRUST HEEL STRAIGHT UPWARD
THRUST UPPER THIGH FORWARD
THRUST CHEST AND ARMPIT FORWARD
KEEP MOUTH SHUT AND FACE RELAXED
KEEP FOOT IN LINE WITH ARM

Hanumanasana 10-30s (138)

a monkey chief

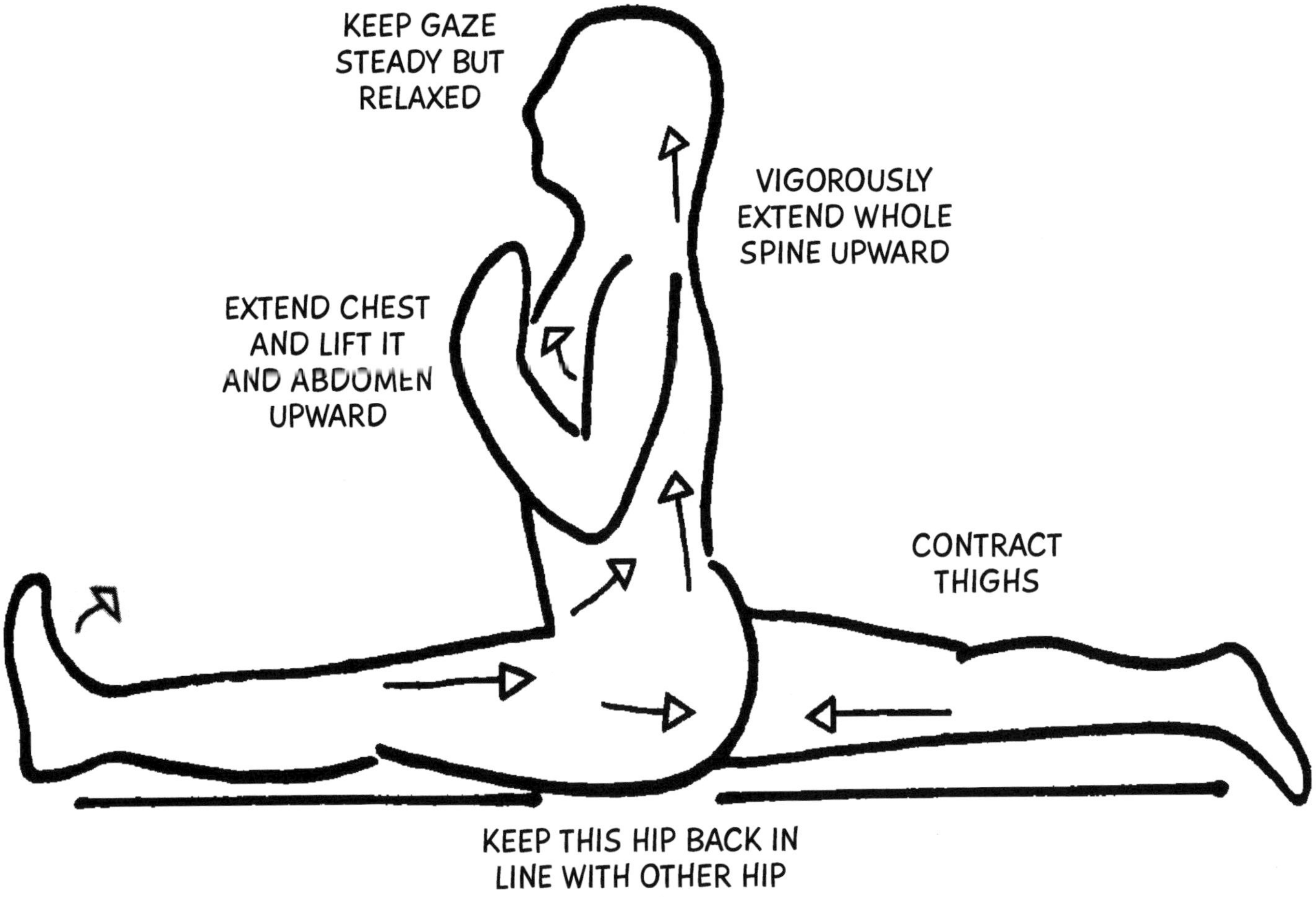
KEEP GAZE STEADY BUT RELAXED
VIGOROUSLY EXTEND WHOLE SPINE UPWARD
EXTEND CHEST AND LIFT IT AND ABDOMEN UPWARD
CONTRACT THIGHS
KEEP THIS HIP BACK IN LINE WITH OTHER HIP

Var: For added challenge, thrust your arms straight out to the side, level with the shoulders. Then raise them above your head.

Twelve Hatha Yoga Cycles

(These postures are arranged in an order that works well for me. Feel free to rearrange them in any way that works best for you!)

STANDING CYCLE (page 72)
Utthita Trikonasana – 3
ParivrttaTrikonasana – 4
Utthita Parsvakonasana – 5
Virabhadrasana I – 6
Virabhadrasana II – 7
Virabhadrasana III – 8
Parsvottanasana – 9
Prasarita Padottanasana – 10
Ardha Chandrasana – 43
ParivrttaParsvakonasana – 44
Uttanasana – 11
Utthita Hasta Padangusthasana – 45
Parigasana – 46

LOTUS CYCLE (page 72)
Padmasana – 40
Tolasana – 41
Baddha Padmasana – 67
Yoga Mudrasana – 68
Simhasana – 69
Garbha Pindasana – 70
Goraksasana – 71
Matsyasana – 42
Vatayanasana – 72

BASIC CYCLE (page 73)
Adho Mukha Svanasana – 18
Urdhva Mukha Svanasana – 19
Chaturanga Dandasana – 20
Nakrasana – 20
Salabhasana – 21
Dhanurasana – 37
Parsva Dhanurasana – 77
Bhekasana – 78
Ustrasana – 22
Lolasana – 49
Virasana II – 23
Virasana III – 24
Virasana IV – 38
Paryankasana – 50
Paripoorna Navasana – 15
Ardha Navasana – 16
Urdhva Prasarita Padasana – 17
Jathara Parivartanasana – 30

FORWARD CYCLE (page 73)
Janu Sirsasana – 25
Parivrtta Janu Sirsasana – 64
Paschimottanasana – 31
Parivrtta Paschimottanasana – 85
Ardha Baddha Padma Paschimottanasana – 32
Triang Mukhaika Pada Paschimottanasana – 65
Krounchasana – 86
Akarna Dhanurasana – 87
Supta Padangusthasana – 88
Upavistha Konasana – 66
Baddha Konasana – 33
Kurmasana – 89
Supta Kurmasana – 90

HEAD CYCLE (page 103)
Sirsasana I – 27
Sirsasana II – 51
Sirsasana III – 52
Parsva Sirsasana – 53
Parivrttaikapada Sirsasana – 79
Eka Pada Sirsasana – 80
Parsva Eka Pada Sirsasana – 81
Padma Sirsasana – 82
Parsva Padma Sirsasana – 83
Pinda Sirsasana – 84
Urdhva Dandasana – 28

SHOULDER CYCLE (page103)
Sarvangasana I – 12
Sarvangasana III – 55
Sarvangasana II – 54
Halasana – 29
Supta Konasana – 56
Parsva Halasana – 57
Eka Pada Sarvangasana – 58
Parsva Eka Pada Sarvangasana - 59
Padma Sarvangasana – 60
Parsva Padma Sarvangasana – 61
Pinda Sarvangasana – 62
Parsva Pinda Sarvangasana – 63
Parsva Sarvangasana – 96
Eka Pada Setu Bandha Sarvangasana – 98
Setu Bandha Sarvangasana – 97

BASIC ARM CYCLE (page 125)
Bhujapidasana – 75
Mayurasana – 76
Adho Mukha Vrksasana – 92
Pincha Mayurasana – 93
Padma Mayurasana – 94
Astavakrasana – 95
Sayanasana – 99
Hamsasana – 100
Vasisthasana – 101
Visvamitrasana – 102

TWIST CYCLE (page 125)
Bharadvajasana I – 26
Bharadvajasana II – 34
Marichyasana III – 35
Ardha Matsyendrasana I – 36
Ardha Matsyendrasana II – 107
Pasasana – 108
Marichyasana IV – 91
Ardha Matsyendrasana III – 129

LEG HEAD CYCLE (page 157)
Eka Pada Sirsasana – 103
Skandasana – 104
Chakorasana – 119
Kalabhairavasana – 118
Ruchikasana – 121
Durvasana – 120
Bhairavasana – 105
Yoganidrasana – 106
Dwi Pada Sirsasana – 127

BACKWARD CYCLE (page 157)
Urdhva Dhanurasana – 73
Setu Bhandasana – 110
Dwi Pada Viparita Dandasana - 111
Eka Pada Urdhva Dhanurasana – 112
Mandalasana – 122
Kapotasana – 123
Viparita Chakrasana – 124
Eka Pada Viparita Dandasana I 135
Lagu Vajrasana – 136
Eka Pada Viparita Dandasana II – 137

ADVANCED ARM CYCLE (page 158)
Bakasana – 74
Eka Pada Bakasana II – 132
Eka Pada Bakasana I – 131
Parsva Bakasana – 113
Koundinyasana – 117
Eka Pada Galavasana – 116
Eka Pada Koundinyanasana I - 133
Eka Pada Koundinyanasana II - 134
Tittibhasana – 128
Galavasana – 114
Urdhva Kukkutasana – 115
Parsva Kukkutasana – 130

KNEE/HIP CYCLE (page 158)
Hanumanasana – 138
Vamedevasana – 125
Yoga Dandasana – 126
Supta Bhekasana – 109

Index to All 138 Hatha Yoga Postures

Form Self Evaluation   Name____________________   Year 20___   Scale: A-F

A self evaluation at any stage, from beginner on, can help you consolidate your practice. This works even if you are an 'F' on most postures. You can attempt them all and evaluate each, or just the ones you currently do. Then, repeat the process a year from now... and so on.

[A] = Looking for fine points now   [B] = It's in sight now, just another year   **[C]** = *'doable'*, though more years needed
[D] = Very difficult, but there is some promise   [F] = No idea when, if ever, a *'doable'* [C] will be possible. Time will tell!

Standing Cycle (About 15 minutes)

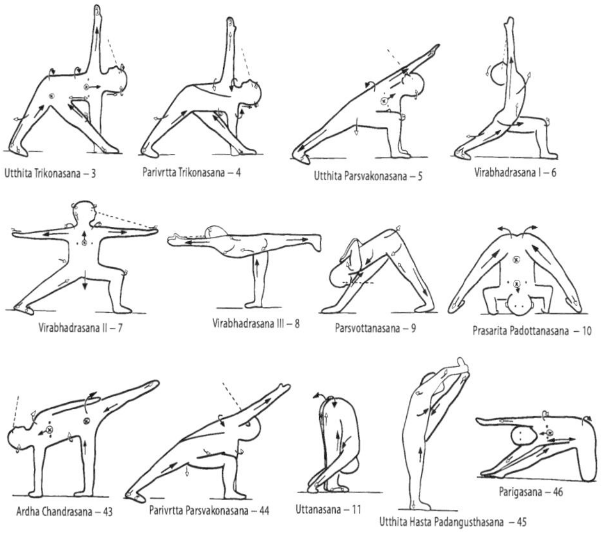
Utthita Trikonasana – 3
Parivrtta Trikonasana – 4
Utthita Parsvakonasana – 5
Virabhadrasana I – 6
Virabhadrasana II – 7
Virabhadrasana III – 8
Parsvottanasana – 9
Prasarita Padottanasana – 10
Ardha Chandrasana – 43
Parivrtta Parsvakonasana – 44
Uttanasana – 11
Utthita Hasta Padangusthasana – 45
Parigasana – 46

Basic Cycle (About 13 minutes)

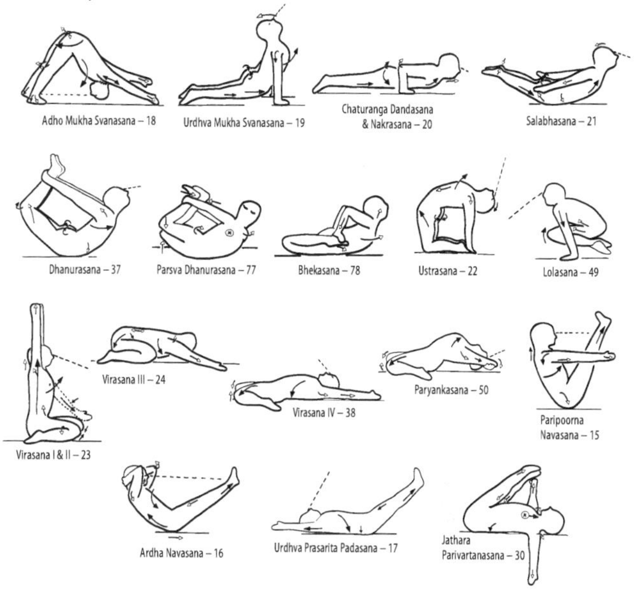
Adho Mukha Svanasana – 18
Urdhva Mukha Svanasana – 19
Chaturanga Dandasana & Nakrasana – 20
Salabhasana – 21
Dhanurasana – 37
Parsva Dhanurasana – 77
Bhekasana – 78
Ustrasana – 22
Lolasana – 49
Virasana I & II – 23
Virasana III – 24
Virasana IV – 38
Paryankasana – 50
Paripoorna Navasana – 15
Ardha Navasana – 16
Urdhva Prasarita Padasana – 17
Jathara Parivartanasana – 30

Forward Cycle (About 20 minutes)

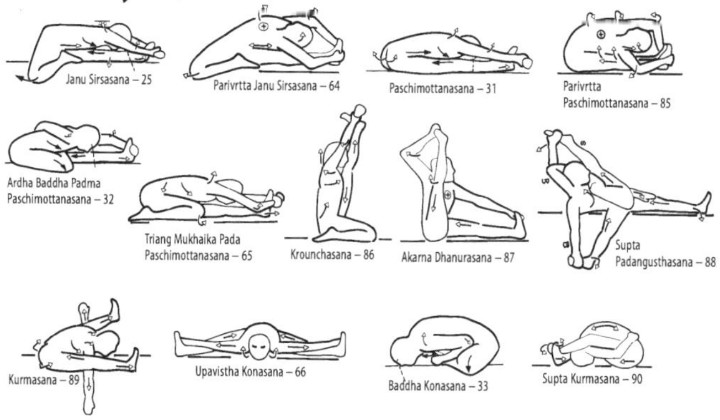
Janu Sirsasana – 25
Parivrtta Janu Sirsasana – 64
Paschimottanasana – 31
Parivrtta Paschimottanasana – 85
Ardha Baddha Padma Paschimottanasana – 32
Triang Mukhaika Pada Paschimottanasana – 65
Krounchasana – 86
Akarna Dhanurasana – 87
Supta Padangusthasana – 88
Kurmasana – 89
Upavistha Konasana – 66
Baddha Konasana – 33
Supta Kurmasana – 90

Twist Cycle (About 14 minutes)

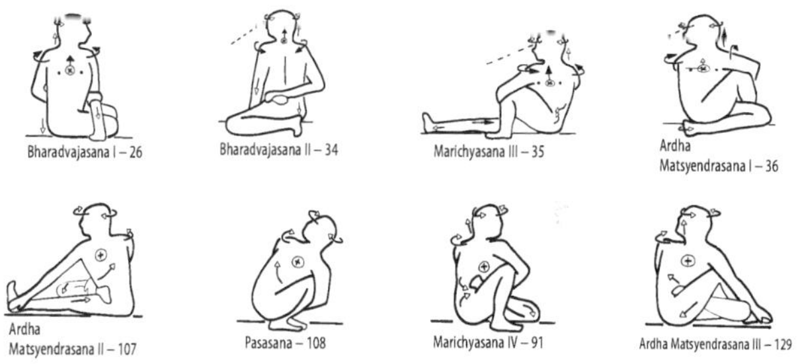
Bharadvajasana I – 26
Bharadvajasana II – 34
Marichyasana III – 35
Ardha Matsyendrasana I – 36
Ardha Matsyendrasana II – 107
Pasasana – 108
Marichyasana IV – 91
Ardha Matsyendrasana III – 129

Lotus Cycle (About 14minutes)

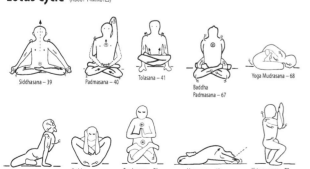
Siddhasana – 39
Padmasana – 40
Tolasana – 41
Baddha Padmasana – 67
Yoga Mudrasana – 68
Simhasana – 69
Garbha Pindasana – 70
Goraksasana – 71
Matsyasana – 42
Vatayanasana – 72

Knee-Hip Cycle (About 6 minutes)

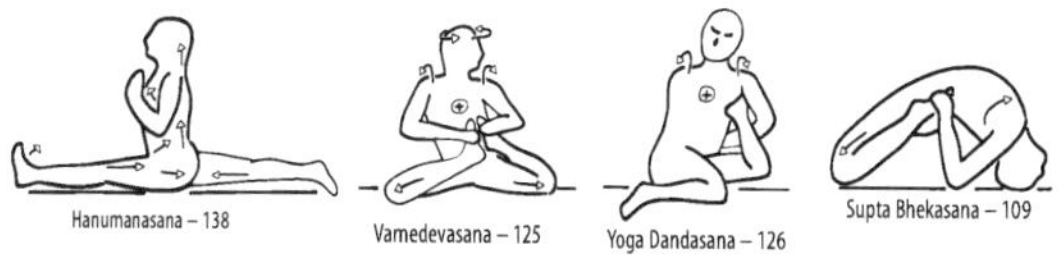
Hanumanasana – 138
Vamedevasana – 125
Yoga Dandasana – 126
Supta Bhekasana – 109

Headstand Cycle (About 11 minutes)

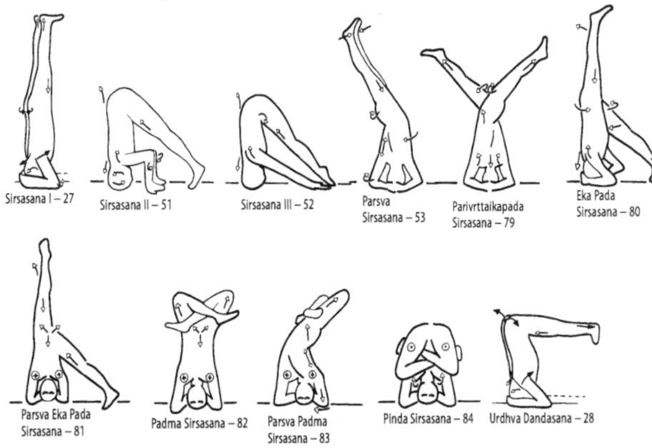

Sirsasana I – 27
Sirsasana II – 51
Sirsasana III – 52
Parsva Sirsasana – 53
Parivrttaikapada Sirsasana – 79
Eka Pada Sirsasana – 80
Parsva Eka Pada Sirsasana – 81
Padma Sirsasana – 82
Parsva Padma Sirsasana – 83
Pinda Sirsasana – 84
Urdhva Dandasana – 28

Shoulderstand Cycle (About 15 minutes)

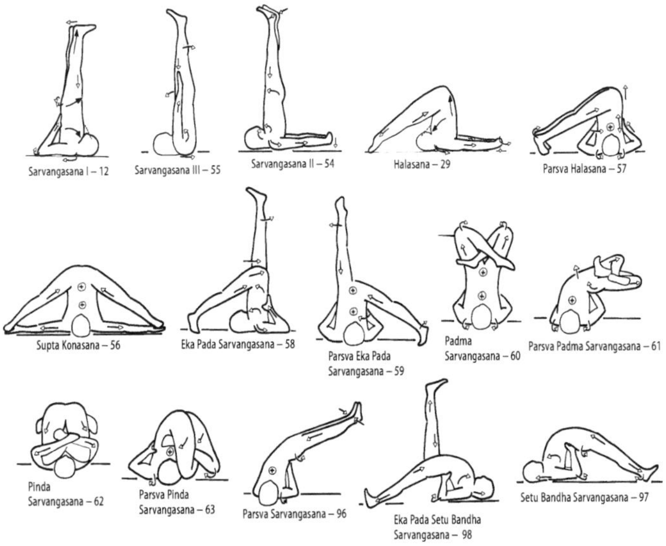

Sarvangasana I – 12
Sarvangasana III – 55
Sarvangasana II – 54
Halasana – 29
Parsva Halasana – 57
Supta Konasana – 56
Eka Pada Sarvangasana – 58
Parsva Eka Pada Sarvangasana – 59
Padma Sarvangasana – 60
Parsva Padma Sarvangasana – 61
Pinda Sarvangasana – 62
Parsva Pinda Sarvangasana – 63
Parsva Sarvangasana – 96
Eka Pada Setu Bandha Sarvangasana – 98
Setu Bandha Sarvangasana – 97

Basic Arm Cycle (About 13 minutes)

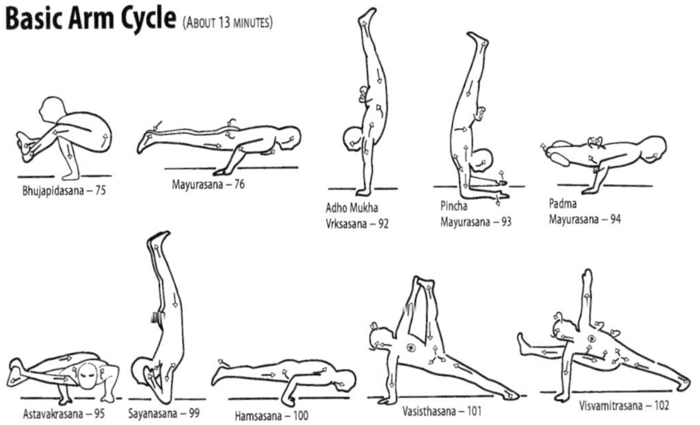

Bhujapidasana – 75
Mayurasana – 76
Adho Mukha Vrksasana – 92
Pincha Mayurasana – 93
Padma Mayurasana – 94
Astavakrasana – 95
Sayanasana – 99
Hamsasana – 100
Vasisthasana – 101
Visvamitrasana – 102

Advanced Arm Cycle (About 15 minutes)

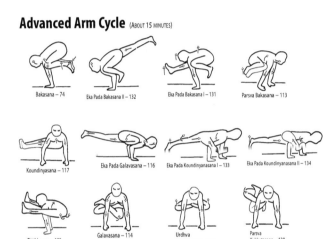

Bakasana – 74
Eka Pada Bakasana II – 132
Eka Pada Bakasana I – 131
Parsva Bakasana – 113
Koundinyasana – 117
Eka Pada Galavasana – 116
Eka Pada Koundinyanasana I – 133
Eka Pada Koundinyanasana II – 134
Tittibhasana – 128
Galavasana – 114
Urdhva Kukkutasana – 115
Parsva Kukkutasana – 130

Leg Head Cycle (About 11 minutes)

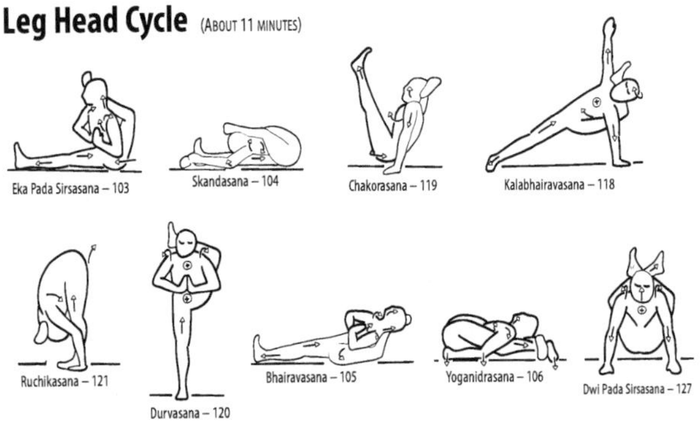

Eka Pada Sirsasana – 103
Skandasana – 104
Chakorasana – 119
Kalabhairavasana – 118
Ruchikasana – 121
Durvasana – 120
Bhairavasana – 105
Yoganidrasana – 106
Dwi Pada Sirsasana – 127

Backward Cycle (About 15 minutes)

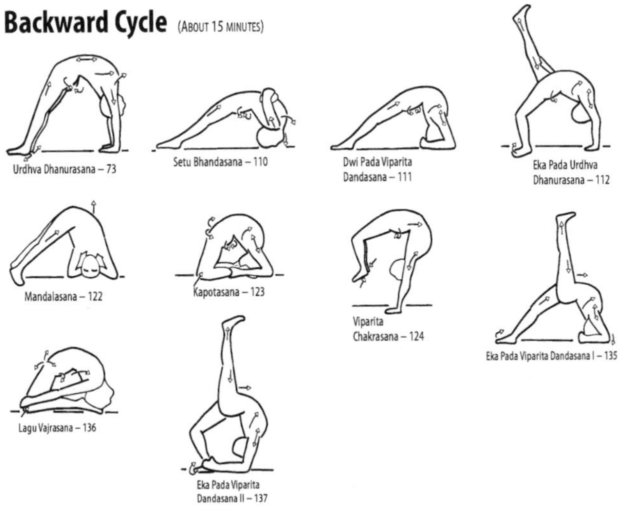

Urdhva Dhanurasana – 73
Setu Bhandasana – 110
Dwi Pada Viparita Dandasana – 111
Eka Pada Urdhva Dhanurasana – 112
Mandalasana – 122
Kapotasana – 123
Viparita Chakrasana – 124
Eka Pada Viparita Dandasana I – 135
Lagu Vajrasana – 136
Eka Pada Viparita Dandasana II – 137

BUDDHA'S FOUR NOBLE TRUTHS

For the past 40 years, I've recited the Four Truths during headstand. Over this time I've gradually plumbed deeper and deeper meaning from them. The words are easy to understand, while the knowing appears to rests deep within and 'bubbles' up into awareness as I mature enough to 'handling' it. I recommend doing something like this long term; you may be surprised at what 'bubbles up'.

The First Noble Truth is the existence of suffering. Birth is suffering; growth, decay, and death are suffering. Sad it is to be joined with that which we dislike. Sadder still is the separation from that which we love, and painful is the craving for that which cannot be obtained.

The Second Noble Truth is the cause of suffering. The cause of suffering is lust. The surrounding world affects sensation and begets a craving thirst that clamors for immediate satisfaction. The illusion of self originates and manifests itself in a cleaving to things. The desire to live for the enjoyment of self entangles us in a net of sorrows. Pleasures are the bait and the result is pain.

The Third Noble Truth is the cessation of suffering. He who conquers self will be free from lust. He no longer craves and the flames of desire find no material to feed upon, thus they are extinguished.

The Fourth Noble Truth is the Middle Path that leads to the cessation of suffering. There is salvation for him whose self disappears before truth, whose will is bent on what he ought to do, whose sole desire is the performance of his duty. He who is wise will enter this path and make an end to suffering. Eight steps on the Middle Path are:

1. **Right Understanding** [*]
2. **Right Mindedness** [*]
3. **Right Speech**
4. **Right Action**
5. **Right Living**
6. **Right Effort**
7. **Right Attentiveness** [*]
8. **Right Concentration** [*]

COMMENTARY

Pleasure and Desire

Desire (thirst, need, lust, crave,...) is central to these Truths (1). In fact, all religions view pleasure and desire as problematic. But why? After all, life would be impossible without pleasure. Indeed, it's not a problem in Nature. It's the circumstances of civilization that make pleasure problematic. For example, the pleasures of high energy food (fats and carbohydrates) guides us to eat healthful food in Nature. Civilized man, however, refines fats and carbohydrates to make pizza and then, driven by desire, overeats.

As naked primates on the savanna, we lived simply with little to cling to but each other, and Nature itself. Civilization began with stone tools and fire, out of a desire to increase our security and comfort. And it continues, for the pursuit of comfort and security ostensibly gives life meaning. As our tools continue to liberate us from Nature's dominion, our ability to pursue pleasure and desire steadily increases, but does life meaning? Maybe religion is simply an attempt to cope with the loss of life meaning caused by our 'liberation' from 'mother' Nature's bosom?

(1) Note: there is an important distinction between innate needs like hunger and thirst, and emergent needs like desire, want, lust, and crave. For example, feeling hunger is a universal need of all living things. Feeling hungry I start to think about what I want to eat. Today I crave to eat at out and deliberate which restaurant, and whether I desire pizza or really lust for something more decadent. What begins as a innate need easily turns into a pursuit of certain desires and the pleasures they promise us.

Stepping back, all I see is this: **Need + Thought = Desire** (want, craving, lust, etc.). It is the thinking part of need which creates problems not found in the rest of nature. Life turns into a struggle between conflicting desires arising from the mind. This surely accounts for Buddha's emphasis on "mind only", as I think he put it.

Self

Clinging to things (objects and thoughts, attractions and aversions...) re-enforces our conception of self. The fleeting sense of security and comfort this gives, lures us in and promises us life meaning. Anything that enhances this is irresistible... and so we cling still tighter. Trapped emotionally in this self perpetuating cycle, we unwittingly adopt a world view that further validates this perception of self. This experience of self is so compelling that it easily overshadows awareness of our innate original Nature.

Truth (Dharma)

Truth is the innate Nature of things, how things are—not how we think they are, nor how we want them to be. A mystery to bear in mind, to paraphrase the Tao Te Ching: 'The Nature that can be spoken of, is not the constant Nature'.

The Eight Steps

Half of the eight steps above relate directly to the mind (indicated by [*]). Our perceptions determine how we react to life's circumstances. So obviously Right Understanding is a critical first step.

Buddha Final Advice

Strive on diligently are reportedly Buddha' final words of advice he gave his disciples before the moment of death. At the end of the day what else can one do but strive on diligently!

Hatha yoga gives us a daily opportunity to train ourselves to *strive on diligently* in an 'uncontaminated' way. Meaning, Hatha yoga is largely free of any social or economic reward that usually drives us to strive on diligently. The challenge to self-integrity, especially as a private practice, is maximal. Here are a few parallels from the Bhagavad Gita:

> *Set thy heart upon thy work, but never on its reward. Work not for a reward: but never cease to do thy work.* 2:47
>
> *Work done for a reward is much lower than work done in the Yoga of wisdom. Seek salvation in the wisdom of reason. How poor those who work for a reward!* 2:49
>
> *This man of harmony surrenders the reward of his work and thus attains final peace: the man of disharmony, urged by desire, is attached to his reward and remains in bondage.* 5:12
>
> *A sacrifice is pure when it is an offering of adoration in harmony with the holy law, with no expectation of a reward, and with the heart saying 'it is my duty'.* 17:11

Action independent of a reward, while biologically unattainable need-wise, is a very useful and liberating approach to practice in terms of desire (i.e., desire = visceral need + cerebral thinking). Taoist parallels of all this are: "The sage desires not to desire", and "he who perseveres is a man of purpose". Occasions of fasting (e.g., food, sex, speech, intoxicants, shopping, whatever one desires—you name it) are another way to confront pleasure's lure and train ourselves to "persevere" and "desire not to desire".

Step By Step Lessons

These Step By Steps were written 30 years ago from my youthful point of view. In those days I made more mountains out of molehills. Still, they hold up fairly well[1].

Introduction

Many people are loathe to follow step by step instructions. It's not for nothing that they say, "When all else fails, read the instructions". I am fairly certain one could learn Yoga just fine using only the full page illustrations of the essential dynamics. That said, these Step by Steps will be useful for some, especially those learning completely on their own from scratch. In any case I'm offering two very different ways to learn so that folks can mix and match to suit their individual learning style.

These lessons give in-depth instruction in the most basic beginning Yoga postures. A solid understanding of these basic postures will be invaluable for the correct and productive practice of the intermediate and advanced postures you will attempt in the years ahead. In fact, all the advanced postures use the same basic approach, but in more challenging ways.

Many people may well prefer learning the postures using the full page illustrations of the essential dynamics rather than following these lessons. Nevertheless, most everyone would benefit by looking over this material, at least somewhat, to see what they may have overlooked.

1 Sure, all this could stand better editing, photos, examples and so on... maybe someday (although I do like the simplicity of those black and white photos). In any case, I feel a careful, occasional review of the first dozen pages of this book would serve most folks even better.

Alphabetical Lesson Index

Directions for the Lessons

As there are many stages to learning Yoga and many aspects to each posture, I have broken the instruction down into five sections. When you begin a new posture, read through these instructions, try doing what you can, and then look over the full page illustration of essential dynamics given for that posture (pages 17-170).

The introduction to each posture:

The suffix of each posture's Sanskrit name is ASANA which means posture, so I've omitted the word "posture" in the translation. Following the translation, I give a short description.

Next, I summarize some traditional views concerning how the posture effects the body. Take these with more or fewer grains of salt. Meaning, while I've found some effects to be very true; others little more than old wives' tales, as I see it anyway.

I. Basic Procedure:

Follow these basic steps initially. When you can perform the posture from memory according to these steps you are ready to study and apply the information given under III. and IV. (Perfecting and Teaching).

II. Variation Procedure:

This shows easier variations of the posture which may be practiced by those too stiff or weak to perform the Basic Procedure. However all students should read over these variations and practice them a few times, as there are points covered here that will benefit.

III. Perfecting Procedure:

Begin this section after a few weeks (or months) working on the Basic procedure. Don't try to absorb all this information in one reading—it can take years to really master. It's more effective to occasionally reread and review this information and integrate it into your practice little by little. Trying to get it all at once makes for a confusing and tense experience! That is not what you've come to yoga for is it?

IV. Teaching procedure:

Here are various teaching and learning techniques, along with additional aspects of the posture. This information is valuable to all, whether you plan to teach or not—in any case, you are teaching yourself! The information given here can enable you to develop your practice without the aid of a teacher, or at least with a minimum of classroom instruction.

It would be also helpful to study Iyengar's book "**Light On Yoga**". Here you will fine further information on the history of the posture, its meaning, its effects, and details of its practice.

> *"In liberty from the bonds of attachment, do thou therefore the work to be done: for the man whose work is pure attains indeed the Supreme".* Bhagavad-Gita 3-19

LESSON I

1. TADASANA

(Mountain)

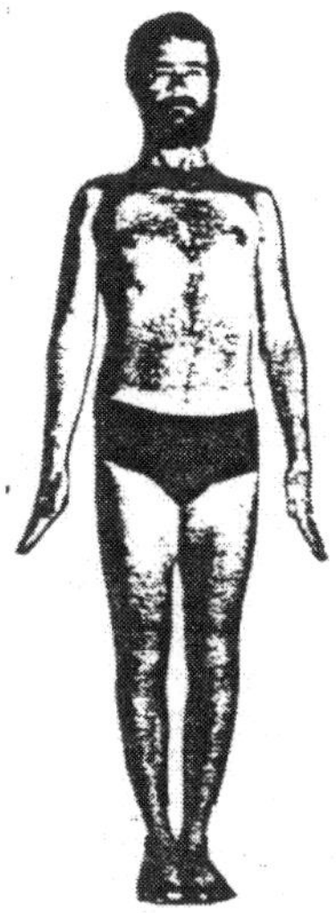

Fig. 1-0

Tada means mountain and sans or asana means posture. Here one learns to stand as firm and stable as a mountain. Mountains never tire in standing and neither do we if we learn active standing. In Tadasana the body feels light so we are able to stand longer periods of time with less fatigue. We stand mindfully and not just hang on our bones.

I. Basic procedure

1. Stand with feet together, toes and ankles touching, and adjust the body weight so it's equally distributed. We often tend to stand with the greatest proportion of our weight either on the heels or on the balls of the feet.

2. Tighten the muscle of the buttock and curl the tail bone in towards the anus. This and contracting and lifting the lower abdominal muscles raise the pubic area, Fig. 3-4

3. Tighten the thigh and calf muscles which will in turn raise the knee cap and lock the legs straight by locking the knee joint, Fig. 3-10. Both this and point 2 above are covered more thoroughly in the next posture.

4. Keep the arms at the sides locked at the elbow as you did with the knee above. Draw the shoulders back and lift the back of the neck backward and upward toward the ceiling. Extend and stretch the spine upward, in effect lifting you up from the spine, Fig. 1-1.

5. Keep the head erect, chin down and gaze to the front.

II. Variation procedure:

This posture may be done with the feet spread one foot or so apart and the hand and arms may be placed where you like. You can practice standing this way at other times of the day, e.g., while standing in a line, brushing teeth, etc. Don't over tighten the muscles; just keep them firm, active and alive.

III. Perfecting procedure:

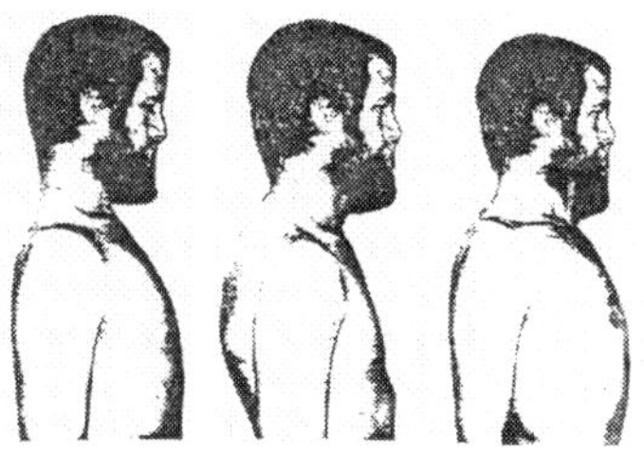

Fig.1-1, Fig.1-2, Fig.1-3

1. Stooped shoulders, hanging head and a floating chin are some of the weaknesses in the posture of modern man. The first and most important point in posture: keep the back of the neck extended upward, which takes care of the head, shoulders, and chin. This can be made easier by imagining yourself dangling from the sky on a string which is connected to and lifting you from the back of the neck at the first thoracic vertebrae, Fig. 1-1.

Maintain this *lift* in most Yoga postures and other activities throughout the day. Physical aspect, like this, can influence mind greatly. Another example of this is how putting a smile on one's face can actually lighten one's frame of mind. Here, this *lift* effects endurance, concentration, and emotional control, all of which will be found lacking to a certain degree when you hold yourself as shown in Fig. 1-2.

2. A more intense drawing back of the shoulders is required in many Yoga postures (Fig. 1-3). Care should be taken not to lift the shoulders as you draw them back. It's just the opposite. Try to roll them down your back toward the buttocks, feeling them somewhat heavy.

Simultaneously extend the front chest (sternum) and the side chest (side ribs near the armpits) forward, outward and upward towards the head. This whole movement causes the shoulder blades to draw in nearer together and the chest to open up.

These points concerning the head, neck and shoulders can be applied in all activities to reduce tension and keep one fresh all day. This will be especially helpful for those who must stand, sit or walk long hours.

3. The ankles are raised and kept perpendicular to the floor, Fig. 1-4, and not allowed to sag or slang as shown in Fig. 1-5. This holds true for all Yoga postures whether the feet are apart or together.

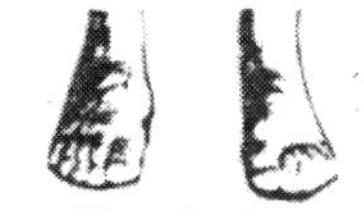

Fig. 1-4

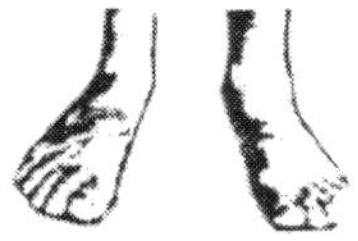

Fig. 1-5

When the feet sag the body weight is borne on only one side of the foot, or on the heel or ball of the foot. The body weight should be distributed evenly over the foot area, from heel to toe and along outside edge. Notice that when the ankles are raised the arches alas are lifted which can lift falling arches and relieve aching feet.

One should continue to maintain this lift on the ankles when walking. Many shoe wearing city folk walk with sagging ankles and their feet angled outward like a duck. This leads to poor weight distribution and they tire out quickly. If this is you, try walking with a parallel stride. This is achieved by the ankle lift and by lifting the big toe (or having it already lifted) when the foot hits the ground. This draws the foot inward slightly correcting the problem. The only difficulty is in remembering to maintain this lift until you replace this bad habit. When one walks barefoot the toes are automatically raised, especially after stubbing them a few times

Developing and maintaining good posture habits requires constant watchfulness. This is true for maintaining anything. In the end, this practice of watchfulness benefits all aspects.

IV. Teaching hints

Most of the principles used in Tadasana are true for ALL standing Yoga postures and most of the other Yoga postures. Look for the similarities and stress them to your student while he is performing other postures.

When teaching this posture, have the student stand with back touching the wall. Press his shoulder and small of the back as close the wall as they will go. This brings the chest and pubic region outward. The head should touch the wall with the student trying to press the back of the neck near the wall as possible. Do with natural muscle tone and not tension keeps the diaphragm relaxed

3. UTTHITA TRIKONASANA

(Three angle-extended)

This posture tones the leg muscles and removes leg and hip stiffness. It gives one a sense of balance, strengthens the whole body and reduces fat. Due to the lateral twist it relieves backaches and awakens the chest. The principles of this posture and Tadasana are basic to all standing postures introduced later on. The standing postures are among the most difficult in Yoga to master but at the same time can be attempted by nearly all regardless of age or physical condition. They develop a stiff and weak body very quickly.

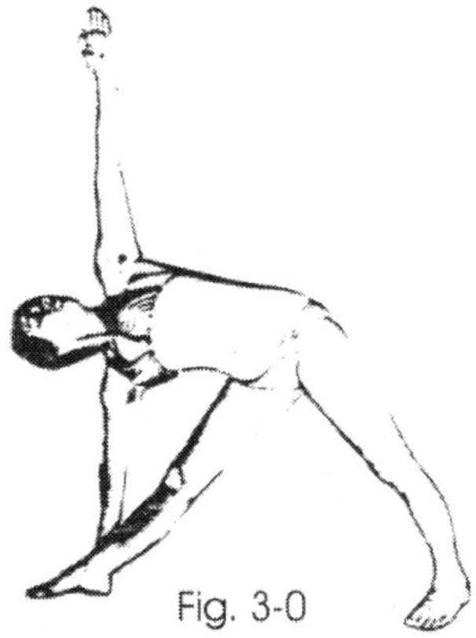

Fig. 3-0

I. Basic procedure:

1. From Tadasana inhale deeply and upon the exhalation jump spreading the feet three feet apart and parallel to each other. Extend the arms to the sides, locked at the elbows, with palms facing downward. Look straight to the front and take several breaths, Fig. 3-1.

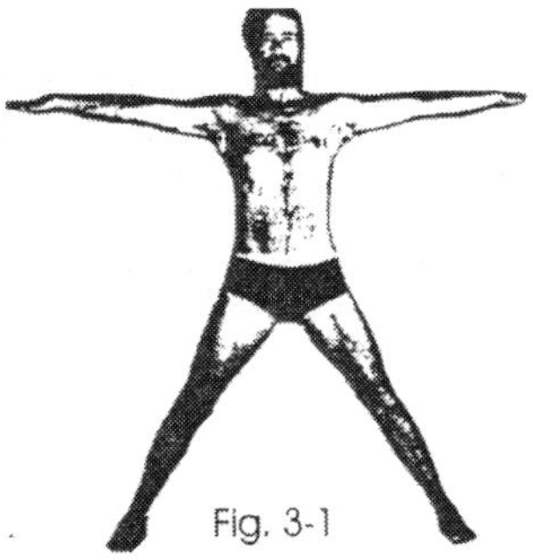

Fig. 3-1

2. Turn the right foot 90° to the right and turn the left foot slightly to the right. Then with an exhalation slowly bend the trunk laterally to the right and place the hand on the ankle (Fig. 3-2) pull left trunk back and then place palm of the right hand on the floor to the right of the right foot.

3. Simultaneously extend the left hand upward toward the ceiling with the left arm firmly locked straight at the elbow. Press the right hand firmly to the floor and bring the trunk in line with the legs, Fig. 3-7.

4. Extend the back of the neck as you did in Tadasana (Fig. 1-1) but turn the head as far to the left as it will go and gaze up past the outstretched left hand. Hold this posture for 30 sec. with full breathing, Fig. 3-0.

5. Then with an inhalation return to the position shown in Fig. 3-1. Repeat steps 2-4 on the left side, turning the left foot left 90° and bending the trunk to the left.

6. After holding the left side for 30 sec. with full breathing return on an inhalation to portion, Fig. 3-1. Then with an exhalation, jump back to Tadasana.

II. Variation procedure:

If you are unable to place the hand on the floor, spread the fingers on the right hand and only place them on the floor.

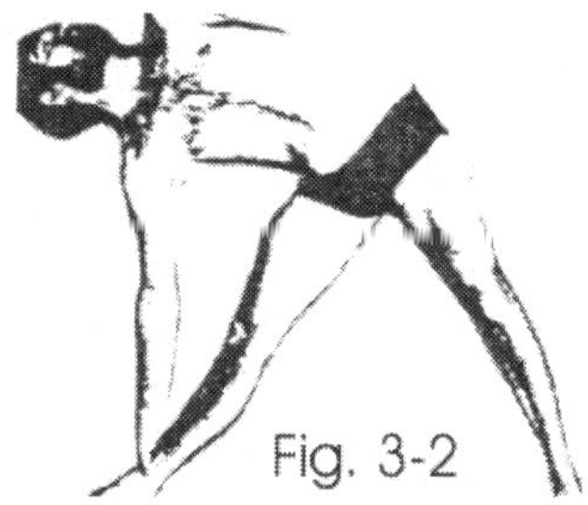

Fig. 3-2

If this too you are unable to do this, then just grasp the ankle as far down on the right calf as possible. Gripping the ankle firmly, move the trunk until it is in line with the legs. On no account are the legs to bend; just go as far as possible toward the floor keeping them locked straight, Fig. 3-2.

III. Perfecting procedure:

1. One cause of backache can be sunken lower spine. When this curve in the spine is great the upper body weight is unevenly distributed on the vertebrae of the lower lumbar and sacral regions of the spine, Fig. 3-3.

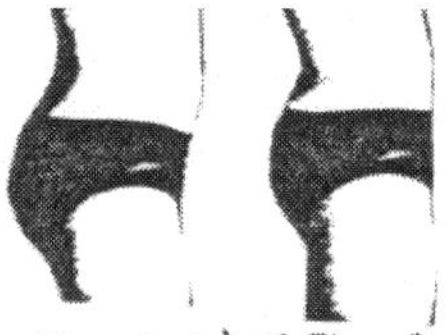

Fig. 3-3 Fig. 3-4

Many Yoga postures work at countering this curve. Contract the lower abdominal muscles and lift them in slightly toward the spine. Simultaneously contract the buttock muscles and roll them in towards the anus which swivels the hip forward and upward slightly raising the pubic region and reducing the lower curve, Fig. 3-4.

2. As you bend to the right, extend the right arm and the right side ribs straight outward—really reach to stretch this. You bend only from the lowest part of the spine, keeping the abdomen, chest, and shoulder in line, Fig. 3-5. Try to feel the right hip dig deep into the side of the trunk. Also as you are bending roll the left shoulder and left side of the chest backwards toward the wall (in Fig. 3-7) and simultaneously push the right shoulder and right side of the chest away from the wall. This action keeps the median line of the right side of the chest in line with the median line of the right leg, Fig. 3-7.

Fig. 3-5 Fig. 3-6

3. Roll the left hip backwards towards the wall (Fig. 3-2) to bring it and the right hip in line with the trunk and the legs. This will bring the nipples in line with and perpendicular to the floor, Fig. 3-7.

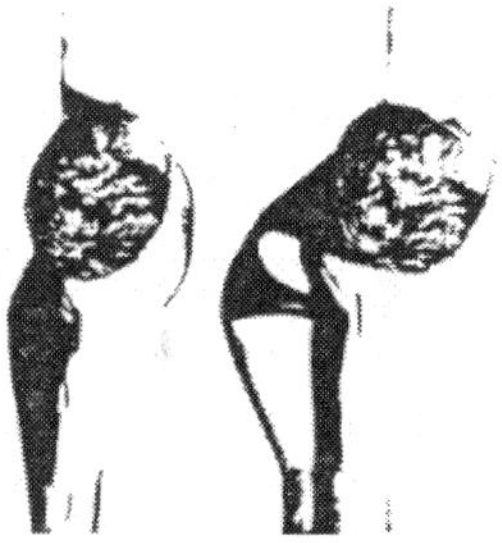

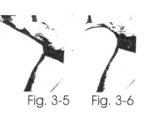

Fig. 3-7 Fig. 3-8

In order to bring the left hip to the rear and in line with the trunk, dig the left rear heal into the floor keeping its ankle raised (Fig. 1-4) throughout. In a sense this is a movement antagonistic to the intense bending on the right side of the trunk. This principle of opposing yet complimentary forces is used throughout Yoga. You challenge of one area of the body with/against another area. Can you see how this challenge is lacking in Fig. 3-8, in Fig. 3-6 and in Fig. 3-3?

4. The right foot is turned 90° to the right from the right hip. The right thigh muscle is pulled up tight and rolled to the right revolving

the whole of the leg around so that it and its knee cap are in line with the right foot.

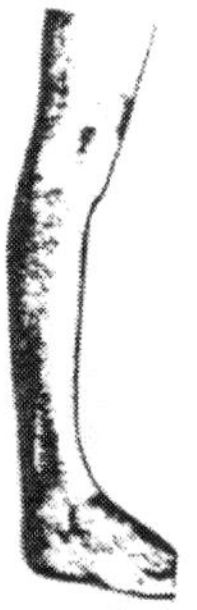
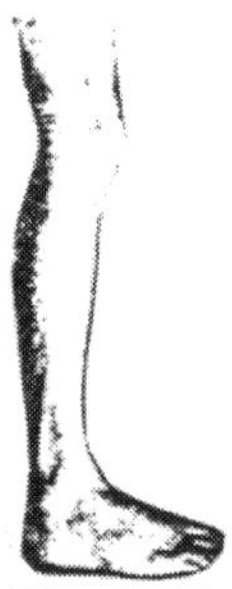

Fig. 3-9 Fig. 3-10

The thigh and calf muscles of the legs are pulled tight enough to raise the knee cap into the thigh. The more this is done, the more the skin on the back of the knees is stretched tight. This locking of the knee is done on all Yoga postures where the leg is supposed to be straight, as in Fig. 3-9, not Fig. 3-10.

As you stay in this posture, (or move into and out of it) maintain an even pressure over the whole of the foot, from toe to heal and from side to side, keeping the ankles raised throughout.

Fig. 3-11

Fig. 3-12

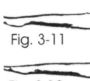

5. In the position shown in Fig. 3-1, extend the arms out to the side stretching them as though you were being pulled apart by two people. Simultaneously keep the shoulders rollled back and the chest extending upward with the back of the neck raised as described in Tadasana [1]. The arms should be locked at the elbows just as the legs are locked at the knee. The fingers are also extended and locked at the knuckles, causing the hands to be somewhat bow shaped, Fig. 3-11. This applies to all standing postures where the arms are extended straight.

Notice in Fig. 3-0, how the left arm is extended towards the ceiling. Turn the head to the left and gaze towards it. The head should turn until you see the thumb of the left hand with the right eye, yet while still keeping the head in line with the rest of the body. The right hand is placed on the floor firmly with the fingers in line with the toes of the right foot making the right arm perpendicular to the floor.

IV. Teaching procedures:

Have the beginner practice the posture first with the left hand on the left hip, with the thumb poking into the back of the hip. Have him use this hand to push the pubic region forward, and concentrate on getting the trunk and the hip in line with the legs as shown in Fig. 3-7.

If the student practices the posture with his back touching the wall you can then push his shoulder against the wall, which brings his trunk in line with his legs.

6. VIRABHADRASANA I

(Warrior I)

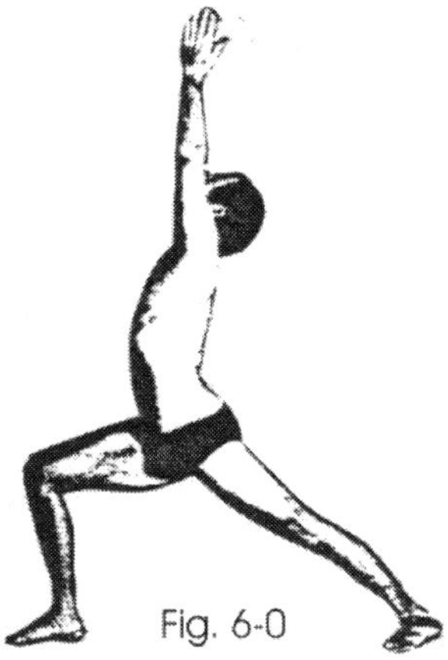

Fig. 6-0

This posture, dedicated to one of Sivas warriors in Hindu mythology, is strenuous when done correctly, or when attempting to do it correctly. It strengthens the body and reduces fat in the hips. It relieves neck, back, hip, and shoulder stiffness and ache. It also tones the ankles and knees and promotes full breathing.

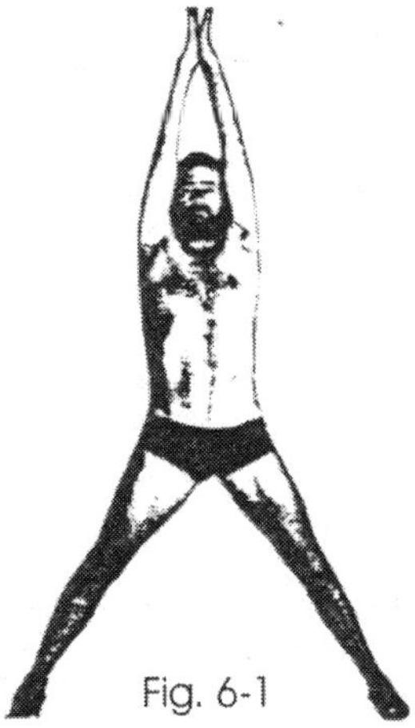

Fig. 6-1

I. Basic procedure:

1. From Tadasana [1], inhale and then on the exhalation jump, spreading the feet 3-4 feet apart (Fig. 3-1). Keeping the shoulders rolled back, revolve the arms from the shoulder until the palms face upwards. Then stretching the arms as though two people were pulling you apart. On an inhalation, raise them above the head joining the palms, Fig. 6-1. Keep the arms as straight as possible throughout.

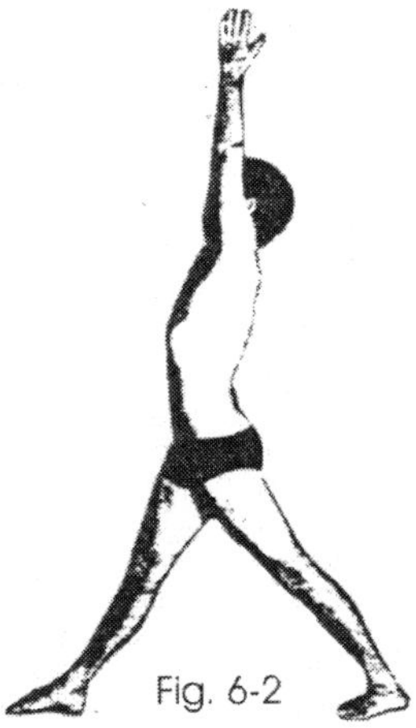

Fig. 6-2

2. Turn the right foot 90º to the right and the left foot slightly to the right. Then on an exhalation revolve the

left hip and trunk as far as possible to the right. The whole trunk from head to pubis should face 90° to the right in line with the right leg, Fig. 6-2.

3. On an exhalation bend the right leg until the thigh is parallel and the calf is perpendicular to the floor. Throw the head back as far as it will go and gaze up toward the palms. Extend the chest and stretch the whole trunk upwards. Hold this posture for 30 sec. with normal breathing. Fig. 6-0.

4. Return to the position shown in Fig. 6-2 on an inhalation and then on the exhalation bring the trunk to the front, Fig. 6-1. Repeat steps 2-4 on the other side, turning the left foot 90° to the left and the right foot slightly to the left, etc. After holding this posture on the left side for 30 sec., return to positions in Fig. 6-2, 6-1, inhale, and jump back to Tadasana [1] on the exhalation.

II. Variation procedure:

If it is too difficult to join the hands above the head and keep the arms rather straight, you can move the palm apart just enough (about 6 inches) to permit you to straighten and lock the arms.

Remember it's more important to keep the left leg straight than to bring the right thigh parallel to the floor, so don't sacrifice the locked straight left leg for any other aspect of this posture.

III. Perfection procedure:

1. The upper chest and shoulders are often not stretched up as much as they should be, but instead sag. Try to feel you are opening up your arm pit. Raise the arms and the shoulders, extending them from the side ribs, so that the side ribs and the nipples are lifted up several inches from there natural position. Move the shoulder blades in towards each other as though you were trying to press them together. Really stretch up toward the ceiling, and simultaneously draw the arms and shoulders backward so they are in line with the trunk, Fig. 6-1, 6-2 6-0.

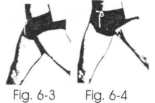

Fig. 6-3 Fig. 6-4

2. While maintaining this upward lift of the trunk, and keeping the knees locked, revolve the hip, screwing the left hip into the right one. Feel like you are trying to touch the left hip to the right thigh. The buttock muscles are tightened drawing the tailbone in towards the anus. Simultaneously dig the left heal into the floor, and using this as leverage, pull the right hip tightly into the abdomen, rotating from Fig. 6-4 into Fig. 6-3.

3. In order to keep the hip rotation you achieved in step 2 above, bend the right leg by sinking the trunk directly down towards and perpendicular to the floor. Avoid slanting the trunk forward.

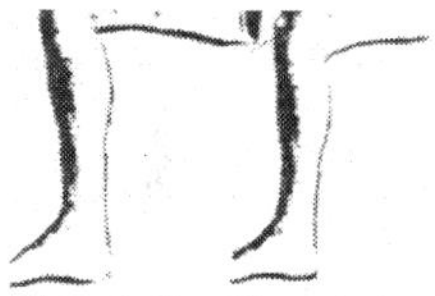

Fig. 6-5 Fig. 6-6

The squaring of the right leg is a problem for most. Bring the knee cap in line with the ball of the right foot Fig. 6-5. The more you bend the right leg, however, the more difficult it is to keep the left one straight. Counter this tendency by pulling the left thigh and calf muscle until it's as firm as stone, and keeping the left ankle lifted (Fig. 1-4), dig the left heal into the floor.

4. A common error for many is leaning the trunk and the arms too far forward once they are in the final position of Fig. 6-0. One must continue applying the principles in point 2 above. Try to bend from the lower part of the lumbar region of the spine, tightening the buttocks and curling the tail bone in towards the anus.

IV. Teaching procedure:

Pressing your thigh into the student's buttock, push his trunk lower to the floor until his right thigh is parallel to the floor. Gently pull his trunk and shoulder / arms back until the trunk is perpendicular to the floor. Check to see that the knee cap doesn't extend beyond the toe of the right foot. You can place their hands on the hip throughout the movement, or just during the preliminary swivel to simplify.

18. ADHO MUKHA SVANASANA

(Downward facing dog)

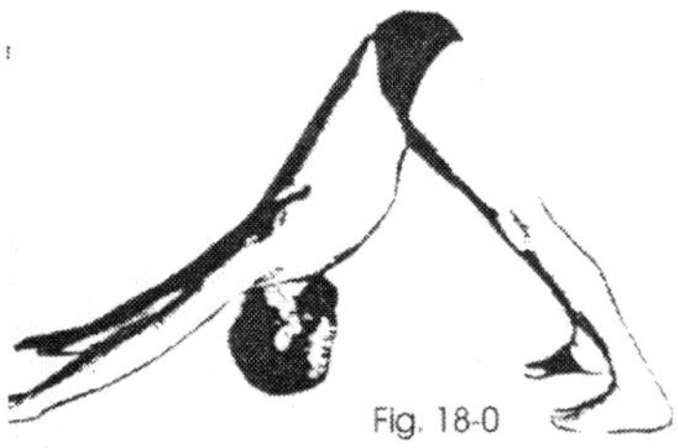
Fig. 18-0

This posture removes fatigue and restores energy. It relieves pain and stiffness in the heels, limbers the shoulder blades and relieves arthritis there. It is beneficial for sufferers of high blood pressure and has restorative effects similar to Sirsasana (headstand)

I. Basic procedure:

1. Lay on the stomach with palms by the side as though you were doing push ups. Place the feet one foot apart and with an exhalation, straighten the arms and lift the buttocks toward the ceiling. Keep the feet and the hands parallel to each other.

2. Move the chest in towards the knees so that the crown of the head rests on the floor, but doesn't press into the floor; it merely touches it.

3. Keep the back straight or a little concave, bending from the base of the spine. Hold this posture for 60 sec. or longer with full even breathing. Gaze should be held at nose level and focused beyond the feet.

From the position shown in Fig. 18-0, the student may move directly into the next posture, Fig. 19-0. On an inhalation, keeping the arms straight, pull and rotate the trunk forward. Rest the tops of the feet on the floor and thrust and extend the chin toward the ceiling.

II. Variation procedure:

Fig. 18-2

Fig. 18-3

The heels may be kept off the floor until the ankle flexibility is better developed. Likewise the head may be kept off the floor until the shoulder flexibility is better developed, but in both cases one continues to aim at touching both these points to the floor.

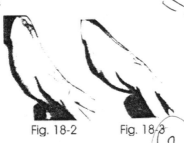

III. Perfecting procedure:

1. For those who can do Uttanasana [11], lesson III. (page 196), move the feet back from Uttanasana 3-4 feet, and spread them one foot apart. Then apply points 2 and 3 above.

2. Keep your heels 2-3 inches off the floor initially, resting body weight on the balls of the feet and palms. Raise and lock the knee caps and push the palms firmly into the floor. Pull the thigh and calf muscles tight as usual but this time roll the buttock muscle outward, opening up the anus area, and raising the tailbone upwards toward the ceiling. This is opposite to the standing postures where we roll buttocks inward tightening the anus area.

Once you achieve the maximum extension possible slowly lower the heels to the floor, keeping the ankles lifted. Push the heel into the floor from the calf.

3. Thrust the sides of the ribs towards the buttocks. Pull the chest to the rear as though you wished to touch it to the knees/thighs. Roll it in towards the abdomen.

Think of opening up the arm pits and rolling the shoulder and shoulder blades backwards and in towards the spine. See Fig. 18-2. Compare this with the insufficient opening up of the arm pits shown in Fig. 18-3. Aim for open - rising buttocks with open lowering chest.

IV. Teaching procedure:

Stand close in behind the student with your right thigh between his legs. Place one end of the loop rope around the student's waste where the thigh meet the pelvis, and loop the other end around your neck. Lift the student's buttocks upward and backward slightly by raising your trunk/neck up. Simultaneously press the students lower mid back region downward towards his feet with both hands.

You may instead just gently press the student's shoulders down towards his feet.

19. URDHVA MUKHA SVANASANA

(Upward facing dog)

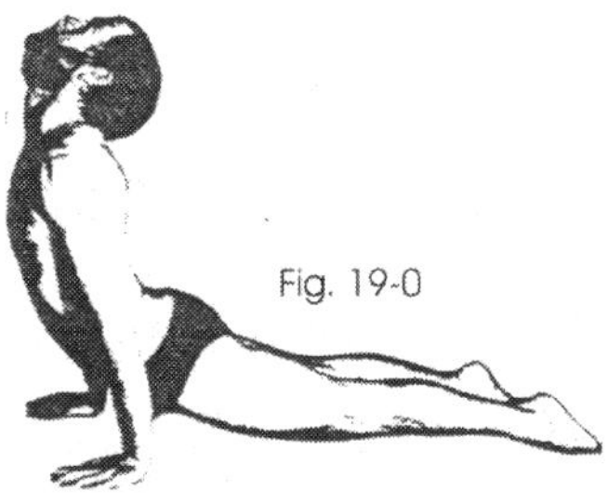

Fig. 19-0

This posture is especially good for people with stiff backs as it rejuvenates the lumber and sacral regions of the spine. It further strengthens the wrists, promotes chest expansion and increases circulation in the pelvic region.

I. Basic procedure:

1. Lie on the stomach with the feet spread one foot apart, and place the palms by the waste as in the previous posture, but with the toes pointing straight to the rear.

2. On an exhalation raise the trunk upward by straightening the arms and pull it forwards (which drags the feet forwards slightly). Keep the legs locked at the knees throughout. Bend from the lower back region and lift the upper chest and shoulders toward the ceiling.

3. Stretch the head back as far as it will go and lock the joints of the elbows. Gazing steady at nose level or upward between the eyebrows, hold this position for 30-60 sec. Breath fully and evenly. Then with an exhalation return to the floor.

II. Variation procedure:

Guard against the tendency to sacrifice the firmly locked knee caps for a small gain in back-bend. As with all Yoga postures the degree of movement is not as important as the correctness of movement. The palms may be placed further up by the ribs if necessary in the beginning.

III. Perfecting procedure:

1. Don't tense the muscles of the forehead and around the eyes if gazing upward between the eyebrows.

2. Its important to place the hand far enough back towards the hip that balance is only possible with a maximum back bend. This is done by sliding the trunk forward and bending it backwards, thus bringing the hips nearer the arms and resting the body weight on the palms and the tops of the feet.

Bend from the lowest part of the spine, keeping the upper part straight. Feel as though you are trying to make space in the lower spine extending it lengthwise as you bend it. This movement is increased by tightening and rolling the muscle of the buttocks inward and by tightening the anus muscle. Simultaneously spread and open out the groin/pubic area. Notice that this is the opposite buttock movement as done in the previous posture

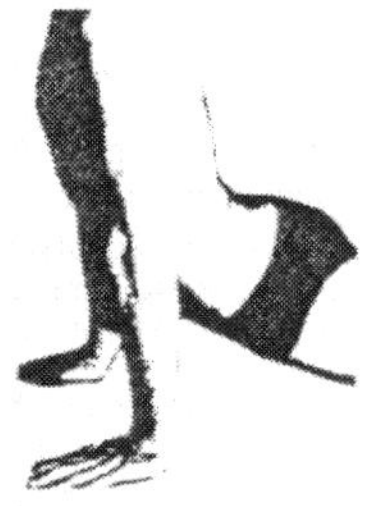

Fig. 19-1

Fig. 19-1 shows insufficient forward movement of the trunk towards the arm. Compare this with the position shown in Fig. 19-0. Elbows are facing outward which weakens the movement. Keep them facing straight to rear as in Fig. 19-0.

3. On each exhalation try for a little more back-bend and chest expansion. Lock the knees and elbows a little tighter and squeeze the buttocks inward-toward the anus a little more. Extend the head back and the chin up a little further.

Giving an extra push on each or every other exhalation intensifies the posture and increases it benefits. This extra push involves tightening muscles to the degree required (as in raising the knee caps to lock the legs) but it also involves relaxing muscles or joints to the degree required to make space in the lower back to bend further, and open up the groin area.

4. Don't sag or hang the trunk down from the shoulders. Raise the trunk, roll the chest outward, roll the shoulders backward and lift the sternum upward.

IV. Teaching procedures:

The student may not achieve much bend in the beginning which is fine. Just insist that he keep his arms and leg lock straight and that he pull his trunk forward as much as possible.

Place the crown of your head against the student's sternum and both hands around his lower back. Pull his trunk forward while simultaneously pushing his chest backward and upward with your head. Put a weight on the buttock (10lbs. more or less)

23. VIRASANA I & II

(Hero)

Fig. 23-0

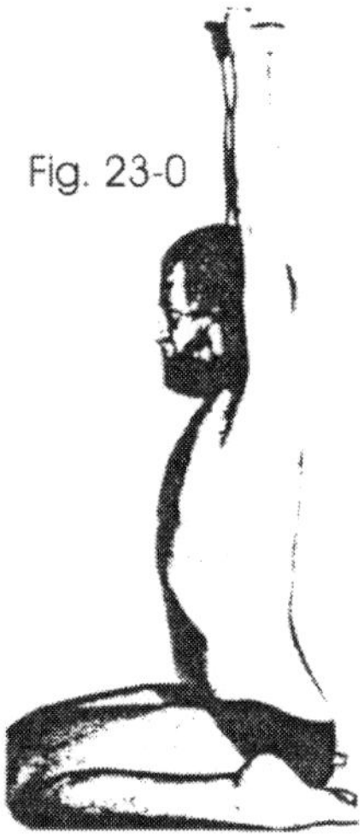

There are four separate movements to this posture. The first two are covered now and the others latter. In general, Virasana develops the knees and can 'cure' rheumatic pains in them if done daily.

The posture in Fig. 23-1 is well suited for meditation [48], pranayama [47], or just sitting. The spine is kept erect eliminating back pain that can come from sitting without back support. The posture in Fig. 23-0, removes stiffness in the shoulders and fingers and wrists, and so is helpful to all office workers.

I. Basic procedure:

1. Sit on the floor with the knees touching and the feet spread 18 inches apart, or just enough so that the buttock can rest between them. Toes are pointed to the rear and pressed flat to the floor.

2. Place the wrists on the knees with the arms locked straight. The ends of the first finger and the thumbs are joined lightly and the other three fingers are extended out straight, Fig. 23-1.

3. Hold this posture for as long as you like with normal breathing. Gaze at nose level, and focus the eyes out past the fingers. This completes the first movement.

4. From the first movement, take the hands off the knees and interlock the fingers so that the thumb of the right hand rests on top of the thumb of the left hand. Turn the palms outward and raise the hands over the heed. Stretch the arms upward and backward as though you were going to touch the ceiling

5. Maintain this stretch with full even breathing for 30 sec. Gazing straight ahead. On an exhalation lower the arms to the knees and then release the finger lock. Interlock the fingers again only this time so the thumb of the thumb of the left hand rest on the thumb of the right hand, and raise the hand over the head and hold for 30 sec.

II. Variation procedure:

If your knees are too stiff to allow you to place the buttocks on the floor, place a folded blanket under them and sit on this. Use progressively less under the buttocks as flexibility improves.

III. Perfecting procedure:

1. When you place the buttock on the floor roll the calf muscle outward away from the thigh to allow greater contact between the buttock and the floor. Hold your trunk as you did in Tadasana [1], rolling the shoulders backward, extending the spine and the back of the heck upward, and extending the chest outward.

2. Keep the arms locked at the elbows, Fig. 23-1. Compare this with Fig. 23-2 where the attention has lapsed. This completes movement one.

3. In the second movement move the arms with an outward thrusting force when raising them upward, Fig. 23-3. This pulls the shoulders backward when the arms come in line with the trunk, Fig. 23-0.

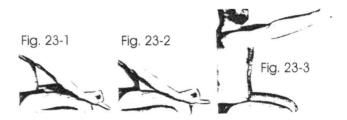

Fig. 23-1

Fig. 23-2

Fig. 23-3

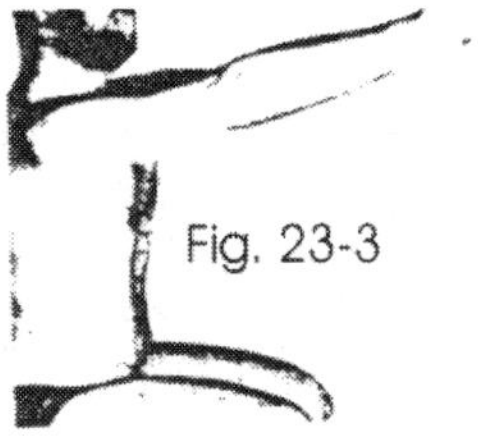

4. When the hands are over the head, stretch them and the shoulders up from the side rids. The side ribs, nipples and shoulders rise two or three inches above their position in Fig. 23-3. This causes the shoulders and the upper arms to push closer in toward the ears. This intensive stretch upward tends to make the facial muscles tighten so deliberately keep them as relaxed as possible.

IV. Teaching procedure:

1. For the first movement, Fig. 23-1, place your knee against the student's lower back and place your hands on his shoulders. Gently push his lower back concave and roll his shoulders backward.

2. For the second movement, Fig. 23-0, also push the lower back in slightly. Next, draw the shoulders and arm back until they are perpendicular to the floor and in line with the rest of the trunk.

3. To get the upward extending of the arms and shoulders place a board of his palms, press it down slightly, and have him push the board upward against your downward pressure.

4. Check to see that he is raising the back of the neck and bringing his head backward so that the back of the head is in line with the upper back. There is a tendency for the head to droop forward. But as the head is brought back facial strain tends to increase so then the student must relax facial muscles, especially around the mouth and in the neck.

16. ARDHA NAVASANA

(Half ship posture)

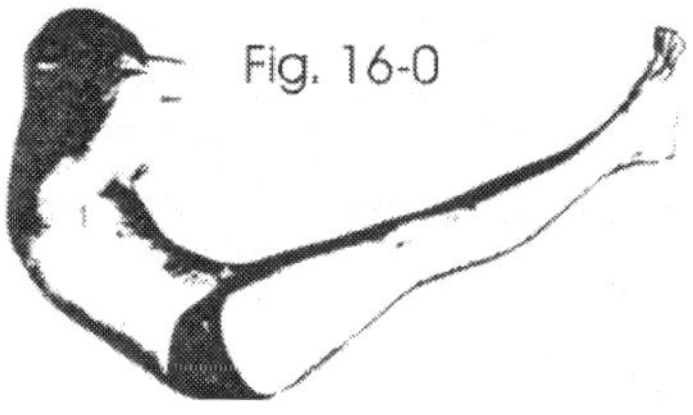

Fig. 16-0

This posture strengthens the abdominal muscles and the back. It also has a beneficial effect on the liver, gallbladder, and the spleen.

I. Basic procedure:

1. Sit on the floor and with interlocked fingers, place the hands behind the head just above the neck. Pull the knee caps up into the thighs and keep the ankles touching

2. On an exhalation, recline the trunk backwards, about 45°, until the feet begin to rise of the floor. Raise the legs until the feet are level with the head, about 18 inches off the floor, forming a very obtuse angle with the trunk.

3. The weight of the body should rest on the buttock and not on the spine proper. Some pressure however will be felt on the tip of the 'tail bone'. With the gaze between the eyebrows and focused beyond the toes, hold this pasture for 30-60 sec. with shallow breathing.

II. Variation procedure

The following posture may be an easier variation for Ardha Navasana [16] for some people. Try it.

17. URDHVA PRASARITA PADASANA

(Up stretched out foot)

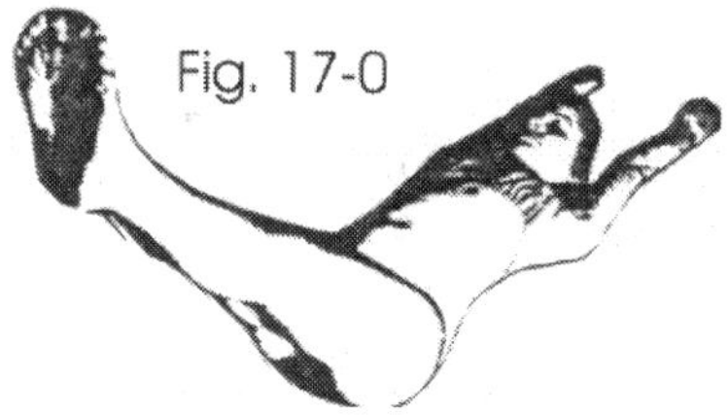

Fig. 17-0

Beginners may find that even a stay of 30 sec. is not possible. You can alternate between Ardha Navasana and the following variation.

1. Lie on the back with arms stretched beyond the head, palms up. Lock the knee caps and touch the ankles together.

2. On an exhalation, raise your legs until they are perpendicular to the floor, then lower them in several stages, holding each stage 15 sec. Above all, be sure to keep your back flat to floor throughout to avoid back strain.

3. Alternately, exhale and lift the legs one foot off the floor and hold for 15 sec. Then, exhale and raise them another foot and hold 15 sec., Fig. 17-0. Next, exhale and raise them until

they're perpendicular to the floor. Hold for 15 sec. Finally, repeat this sequence in reverse order as you lower the legs to the floor.

III. Perfecting procedures:

1. In Ardha Navasana, instead of raising the sternum and extending the chest as in the previous posture, depress both inward into the chest cavity. Push the ribs of the frontal chest into the abdomen keeping the back convexly curved as possible. Roll the upper chest and shoulders towards the feet without lifting the trunk any further off the floor. This action makes only shallow breathing possible which increases the postures effects.

The trunk should be reclined to the point where the body weight begins to fall on the end of the spine. Rise up just a little and hold the trunk at this angle, just on the "edge". Balance can be difficult in the beginning.

2. After the trunk is in position, raise the legs until the feet are in line with the head. Be sure to keep the feet high enough by looking directly ahead to the ankle. The elbows tend to drift in toward each other, therefore keep the tips of the elbows in line with the forehead.

IV. Teaching procedure:

Keeping the back convex with the chest depressed into the abdomen can be difficult while in the pose due to balance fatigue. To free the student to concentrate on the movement described in point 1 of the Perfecting procedure, have him keep the legs on the floor. Start with legs to floor and slide palms down along the thighs. You can also stretch hand out.

Next the student does a partial sit up by raising the trunk until the shoulders are 5—12 inches off the floor. Extends the arms straight towards the feet with palms on the leg. He tries to touch his hands as far down the leg as possible toward the feet without raising the trunk any further. Instead he must focus on curving the back and shoulders as convex as possible. Make sure he doesn't hold the breath at any time during this or during the proper posture.

26. BHARADVAJASANA I

(This posture is dedicated to the father of an ancient Indian hero.)

Fig. 26-0

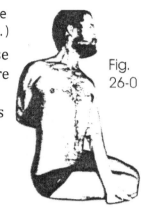

This posture prepares those with stiff backs for the more advanced lateral twisting postures latter on. It makes the back supple and helps those with arthritis.

I. Basic procedure:

1. Sit on the floor with both legs to the right of the hip. Place the right ankle of the instep of the lower left foot, as shown in Fig. 26-1.

2. With an exhalation turn the trunk to the left as far as it will go and place the right hand palm down, under the knee of the left leg just above the knee. Then on the next exhalation swing the left arm behind the back and grasp the right arm just above the elbow.

3. Once a firm grip is established straighten out the right arm as much as possible and continue twisting the trunk to the left as far as it will go.

4. Turn the head to the right and gaze over the right shoulder. Hold the posture for 30 sec. with full breathing. Release the grip and turn back to the front on an inhalation. Repeat the posture on the other side.

II. Variation procedure:

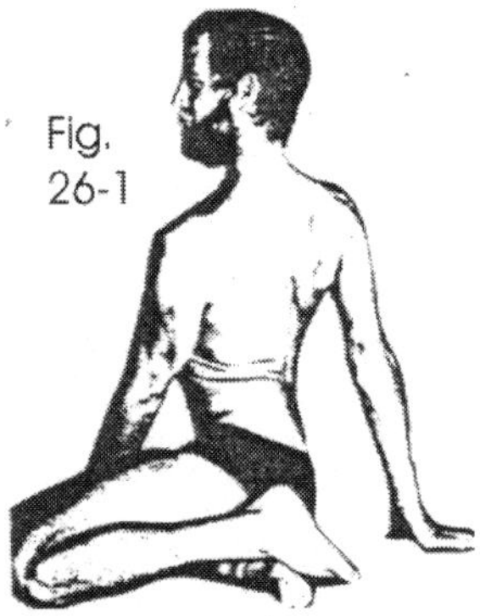

Fig. 26-1

If it's difficult to rest the buttock on the floor with the legs to the side you can place a blanket folded several times or a pillow under the buttocks.

Beginners usually can't twist around enough to grasp the right arm with the left hand. They may follow the same procedure principles above but instead of grasping the arm they can place the arm about 8—12 inched behind them, pressing it firmly into the floor. Move this left arm as far to the right side of the body as it will go and lock it at the elbow, Fig. 26-1.

Another variation is to do the posture facing a wall or table and with your hands, use this wall or table for leverage to help you twist yourself around.

Yet another variation is simply sit with straight legs. Then, grasping the left leg with the right hand and twisting the trunk to the left, place the left hand behind on the floor. Now continue rotation as described in step 3 and 4 above.

III. Perfecting procedure:

1. Extend the chest and lift the sternum as shown in Fig. 26-2. Fig. 26-3 shows the chest with too little "life" in it. This chest extension and lifting of the sternum gives a "proud" character, beauty to the pose and intensifies its effects. This is the type of extension aimed for in most Yoga postures.

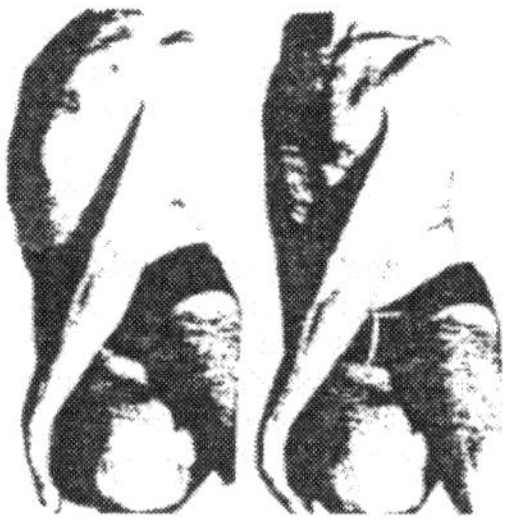

Fig. 26-2 Fig. 26-3

2. Draw the left shoulder back and roll it downward while simultaneously extending the right shoulder to the right. This screwing action of the shoulders is similar to that of the hips in Virabhadrasana I [6].

3. Keep the ears on a parallel plain to the floor by not allowing the head of tilt to either side, nor to the back or front. To do this, maintain the extension at the back of the neck as described in Tadasana [1] while you twist your head as far as it will go to the right until you are looking directly over your right shoulder.

IV. Teaching procedure:

The teacher can place his knee on the student's lower middle back and his hands on the student's shoulders. Push the back in concave and simultaneously pull the shoulders back and twist them around.

13. SAVASANA

(Corpse posture)

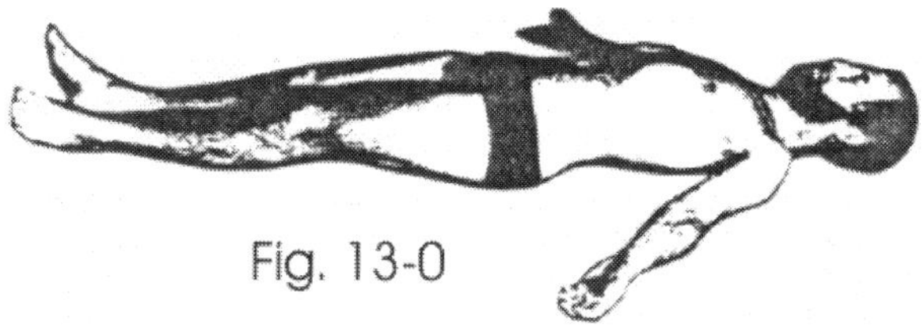

Fig. 13-0

Here you imitate a corpse. Keeping the body and the mind at this degree of stillness while maintaining full consciousness invigorates and refreshes mind and body.

In Savasana you learn to consciously relax—a difficulty invaluable in our stressful modern world. This posture relieves fatigue quickly and when done with steady, smooth, and full breathing soothes the entire nervous system and calms the mind.

I. Basic procedure:

1. Lie flat on a firm surface, face up, with the whole body from head to toes in a straight line. You can place a folded cloth over the eye to keep out light. Place the arms at a 45° angle to the body with the palms turned up. Keep the heels together with the toes apart.

2. Gaze downward at nose level with eyelids shut and eyes focus to infinity. The jaw should be just firm enough that the teeth touch each other just slightly. The tongue is kept passively resting on the lower palate.

3. Consciously feel the whole body, part by part. Relax each part in turn until the whole body is felt heavy and still. Especially important parts to relax are the face, hands, and shoulders as these store much tension.

Aim at getting all parts of the body symmetrical i.e. the hands equally opened, the left leg as relaxed as the right, the left side of the back in contact with as much of the floor as the right, etc.

4. Now that the body is symmetrical and relaxed you begin to soothe the nerves by rhythmic breathing. Start by breathing deeply

for a minute or two, then begin to slow the rate of breath down gradually so that eventually you have such slow even respiration that no air is felt moving through the nostrils.

5. The exhalations may be made longer and smoother than the inhalations. If the mind continues to wander, pause breathing for a few seconds, without strain, after each exhalation. It can also help to count the breaths, which loosens the "mind" from the "thoughts".

Your consciousness will drop thought as it feels and follows the breath. We begin by having the mind "control" the breathing, but this gradually reverses and we find ourselves letting the even breath "control" our mind, calming and soothing it.

Stay in Savasana for 51 to 20 min. with normal gentle breathing as described above or with Pranayama [14] breathing. Remember that even a few minutes in this posture when done correctly will invigorate the mind and body substantially.

II. Variation procedure:

Those who have trouble relaxing can try this simpler variation. Here the body is positioned the same as above but one aims only at relaxing every thing. The gaze is not held a nose level, but relaxed and rest still where it wants. The jaw is completely relaxed but the lips are still kept touching and closed lightly.

One feels every part of the body as though it were melting stone. Often the facial muscles are tensed unconsciously. Feel the skin of the face; let it sag down towards the floor. Open up the eyebrows, temple, and forehead area. Apply points 3, 4, and 5 above to this posture.

III. Perfecting procedures:

1. To insure that the body is in a straight line, lift the head and line the body up straight, Fig. 13-1. Lower the head with the back of the neck 'rising' as in Tadasana [1]. If the head tilts back so that the neck arches further off the floor making the chin roll upward, concentration drifts.

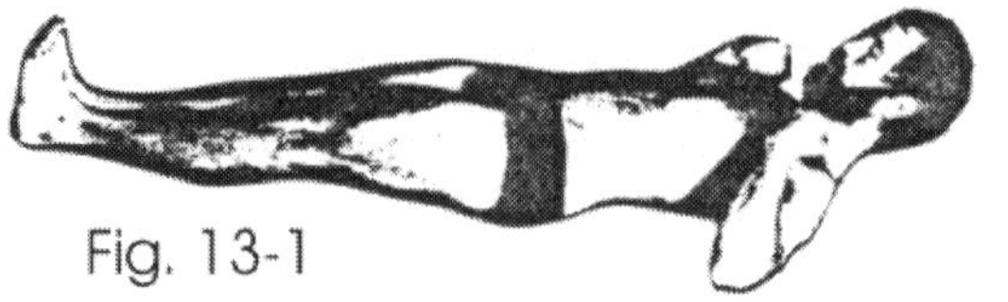

Fig. 13-1

2. The legs are stretched from the heels like you are trying to push some objects (the opposite wall for example) with your heels. Toes, heel, and ankle bone are joined. After a few seconds of intense stretching relax the leg completely and let the toes and ankles separate. Now, the legs should feel slightly stretched out from the leg sockets.

3. Simultaneously bend the arms at the elbows with tightly clenched fists, Fig. 13-1. Stretch the upper arms from their sockets in the shoulder by trying to touch "the opposite wall" with the elbow. Then straighten the arms out and relax them completely. Now the skin on the back of the arms should feel slightly stretched.

4. Open the hands, palms up, as you straighten the arms, stretching them as much as possible, Then relax them completely allowing the fingers to curl into their natural position, Fig. 13-0. One may straighten out the fingers in a similar but more relaxed manner a few times to get as open a hand as possible in a relaxed condition and so releasing any tension stored in the hands. Open the mouth like you are screaming, stretch face muscles in monster face and then relax it completely.

5. Feel the whole body in a creative way. Ask yourself if this part, or that part, is tense or not. Ask yourself if the legs are touching the floor at the same spot with the same degree of "heaviness". Feel the shoulders heavy, and sagging into the floor, with as much of the shoulders touching the floor as possible in the relaxed condition. The chest then feels open and free.

6. The tongue lies passively with a relaxed lower jaw and the muscles around the mouth soft and relaxed. Feel the cheeks as heavy lumps of clay, letting them sag down to the floor. Feel the whole face, letting the skin there fall away from the skull and sag to the floor. Guard against

tightening the eyebrows and forehead area—not only in Savasana, but throughout the day. Much tension is stored here unconsciously. Open up the furrows of the skin between the eyebrows and raise the eyebrows slightly then relax them completely. Feel the eye sockets and relax the muscles and skin surrounding them. Now everything, every part of your body should be completely relaxed. Even the inner organs are felt heavy and sagging down towards the floor.

7. You can remain relaxed in this way with normal light breathing or practice pranayama [14] first to soothe down the nervous system and then go to normal breathing. Applying the procedures above on exhalations works best. For example: as you exhale feel the finger and palms open up and relax. On the next exhalation, feel the legs and arms heavy, and on the next feel the facial muscles sag , and so on.

Finally surrender the self. Expel all thoughts, pride, ego, vanity, etc., along with the exhaled air. Just as each exhalation rids the body of stale air and C0² let it also help rid the mind of its stale thoughts and expectations. Exhale the "self" with the air of each exhalation until you are nothing in a dark empty void. Feel as though the air in each exhalation is blowing yourself out of yourself, your body, releasing you into the infinite universe. See Meditation [48] and Pranayama [14, 47].

IV. Teaching procedure:

To help the student relax, etc.,
try some of the following;

1. Press his shoulders down to the floor and hold them there with your palms applying 10-20 lbs. pressure for a minute or so. Then pull the arms out from the sockets of the shoulders slightly and press the palms and the fingers to the floor. In some cases a light weight may be placed on the fingers and palms to keep them open. Pull the students head away from the shoulders so that the neck comes closer to the floor and the chin rolls in toward the throat.

2. Press down lightly on his closed eyes with your fingers, then rubbing with the fingers, stretch the skin of his forehead from the eyebrows down to the temples Do the same for any other part of the body that seems to be tensed. Sometimes placing a heavy weight (10-50 lbs) on tense places relaxes them, if left on for several minutes or longer, i.e., 20-30 lbs. on the thighs, 10-20 lbs. on the shoulders, etc.

3. Spend the first few minutes of Savasana speaking to the student on the different points covered in the basic and perfecting procedure above to remind him of what he is aiming for.

The following can help students doing pranayama [14] in this posture:

1. Fold a blanket so it's about 8-12 inches wide, more than 36 inches long, and 1-2 inches deep. Place this under the student from the bottom of the lower lumber vertebrae to and including the top of the head, or place a wood plank (or book) about 8" x 12" x 2" under the upper trunk from the shoulders to the lower rib and place a folder blanket or another block under the head raising it to the same (or slightly higher) height.

Either of these techniques allows the arms to fall away from their sockets in the shoulders, raises the chest and opens it up for freer breathing.

2. Lift the student up slightly by placing your hand around the lumber region in order to get more of his neck and shoulders on the floor. This makes the lower back a little more concave. Pulling and rolling the students hips downward toward the feet will get similar results.

Conclusion - Lesson I

If, after a month of daily practice, you can do all but one or two of the nine postures covered in lesson I, continue on to lesson II if you like. Otherwise, continue working on these postures until you feel ready to go on.

There is no time restrictions on how many weeks or even years you stay on a particular lesson. Although 3-4 weeks per lesson probably suits most people with the interest to go to the end of this course. On the other hand one need never go beyond lesson one. You can stop at any lesson and practice it daily or when you want and continue to the next lesson only if and when you want to. Each lesson gives the body a balanced workout.

LESSON II

3. UTTHITA TRIKONASANA
30 sec.. each side with full even breathing

5. UTTHITA PARSVAKONASANA

(Side angle posture)

This is an good strengthening and reducing exercise. It relieves sciatic and arthritic pains, tones the ankles, knees, and increases peristaltic activity.

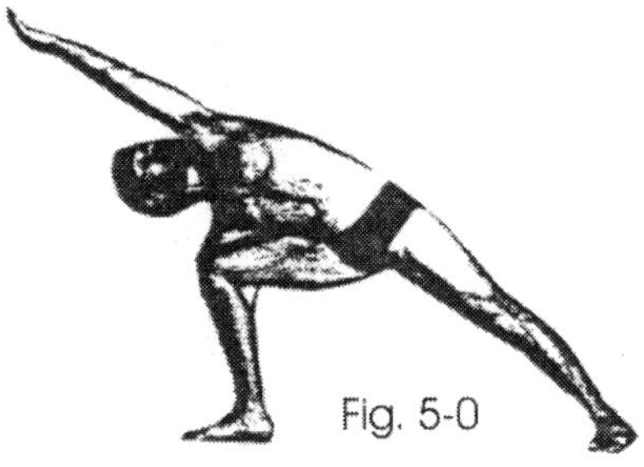
Fig. 5-0

I. Basic procedure:

1. From Tadasana [1], inhale and on the exhalation jump, spreading the feet 4 feet apart, about a foot more than for Utthita Trikonasana, similar to Fig. 3-1. Turn the right foot 90° to the right and the left slightly to the right.

2. On the exhalation, bend the right leg at the knee until the thigh is parallel to the floor. The knee cap shouldn't extend beyond the right toes.

3. On the next exhalation, stretch and bend the trunk to the right laying the right side ribs along the right thigh and covering the outer part of the right knee with the right arm pit. Place the right palm on the floor next to the right foot and extend the left arm out straight over the left ear.

4. Stretch the back part of the body (upper side) from the fingers of the left hand to the heel of the left foot as if there were two people stretching you apart. Feel the skin along the side ribs draw tight. Turn the head and gaze upward pasted the left arm toward the ceiling, holding this posture for 10 sec. with full breathing. Then on an inhalation return to the initial position (similar to Fig. 3-1), and repeat the posture on the left side.

II. Variation procedure:

This posture is made a little easier by placing the left hand on the left hip instead of stretching it out over the ear. Place the hand so the thumb digs in towards center of the spine near the pelvis. Then as you stretch the trunk and the left leg use this hand to push the hip downward and the left side of the trunk backward. Then the arm may be briefly stretched out over the left ear or extended straight up as in Trikonasana [3] Fig. 3-0.

If the distance between the feet is decreased the thigh will not come parallel to the floor. The posture will thus be less challenging and effective, but will allow you to build up your strength more gradually.

III. Perfecting procedure:

Fig. 5-1 Fig. 5-2

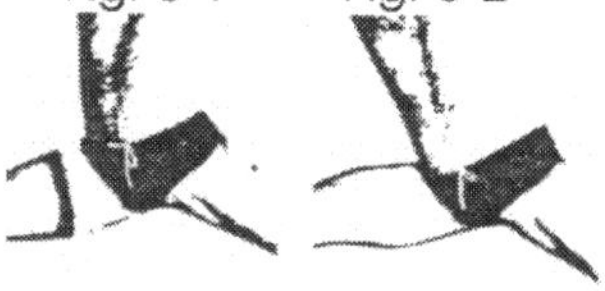

1. Keep the trunk, from the navel to the sternum, perpendicular to the floor as you bend the right leg. This is done by sinking straight down, drawing the chest area back and pulling it upright. Simultaneously push the left hip into the left side ribs, making the angle of the hips the ribs as acute as possible, Fig. 5-1. Remember to raise the pubic region as show in Fig. 3-4.

Fig. 5-3 Fig. 5-4

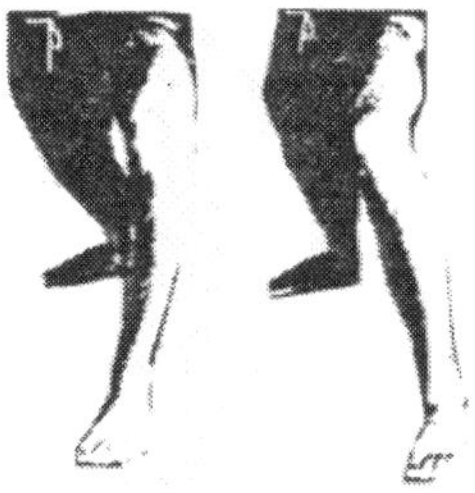

2. There is a certain antagonistic force in the direction of movement of the two legs. While bending the right leg during the posture, the bending right knee is moved and held outward, Fig. 5-3., so the knee cap is directly in line with the foot rather than tilting inward, Fig. 5-4. Simultaneously push the left leg hard to the rear, pressing the left foot flat to the floor and locking the knee cap. To keep the ankle lifted imagine that you are lifting and stretching the left calf to touch the wall to the rear.

3. When the right leg is bent 90°, lower the right side of the chest to the right thigh. As you lower the chest to the knee rub it along into and across the right thigh, with the rubbing pressure felt running from the outside to the inner side of this thigh. Simultaneously with the same twisting movement rooted in the lower waste, roll the left side of the chest and ribs backward.

4. The buttock muscle is rolled in toward the groin such that the groin skin is stretched and extended towards the navel. Keep the left hip down, rolled backward and straight in line with the rest of the left side of the body. With the proper bending and twisting movement above the body will be in a line similar to that showed in Fig. 3-7, with the nipples perpendicular to the floor and both hips in line with both shoulders.

5. The head is kept straight in line with the body and turned enough so that the left arm may still be seen by the right eye if the left one is shut momentarily. Keep this outstretched left arm in line with the rest of the body not letting it swing up or down, or side to side.

6. An intense alternative: Place the right shoulder on the left side of the knee rather that of the right side. This enhances leverage where the upper arm and inner knee press each other.

IV. Teaching procedure:

Insist on students performing each step perfectly whenever his ability allows. i.e. when jumping 4 feet the feet should be parallel or even slightly turned inward, hands locked at the knuckles, Fig. 3-11, knees locked, Fig. 3-9, etc.,

This and some of the other standing postures can be done with the rear foot touching the wall. Have the student press the heel to and extend his calf toward the wall as covered in point 2 above. This raises the rear left ankle slightly putting 'life' into it, and pressing the foot flat to the floor.

6. VIRABHADRASANA I

30 sec. on each side with full breathing.

10. PRASARITA PADOTTANASANA I

(Spread leg stretching posture)

This posture develops the hamstring and abductor muscles of the leg. It is a semi inverted posture and so has some of the effects as Sirsasana (headstand). Circulation is increased in the trunk and head and the digestive powers are increased.

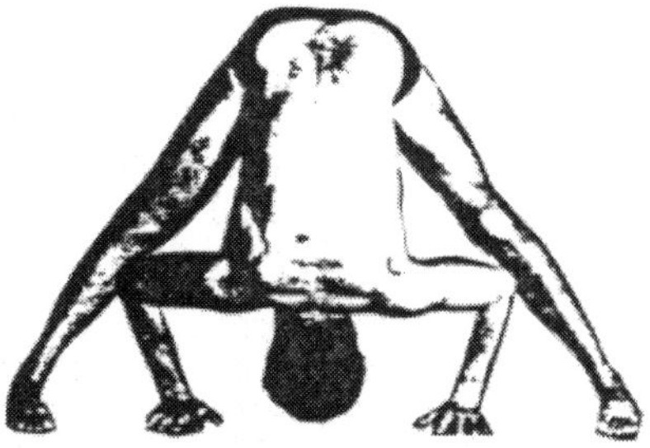

Fig. 10-0

I. Basic procedure:

1. From Tadasana [1] jump on an exhalation and spread the feet 4-5 feet apart. Raise both hands over the head and stretch backward and upward, Fig. 10-1. Inhale deeply and then on the exhalation bend forward placing the palms on the floor, and looking straight to the front, Fig. 10-2. Remember to keep the knee caps lifted up into the thigh.

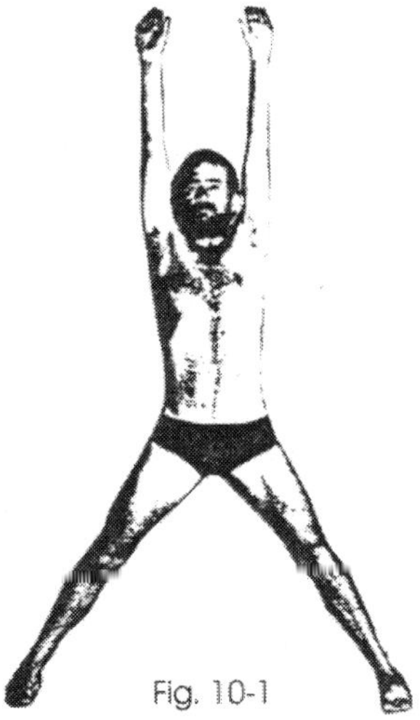

Fig. 10-1

Remain in position shown in Fig. 10-2 for 15 sec. with full even breathing. Then in an exhalation lower the trunk further to the floor until the head touches it lightly resting directly between the feet. Now move the palms in until they too are in line with the head and the feet. Fig. 10-3

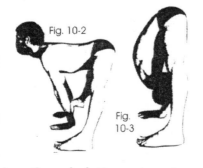

2. Stay in this pasture for 30 sec. with full breathing gazing straight to the rear. Then on an exhalation raise the trunk up to position in Fig. 10-2, inhale deeply and on the exhalation return to position in Fig. 10-1 and jump back to Tadasana.

Fig. 10-2

Fig. 10-3

II. Variation procedure:

In the beginning one probably can't touch the head to the floor, but you can aim it towards the floor. The very stiff beginner can grasp the ankles, shins, or knees, instead of putting his bands on the floor. He should bend as far as possible always making sure that the legs are locked - this is far more important than the degree of bend you attain.

One can also place the hands on the hips and bend. Any variation is as good as the basic posture if it is your maximum ability and if you do it with the greatest degree of watchfulness of which you are capable.

III. Perfecting procedure:

1. The feet are kept parallel to each other throughout the whole movement. Have the toes slightly turn in toward each other, which lift the arch and the ankle, Fig.-10-0.

2. When bending into the position in Fig.10-2, extend the chest outward to the front while pulling the shoulders and arms backward and upward. Doing this help keep the back straight so that you bend only from the lower lumbar region. If the hands are allowed to drop faster than the head when moving then one bends from the wrong part of the spine, Fig. 10-4.

3. As you bend into position in Fig. 10-2, extend the chin upward so you continue to gaze to the front. The back should be kept as concave as possible throughout the bending movements. Compare Fig. 10-2 with the same done incorrectly in Fig. 10-4, where the bend is occurring at the mid back region.

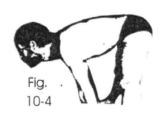

Fig. 10-4

IV. Teaching procedure:

Have the students thrust the hands upward, and stretch backward before bending forward to help loosen the spine for the bend. This posture has the same buttock movement as in Adho Mukha Svanasana [18]. The buttocks are rolled outward and upward towards the ceiling; this opens up the groin and anus area. Slap or tap the student's thighs upward to re-enforce this awareness and 'brush' them outward. Slap or tap the back to re-enforce awareness to the concaveness to aim for.

18. ADHO MUKHA SVANASANA
    50 sec. with full breathing.
19. URDHVA MUKHA SVANASANA
    60 sec. with full breathing.

24. VIRASANA III

(Hero)

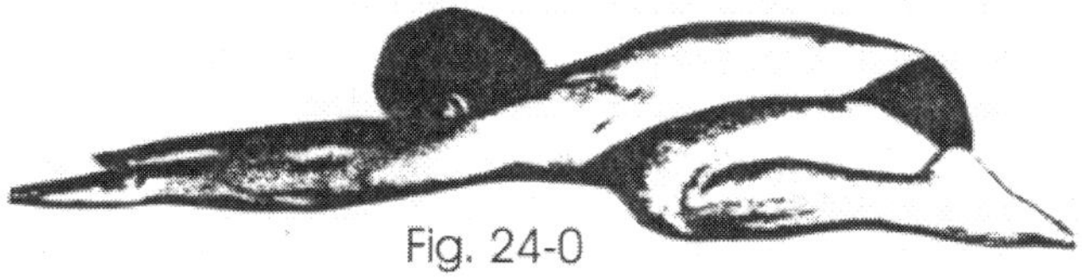

Fig. 24-0

Stay in the first movement, Virasana I. Fig. 23-1, as long as you like with normal breathing. Stay in the second movement, Virasana II. Fig. 23-0, for 60 sec. with full breathing. Now do this third movement, Fig. 24-0, as described below. The third movement stretches the shoulders. It opens up the pelvic region and removes stiffness in the lumbar and sacral regions of the spine.

<u>I. Basic procedure:</u>

1. From the second movement, Fig. 23-0, release the finger lock and turn the palms to face the front. Spread the knees apart as far as possible

2. On the exhalation bend trunk forward, placing your chest and abdomen between the thighs as close to the floor as possible.

3. Stretch your arms out in front of you as far as they will go, and stretch the head back so the chin rubs the floor, extending toward the hands. Gaze between the eyebrows towards the hands. Stay in this posture for 30-60 sec. with normal even breathing.

4. On an inhalation, return to the position in Fig. 23-1

<u>III. Perfecting procedure:</u>

1. As you bend forward maintain as much of the upward extension of the arms and shoulders of the second movement, Fig. 23-0, as possible. The arms are lifted high and lowered to the floor along with the head and trunk.

2. Sink your chest and abdomen down to the floor pressing as much of them on the floor as possible, This is done by relaxing the pelvis / leg joints and opening them up, and by rolling the buttock muscle outward as in Adho Mukha Svanasana [18].

Simultaneously continue extending and stretching your arms to the front as far as they will go. Open up the armpits.

<u>IV. Teaching procedure:</u>

Push the lower back down toward the floor, as this is where the bend must come from. Try place the student's palms on blocks (or books) 2-6 inches high off the floor in order to increase his awareness of the need to keep the back and arms as straight as possible.

16. ARDHA NAVASANA
    30-60 sec. with shallow breathing.
26. BHARADVAJASANA I.
    30 sec. each side with full breathing
13. SAVASANA
    5-15 min. with normal breathing or pranayama [14]

LESSON III

3. UTTHITA TRIKONASANA
   30 sec. each side with full breathing.
5. UTTHITA PARSVAKONASANA
   30 sec. each side with full breathing.
6. VIRABHADRASANA I
   30 sec. in each direction with full breathing.
10. PRASARITA PADOTTANASANA I.
   30 sec. in each position with full breathing.
18. ADHO MUKHA SVANASANA
   50 sec. with full breathing
19. URDHVA MUKHA SVANASANA
   50 sec. with full breathing

21. SALABHASANA

(Locust posture)

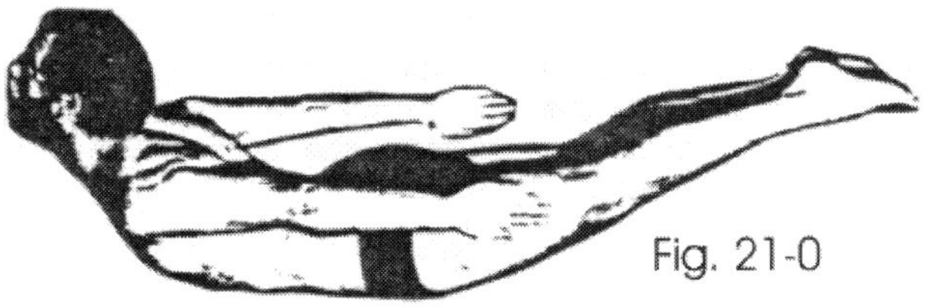

Fig. 21-0

This posture develops the sacral and lumbar regions of the spine, and strengthens the abdominal and leg muscles. The pressure on the abdominal area aids digestion and relieves gastric trouble. The prostate gland and the bladder are also benefited.

I. Basic procedure:

1. Lie face down on the floor with the ankles touching and the hands by the hip.

2. With an exhalation lift the head, chest, and legs (simultaneously) as high as possible off the floor and extend the arms straight to the rear.

3. Stay for 50 sec. with normal breathing and gaze between the eyebrows. Then lower the feet and chest to the floor slowly and rest.

II. Variation procedure:

Beginners should follow the same procedure as above but for a shorter time, and with a smaller degree of leg and chest lift. If this is still too strenuous you can place the hands down on the floor and raise only the head and the legs. An even easier variation than this is to lift only one leg at a time and hold for 10 sec. while the other leg remains on the floor.

III. Perfecting procedure:

1. The chin is extended outward, and raised upward, which stretches the neck. The ribs are lifted until they are almost entirely off the floor. Aim at resting the body weight on the lower abdomen area between the navel and the pubes.

2. Contracting the buttock muscle and rolling it in towards the anus brings added lift to the legs. The thigh muscle is stretched and the legs extended, locked straight, and touching at the thighs, knees, and the ankles as possible. Lock the arms at the elbows, and hands at the knuckles.

Fig. 21-1

Fig. 21-2

Compare Fig. 21-1, which shows correctly locked knees, elbows, and knuckle joints to the same area done with less attention, as shown in Fig. 22-2.

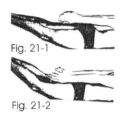

3. The shoulders are lifted and rolled back towards the feet. Feel as if you are trying to pull the shoulder blades inward in order to touch each other.

IV. Teaching procedure:

Have the student try to get a maximum chest lift by allowing him to leave the legs on the floor. You can hold them down for him, while he tries to lift his ribs and chest off the floor. Then hold the students legs up 6-10 inches off the floor and have him lift off again according to the Basic procedure for this posture.

Next, have him aim for a maximum leg lift by allowing him to keep the trunk on the floor, with the arms at the sides.

One can also do the posture with legs bent at the knee, the thighs 6 inches apart, and the shins perpendicular to the floor. On an exhalation, lift the chest and legs as in the basic posture. Brings the legs together, attempting to touch the knees while maintaining the same degree of lift. You can pull students arms back.

23. 24. VIRASANA
Stay in the first movement Fig. 23-1, as long as you like with normal or Pranayama breathing. Stay in the next two movements, Fig. 23-2, Fig. 24-0, for 60 sec. each with full breathing.

15. PARIPOORNA NAVASANA

(Entire boat posture)

This posture strengthens the back and the stomach and helps reduce fat around the waste. It works on the intestines and relieves the bloating sensation in the abdomen.

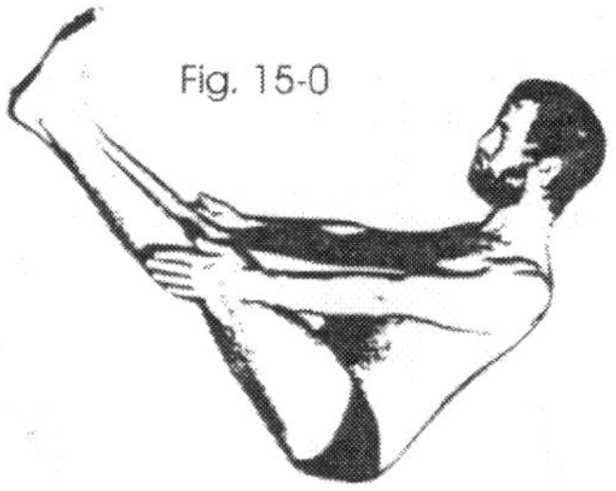
Fig. 15-0

I. Basic procedure:

1. Sit on the floor with palms by the side, legs locked at the knee, and arms locked at the elbow. Extend the chest and lift the back of the neck. This is a Yoga posture called Dandasana (staff posture). Fig. 15-1

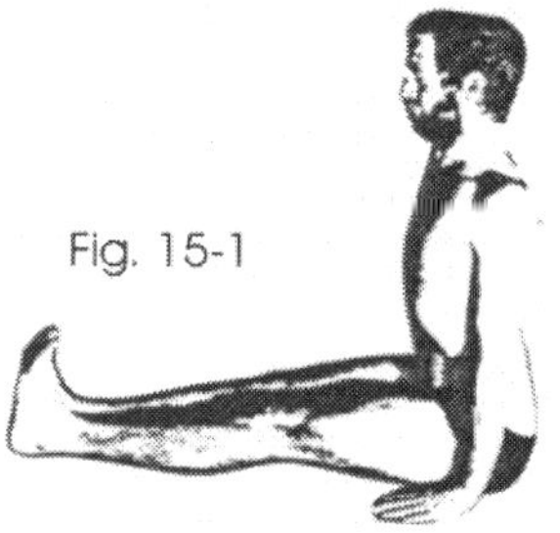
Fig. 15-1

2. With an exhalation recline the trunk backwards and raise the legs until the feet are a foot or so higher than the head and touching at the ankles. Now aim at balancing on the soft part of the buttock only so that no part of the lower spine touches the floor.

3. Extend the arms straight passed the knee, parallel to the floor, with the palms facing each other. Extend the arms as far passed the knee as possible by raising the trunk and legs further and pulling them in towards each other.

4. Hold this position for 30 sec. with normal breathing, gazing toward the feet. Increase the length of stay to 60 sec., then return to Dandasana.

Or, go directly into the next posture Ardha Navasana [16] by lowering the legs to 18 in. off the floor, curving the back and lowering the trunk. Finally, place the interlocked hands behind the head.

II. Variation procedure:

Beginners may be unable to position the palms by the knees let alone past them, or raise his legs higher than his head, but he should always aim for this. Whatever the degree of leg lift possible etc, ensure that the back, arms and legs are kept straight and balance is on the soft part of the buttock.

III. Perfecting procedure:

The back of the neck is lifted and extended backward (Tadasana [1]) and the back is kept some-what concave . The sternum is lifted and the chest extended towards the feet, while the shoulders are rolled backward, Fig. 15-2. This is opposite to the movement done in Ardha Navasana, Fig. 15-3.

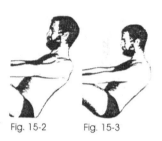

Fig. 15-2

Fig. 15-3

IV. Teaching procedure:

Place a chair under the student's calves to support his legs, thus freeing him to concentrate on getting the correct type of lift of the trunk and the proper chest expansion.

16. ARDHA NAVASANA
10 sec. with normal breathing.
26. BHARADVAJASANA I
Stay 10 sec. each side with full breathing.

11. UTTANASANA

(intense stretch posture)

This posture benefits the nervous system. The spinal nerves are rejuvenated and mental depression relieved if the posture is held for longer than 3 minutes. Those who are easily excitable will find this relaxing.

Discomfort felt by beginners in the head stand may be relieved by doing this posture before and after doing a head stand. It relieves menstrual pains and aids digestion.

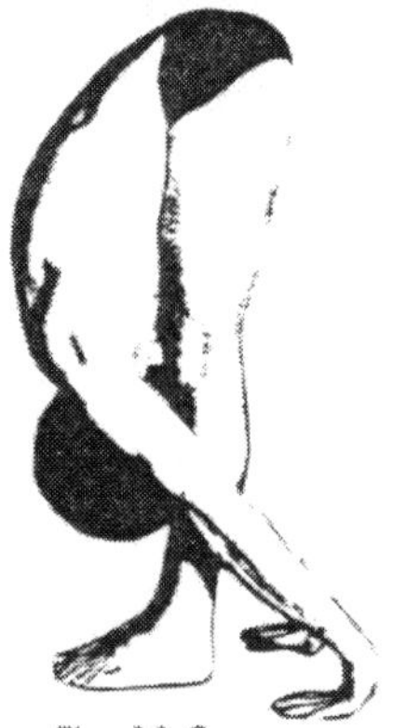

Fig. 11-0

I. Basic procedure:

1. From Tadasana [1] raise the arms over the head on an inhalation and stretch them upward towards the ceiling and thus expanding the chest. Fig.11-1

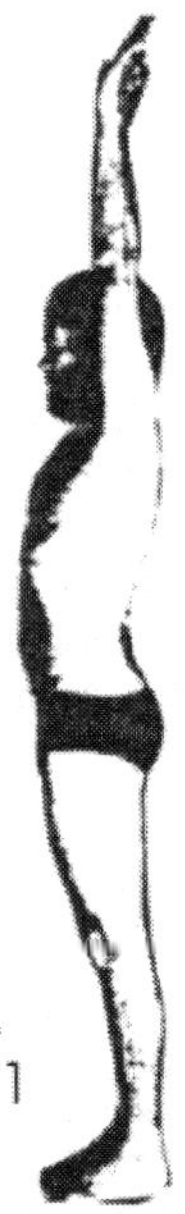

Fig. 11-1

2. On an exhalation swing the trunk and the arms radially outward and downward in a semi-circle arc. Then place the hands palms down, on the floor behind you as far as they will go until the chest is pressed flat against the thighs.

3. Place the head on the shins and rocking forward slightly on the balls of the feet. Move the hips forward so that the legs are perpendicular to the floor. Stay in the posture for 1-5 minutes with full breathing. Maintain the lock on the knees and the elbows and gaze either between the eyes or at nose level

4. Return to Tadasana in two steps. First upon an inhalation lift the head off the shin and raise the chin as high as it will go without lifting the palms. Then on the following exhalation raise the palms off the floor and raise the trunk back to Tadasana.

II. Variation procedure:

Mainly concern yourself here with maintaining a concave back during the forward bend. Keep the legs locked, arms extended outward and lifted along with the shoulders. Turn the head up so the chin extends towards the outstretched hands.

One should not be concerned with "touching the floor" as this only encourages incorrect bending. Instead, think of getting an expanded chest as close to the thighs as possible. On no account should the legs ever bend, even the slightest in order to get you lower to the floor. Such cheating only cheats yourself.

III. Perfecting procedure:

1. Keep the back concave while bending, Fig; 11-2. Extend the arms, chin, and chest outward and lift the shoulders keeping all in line with the trunk. Concentrate on moving from the lowest part of the spine,

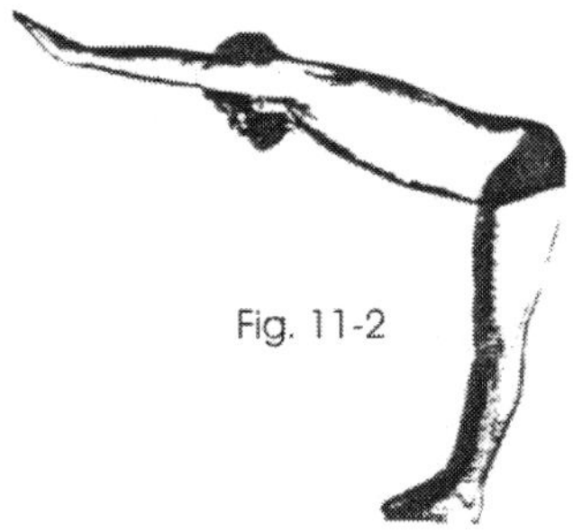

Fig. 11-2

2. After you are in the final position, adjust the body weight and spread it evenly over the feet, from toes to heels, and from big tow to small toe. In order for the legs to be perpendicular to the floor there may be a little added pressure on the balls of the feet. People often tend to stand with more weight on their heels.

3. When the thighs are pulled tight the skin of the leg feels like its being drawn upward and inward. Simultaneously stretch the side ribs and shoulders down towards the floor, rubbing the thighs with the chest. The skin of the ribs should feel like its being pulled down wards. This challenging (or antagonistic) action is common throughout Yoga; here the movement on the thighs being upward and on the trunk being downward. Keep shoulder relaxed and abdomen firmly in.

II. Teaching Procedure:

The posture may be done with the arms fold over the head, but using the same principles of movement as above. This eliminates the tendency to "touch the floor" and so one can concentrate on extending the trunk.

As a variation have the student place his feet 6 inches apart with arms folded. This is used as a rest posture to catch ones breath after strenuous postures. You can have him stand with feet 12 inches away from a wall and with his buttocks resting on the wall, which leaves the student free to concentrate on the upward pull of the thighs and the downward stretch of the ribs and shoulders.

Get the student to open up the buttock, rolling the muscle of the buttock outward and away from the anus raising it upward as done in Adho Mukha Svanasana [18]. If the posture is done against the wall the student can pull his buttock muscle upward with his hands and then maintaining this lift he should rest this raised buttock back on the wall

Have student grasp his ankles first and pull himself, his trunk, in towards his thigh as much as possible before he places his palms on the floor behind him.

Watch out for caving-in ankles and the resulting falling insteps (Fig. 1-5). Have the student turn his toes inward until they touch while keeping his heels apart, as a variation that lifts the ankles and helps lock the knees.

13. SAVASANA
5—15 minutes with normal or Pranayama breathing.

LESSON IV

3. UTTHITA TRIKONASANA
30 sec. each side with full breathing.

4. PARIVRTTA TRIKONASANA

(Three angle posture revolved)

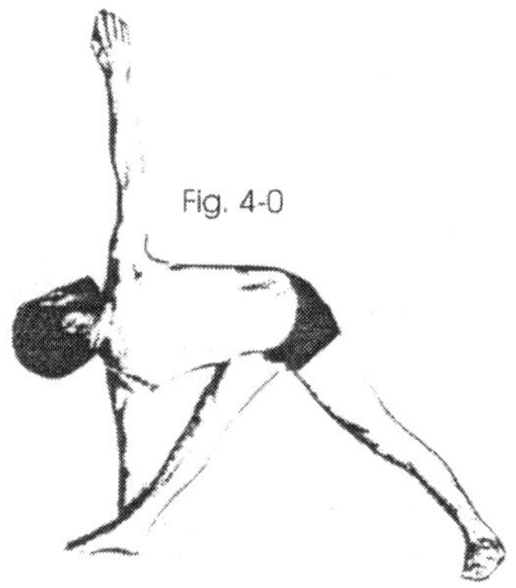

Fig. 4-0

This posture gives a good lateral twist increasing blood supply in the lower parts of the spine, which helps relieve pains in the lower back. The muscle of the back, hip, thigh, calf and hamstrings are strengthened and toned. It has an invigorating effect on the abdominal organs and promotes full chest expansion.

I. Basic procedure:

1. From Tadasana [1] inhale deeply and exhaling jump spreading the legs 3-4 feet apart. Turn the right foot 90° to the right and move the left foot slightly to the right.

2. Simultaneously revolve the trunk and bend to the right and place the left hand, palm down, outside the right foot, with the fingers in line with the toes.

As the left hand is brought to the floor the right one is raised and thrust toward the ceiling and held stretched perpendicular to the floor, Fig. 4-0.

3. The legs and arms are locked and the trunk is twisted to the right as much as possible. Stay in this posture for 30 sec. with normal breathing, gazing upward past the right hand. Then on an inhalation return to position similar to Fig. 3-1. Repeat on the left side.

II. Variation procedure:

If you are still too stiff to place the hand on the floor, grasp the ankle. You can also move the feet closer together and place the right hand on the hip instead of stretching it upward. This makes the balance easier. Use the grip of the hand on the hip to push the right shoulder backwards. Use the grip of the hand on the ankle to pull the left shoulder in line with the right foot.

You can also place your left hand on the inside (instep side) of the forward foot on the floor as close to this foot as possible, and still keep balance.

III. Perfecting procedure:

1. The whole of the right leg should be turned 90° to the right along with the right foot. Both right and left feet should touch the floor completely. The left leg is extended hard to the rear which pushes the outer side of the left foot firmly to the floor.

2. The firm extension of the left foot to the rear gives leverage to the twisting action of the lower spine via the left hand which also presses hard into the floor.

Pressing hard into the floor, using the left arm as a lever, screw the left shoulder to the right. At the same time, thrust the upper right shoulder backward.

This results in the arms, shoulders, and the trunk held in a perpendicular line to the floor, which allows the head to be turned enough so that the extended right hand (thumb) can still be seen when the right eye is shut momentarily, Fig. 4-1. Compare this with insufficient twisting of the trunk and shoulders shown in Fig. 4-2.

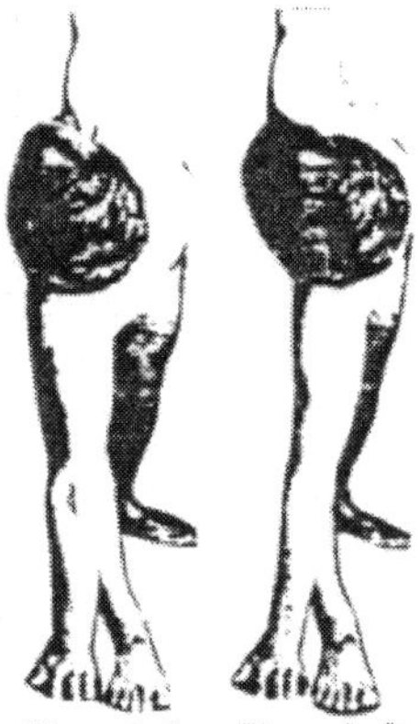

Fig. 4-1 Fig. 4-2

IV. Teaching procedure:

Always have the student take a deep inhalation in Tadasana [1] before jumping on an exhalation. Follow up on the breathing, insuring that extension movements are done on an exhalation and return or recovery movements are done on the inhalation. Encourage him to breathe as evenly as possible, and not hold his breath at any time.

Instead of placing the hand on the floor, have the student place his hand on his shin bone, or rest it on a bench. He then turns his trunk until his shoulder is directly over his foot and the arm is perpendicular to the floor. This gets the student more aware of the twisting of the trunk that is aimed for when the hand is place on the floor.

5. UTTHITA PARSVAKONASANA
   10 sec. on each side with full breathing.
6. VIRABHADRASANA I
   10 sec. on each side with full breathing.
10. PRASARITA PADOTTANASANA I
   10 sec. in each position with full breathing.

25. JANU SIRSASANA

(Knee head posture)

The abdominal organs are toned through doing this posture regularly.

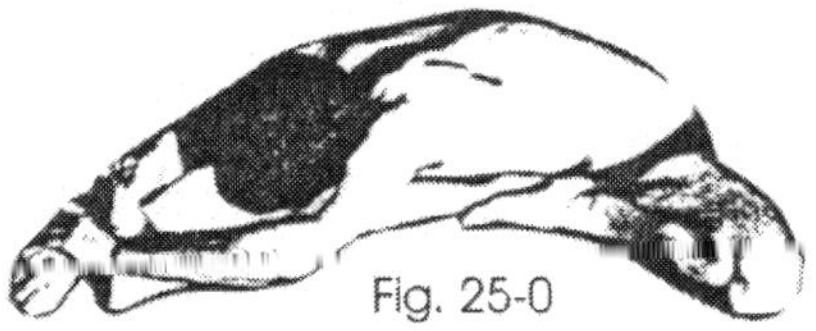

Fig. 25-0

The effect is especially pronounced on the kidneys. This posture develops frontal flexibility and tones the shoulder muscles.

I. Basic procedure:

1. From Dandasana [15] Fig. 15-1, place the left heel at the junction of the thigh and the groin, with the big toe of the left foot touching the inner side of the right thigh. Push the bent left knee as far back as you can, forming an obtuse angle between the left shin bone and the extended right leg. Place the left hand on left knee and the right hand by right hip.

2. Draw the shoulders back, raise the sternum, and extend the chest.

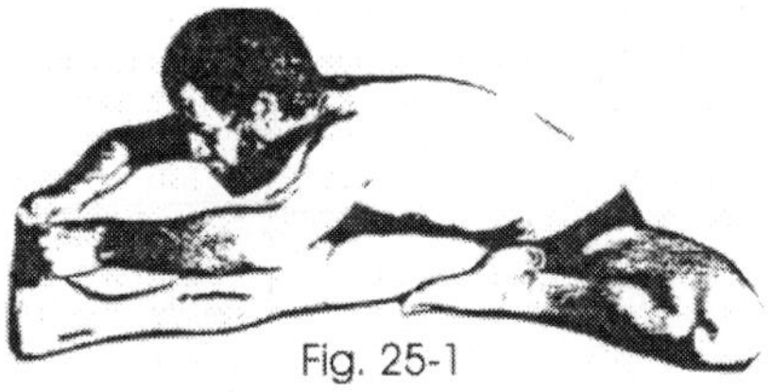

Fig. 25-1

Stretch the spine upward and forward, and lift the back of the neck. Then, bending forward, extend the arms and grasp the bail of the right foot. Fig. 25-1

3. Bend further forward on your following exhalations until the chin rests beyond the knee. Now exhale deeply and extend the arms past the right foot and grasp the wrist of the right hand with the left hand, Fig. 25-0

4. With each exhalation push the chest further downward rubbing it along the center of the thigh. Gazing between the eyebrows towards the feet, hold this position for 30 sec. with full breathing.

Then with an inhalation raise the head and chest off the leg, stretch the chin upward gazing toward the ceiling, and extend the spine making it concave again. Straighten up on the exhalation and repeat on the other side, this time grasping the wrist of the left hand with the right hand.

II. Variation procedure:

Those who are not able to reach the toes can grasp the extended leg with both hands as far down towards the foot as possible. The principle of movement here is the same as for Uttanasana [11], Fig. 11-0. One doesn't aim at touching the feet but instead tries to extend the whole trunk forward, Fig. 25-2.

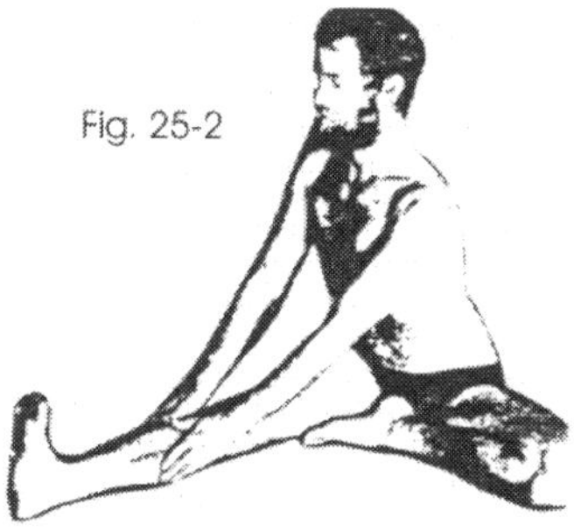
Fig. 25-2

Maintain a lifted and extended chest and concentrate on bending from the lowest part of the spine, near the sacral region, keeping the rest of the back from lumbar to the neck concave or as flat as possible.

III. Perfecting procedure:

1. When the angle between the shin of the bent leg and the straight leg is as obtuse as possible, place both hands on the floor by the hips and lift the buttocks slightly off the floor. Simultaneously rotate the hip slightly so the trunk faces forward. Increased pressure on the left hip will now be felt due to the obtuse angle of the left shin/leg challenging the forward facing trunk.

2. Throughout the movement the knee cap is pulled so tight (locking the right leg) that the skin on the back of the knee touches the floor. Keep the right foot perpendicular to the floor, not allowing it to slant either side to side or front to back. Extend the heel from the calf and curl the toes in slightly towards the head, keeping the toes in a line parallel to the forehead.

3. Raise the ribs, lift the center of the chest and chin and extend them upward and outward throughout the bending movement. Much of the bending force comes from this frontal area, and if properly applied the vital lower back bend will follow naturally. One extends the floating ribs and sternum and aims at "touching the feet with them". This eventually results in the chest being rubbed down the thigh towards the feet, with the center of the chest touching the center of the leg.

4. Bend forward gradually, inch by inch. You will find this bending coming best if done on the exhalations. First grasp the toes, then the balls of the feet, then clasp the hands past the feet, and finally grasp the wrist beyond the feet. When your own maximum bend is reached, relax the chin and rest it on the shin.

5. Don't let the elbows and shoulders droop to the floor as show in Fig. 25-3. Lift the shoulders throughout the posture, pushing the shoulder blades in towards each other and keep the elbows level with the toes of the right foot, as shown in Fig. 25-0, 25-1.

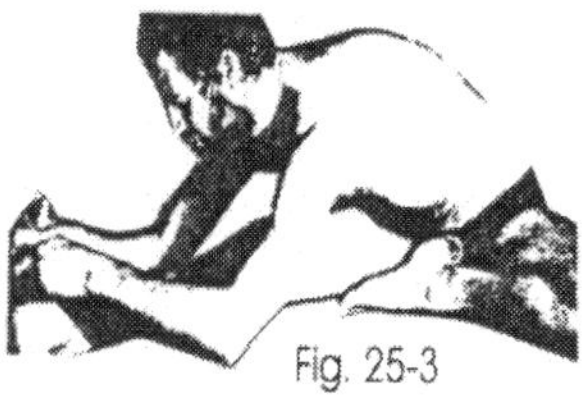
Fig. 25-3

6. Put special attention on pulling the ribs on the side of the body of the bent left leg down toward the floor, Fig. 25-1, and extend the shoulder on this side towards the straight leg on the other side. This helps keep the back level where otherwise it tends to slant.

7. For that extra bit of bend, one can pause breathing momentarily at the end of each exhalation. After a year or two of practice one will be able to grasp the wrists Fiq. 25-0. Here the hand on the same side of the body as the straight leg is clenched firmly into a fist (not overly tight please) and its wrist is then held firmly by the hand on the bent leg side of the body. Remember to change wrists when repeating the posture on the other side.

IV. Teaching procedure:

Place a folding chair in front on the student, and have him place the toes of his straight leg on the lower cross tubing of the chair. He then grasps the legs of the chair instead of his foot and this helps him keep his back level while bending forward.

You can also help by pushing the side of the trunk on the bent leg side of the body towards the floor, and lift up any drooping elbows.

Students who can't reach their foot may loop a towel or rope around the extended right foot and grasping both loose ends, pull their trunks forward.

18. ADHO MUKHA SVANASANA
60 sec. with full breathing
19. URDHVA MUKHA SVANASANA
60 sec. with full breathing
21. SALABHASANA
30-60 sec. with normal breathing.

22. USTRASANA

(Camel posture)

In this posture the spine is stretched backward and toned while the pelvis is thrust forward. A flexible spine is one of the the best insurance against the feebleness that comes with old age.

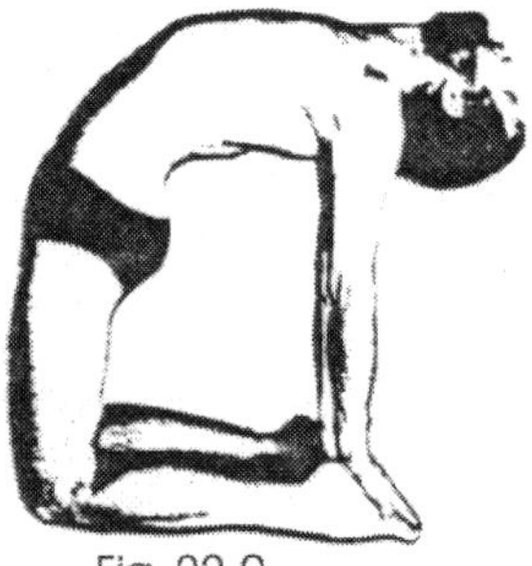

Fig. 22-0

I. Basic procedure:

1. Kneel on the floor with the thighs and feet touching, and place the palms on the hips with the thumbs pressing into the lower spine, Fig. 22-1,

2. On the exhalation curve the trunk backwards and place the palms on the soles of the feet, Fig. 22-0. Simultaneously stretch the chest upward and the thighs forward

3. Press the feet with the palms, throw the head back as far as it will go, and push the lower spine towards the thighs. This movement, plus the upwards and forward stretching of the thighs, pushes the pelvis forward away from the feet.

4. Hold this posture for 10 sec. with normal breathing, gazing between the eyebrows at the wall behind you. Release the hands one by one and straighten the trunk.

II. Variation procedure:

The bend will come a little easier for beginners if the legs are kept 8-12 inches apart at the knees and feet. After completing one bend with knees apart repeat the posture with the knees and feet touching.

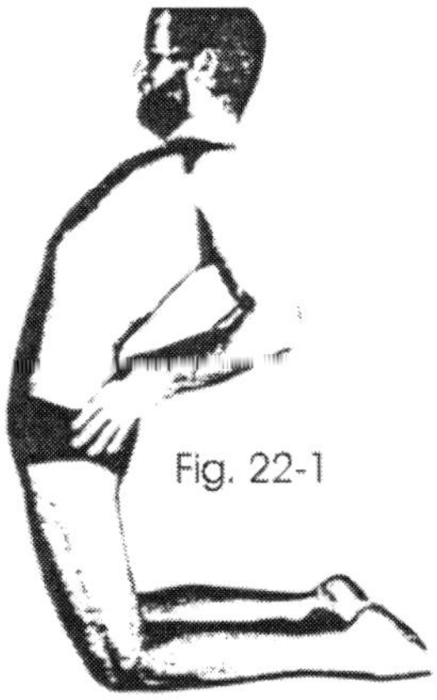

Fig. 22-1

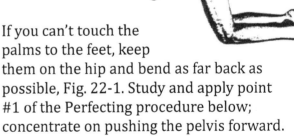

If you can't touch the palms to the feet, keep them on the hip and bend as far back as possible, Fig. 22-1. Study and apply point #1 of the Perfecting procedure below; concentrate on pushing the pelvis forward.

III. Perfecting procedure:

1. The palms are placed with the thumbs resting on the spine. Dig the thumbs into the spine at the point of bend and thrust the pelvis forward while bending the trunk backward. Open up the lower spinal vertebrae with massaging pressure from the thumbs.

2. Roll the buttocks in toward the anus, tightening the anus and opening out the groin area. This movement feels like one is curling the tailbone inward and simultaneously spreading

open and lifting the groin. This is very important for achieving advanced back-bends later.

3. Raise the sternum and open up the chest by pulling the shoulder blades in towards each other. The lower floating ribs however are pushed downward toward the pelvis. Simultaneously move the lower lumbar part of the spine upward towards the navel and thrust the thighs and the buttocks forward until the thighs are perpendicular to the floor

4. The ankles can be grabbed to give leverage for pulling the shoulders downward toward the feet. The chin is stretched to the rear with the head thrust back as far as it will go.

IV. Teaching procedure:

The teacher faces the student and leaning over him places his hands on the students lower back, or alternately hoop a rope under this area and hold the ends. Have the student grasp the ankles firmly while you lift and draw his ribs and pelvis forward.

Encourage the student to open up the groin, tighten the buttock muscle, and curl it and the tailbone in toward the anus. Simultaneously have him "make space" in the lower lumbar region by stretching the lumbar vertebrae laterally during the bending movement. This develops the bend in the proper area of the spine instead of higher up on the spine as often occurs.

23. VIRASANA
    Stay as long as you like with normal breathing.
23. 24. VIRASANA II. and III.
    60 sec. each with full even breathing.
15. PARIPOORNA NAVASANA
    60 sec. with normal even breathing.
16. ARDHA NAVASANA
    30-60 sec. with normal to shallow breathing.
26. BHARADVAJASANA I.
    30 sec. each side with full breathing.
11. UTTANASANA
    1 to 5 minutes with full breathing.
13. SAVASANA
    5-15 minutes with normal breathing or pranayama.

LESSON V

3. UTTHITA TRIKONASANA
    10 sec. each side with full breathing.
4. PARIVRTTA TRIKONASANA
    30 sec. each side faith normal even breathing.
5. UTTHITA PARSVAKONASANA
    30 sec. each side with full breathing.

8. VIRABHADRASANA III

(Warrior posture)

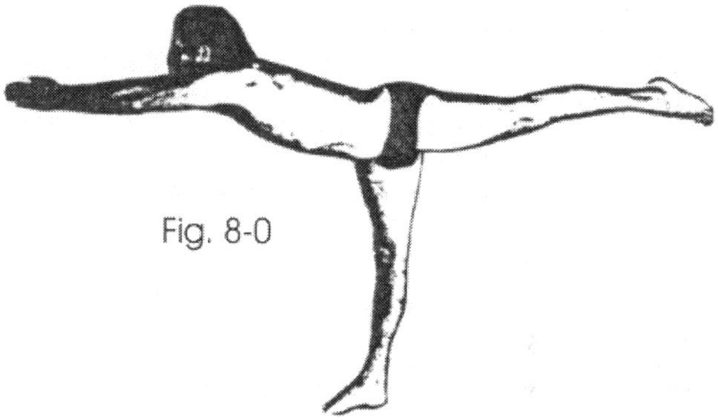

Fig. 8-0

This posture improves ones sense of balance and increases poise by developing power and agility. It strengthens the shoulders, abdominal muscles, back, hip, and leg muscle and it develops firm ankle support.

I. Basic procedure:

1. Inhale deeply and with an exhalation jump, spreading the legs 4 feet apart. Do Virabhadrasana I [6] Fig. 6-0, on the right side briefly.

2. On an exhalation, lower the trunk to the thigh, Fig. 8-1, and take several full breaths. Then, on an exhalation, lift the trunk off the thigh and raise the left leg as you straighten and lock the right one.

3. Lift and extend the arms forward and the left leg backward until the whole body is parallel to the floor, Fig. 8-0. Stretch yourself out horizontally as though two people were pulling you apart, one at each end.

4. Gazing out beyond the extended hands, hold the posture for 20-10 sec. with full breathing. Return to posture in Fig. 8-1 on an exhalation and inhaling return to Virabhadrasana I [6] and repeat on the other side.

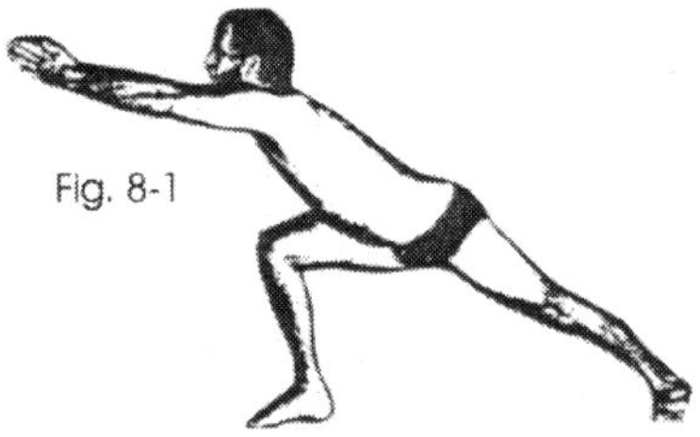
Fig. 8-1

II. Variation procedure:

If the balance is too difficult or the posture too strenuous you can try the posture with the hands placed on the waste, thumbs pointing toward the spine. This helps you feel where your hips are, whether they are level and parallel to the floor as they should be, or slanted to the floor as explained below.

III. Perfecting procedure:

1. Many tend to lock the thumbs of the joined hands either in this posture or in Virabhadrasana I [6], Fig. 8-2. Instead, rest the thumbs side by side as shown in Fig. 8-3. Guard against tilting the hands up, down, or to the side; just extend them to the front. The same applies to the rear foot. It should be in line with the left leg with the toes pointing directly to the rear.

Fig. 8-2

Fig. 8-3

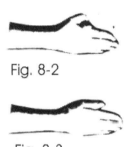

2. Keep the sternum raised with the chest stretched outward and forward throughout the lifting movement. The lifting of the body off the floor is accomplished by a shifting forward of the body weight and not just by lifting upward: the arms and chest are thrust forward as the right leg is straightened, thus swinging the body slightly forward as it is raised.

The degree of lift possible on the left rear leg is partly determined by the extent of tightening of the right leg, so raise the left leg further by pulling the right knee cap up into the thigh.

4. Though the left leg is held high, the left hip is kept down level with the right hip and parallel to the floor. Fig. 8-4 shows the left hip raised too high, compare this with the same hip correctly rolled downward and inward toward the right leg as shown in Fig. 8-0.

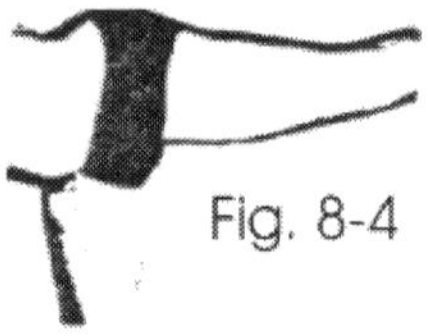
Fig. 8-4

5. Balance is often made more difficult when the ankles are loose. Concentrate on firming them and the rest of the right legs such that the whole leg from the bottoms of the right foot to the hip is felt to be the trunk of an oak tree rooted firmly in the ground.

IV. Teaching procedure:

Slap or tap any rising left hips down so the students remember to keep it rolling downward into the right leg. Encourage the student to keep the abdominal muscle firm so the belly doesn't hang down. Check to see that their faces are relaxed. This is especially true for this and all other strenuous postures.

You and an assistant can stretch and lift the arms and left leg of the students momentarily to increase his awareness of the height and stretch aimed for in the posture. Then let him continue alone aiming for that.

9. PARSVOTTANASANA

(Side stretching posture)

This posture developes flexibility in the wrists and tones the muscles of the forearm. It helps to correct drooping shoulders, drawing them back, which helps develop fuller breathing. Flexibility and elasticity are increased in the hips and spine.

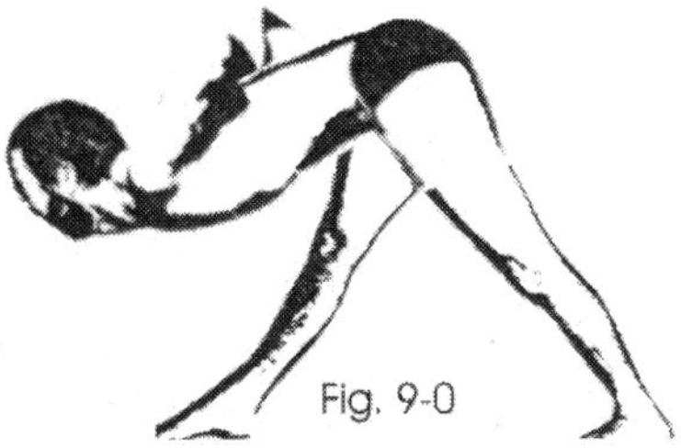
Fig. 9-0

I. Basic procedure:

1. Stand in Tadasana [1] and on a full exhalation, join palms behind the back. The fingers should be on the level of the shoulder blades with the palms touching as much as possible. Fig. 9-1

2. On an exhalation jump, spreading the feet 3 ft. apart or less. Turn the right foot 90° to the right and the left foot 70° to the right. Lock both legs firmly by pulling the knee caps up into the thighs. Rotate the trunk 90° to the right. Then inhaling fully, throw the head back as far as it will go, extending the chin and shoulders to the rear. Fig. 9-2

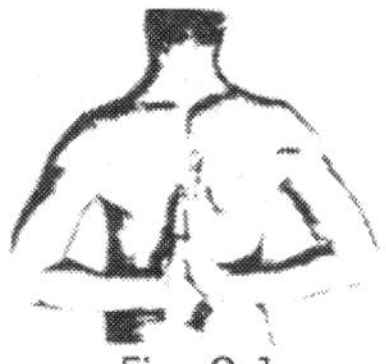
Fig. 9-1

3. On a full exhalation bend the trunk forward halfway, take a full breath and exhale and bend until the abdomen rests flat on the right thigh. Then place the chin on the shin bone of the right calf. Fig. 9-0

4. Stay in this posture for 30 sec. with normal breathing, holding the gaze between the eyebrows and focused toward the feet. With a full inhalation, raise the trunk up. Turn the left foot 90° to the left, etc, and repeat the posture on the left side, then jump back to Tadasana [1] and finally release the palms from behind the back.

5. Keep the lower teeth touching lightly on the upper teeth throughout the movements, especially when stretching backward, Fig. 9-2. This hold true for the other postures in Yoga: keep a firm un-clenched jaw.

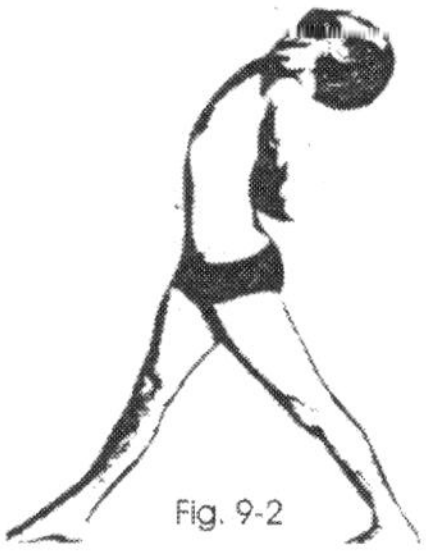
Fig. 9-2

II. Variation procedure:

You won't be able to achieve a maximum bend with your trunk pressed right against your thigh for a few years at least, so be patient. Don't be concerned at all with touching the head to the knee or the chin to the shin for this will lead to faulty bending techniques. Just bend as much as you can while keeping the back as straight as you can, always thrusting the trunk forward and aiming it toward the center of the thigh.

The joining of the palms behind the back is usually difficult in the beginning and one may only be able to touch the fingers. Do whatever you can; increased flexibility will come slowly by surely. The wrist could be grasped by the hand behind the back or the hands place on the hips for awhile until wrist flexibility improves.

III. Perfecting procedure:

1. It is easier to press the palms flat behind the back if you exhale very deeply, lift the chest and stretch the shoulders and elbows back fully.

2. The hips are turned to face the front. One imagines screwing the left hip of the rear leg into the right hip of the forward leg. This squaring of the hips to the front is achieved by digging the rear leg into the floor and using it as leverage to propel its hip forward. Simultaneously dig the front leg into the floor and using it as leverage, push its hip backward toward the rear foot. Initially, keep the pubic area rising when you bend backward.

3. With an exhalation bend forward from the lowest part of the spine (sacral). Suck the abdominal area near the navel in towards the spine as you exhale and extend the chest and the trunk outward and forward, Fig. 9-3. This action helps maintain the concave bend in the lower back. The diaphragm is moved down toward the leg but at the same time is elongated and thrust forward. Keep the center of the chest in line with the center of the thigh as in Janu Sirsasana [25].

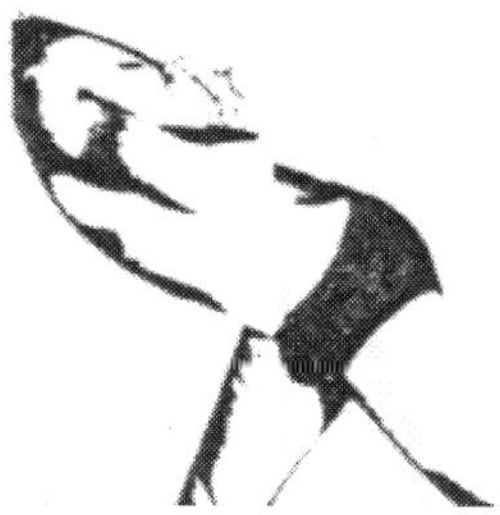
Fig. 9-3

4. In the bending movement, push the right leg deep into the right hip, making this hip/leg junction as acute as possible, as was done in Trikonasana [3]. Simultaneously revolve the other hip, and imagine that you're aiming to touch it to the right leg.

5. Keep extending the chin outward and upward during the forward bend movement. Only after you have achieved the fullest bend possible, for you, can you lower your chin to the leg.

6. Tighten and lengthen the muscle on the inner thigh and calf, turning the right thigh and knee cap well to the front. Use the antagonistic force of the thighs to give maximum rotation of the hip, while insuring that the body weight is evenly distributed over the entire foot.

IV. Teaching procedure:

Make sure the legs are pulled tight at the knees and that the student is aiming to press the chest to the thigh, rather than the head to the knee.

Have the student place his hands on his hips and push them until the hips face the front.

For the first several months to a year have the student do this posture keeping his chin extending upward and outward. Once he has attained enough strength and flexibility to press some of his abdomen on his upper thigh, he may lower his head towards the leg.

10. PRASARITA PADOTTANASANA
10 sec. each position with full breathing

12. SARVANGASANA

(Supported whole body posture)

The Sarvangasana posture is the mother of yogic postures. It has a curative effect on most common ailments, especially those of the head and chest area, i.e. asthma, bronchitis, palpitations, breathlessness, and sore throats. Regular practice of this posture reduces common colds and sinus problems. It soothes the nerves and thus benefits sufferers of epilepsy, hypertension, insomnia, those with nervous breakdowns, and those prone to be easily irritated. Due to the inversion of the body the abdominal organs are activated, relieving pains in this area and causing the bowels to move freely. It also helps to relieve urinary and menstrual disorders. Regular practice twice a day relieves anemia and brings new vitality, especially to those recovering from a long illness.

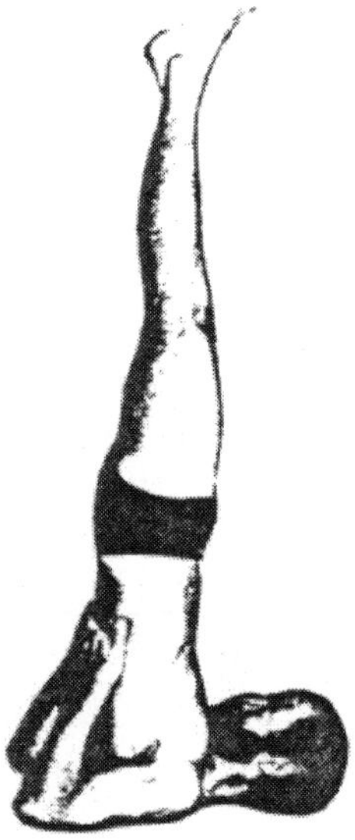

Fig. 12-0

Those with high blood pressure should do Halasana [29], for several minutes before doing this posture.

I. Basic procedure

1. Lie flat on the floor with the hands, palms down, by the side. On an exhalation raise the legs until they are perpendicular to the floor, Fig. 12-1. On the next exhalation, with legs lock straight, lift the lower trunk off the floor by pressing down on the floor with the palms, and roll it and the legs over the head until you are balanced on your upper back.

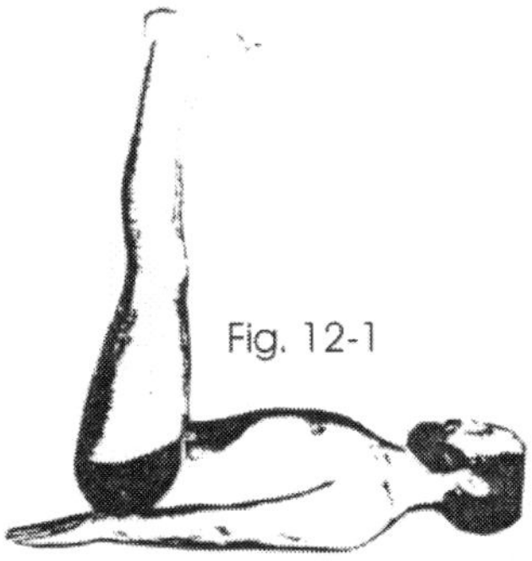

Fig. 12-1

2. Bend the arms at the elbows and, placing the palms on the back of the ribs, push the trunk and legs further forward toward and over the head. Simultaneously lift the legs up vertically over head. The hands should press the trunk toward the chin until the shoulders are lying well on the floor supporting the body weight, and the breast bone is firmly pressed to the chin, Fig. 12-0.

Now only the head, neck, shoulders and arms rest on the floor; the rest of the body is thrust upward perpendicular to the floor.

3. Stretch the shoulders away from the neck so that the lower back part of the neck can be pressed firmly to the floor (similar to the extension of the back of the neck in Tadasana [1]). Then bring the elbows in toward each other until the space between them is not more than the width of the shoulders.

4, Stay in this posture for 5-15 minutes with normal breathing. Gaze at nose level focusing on the center of the chest. Then release the hands and return slowly in the reverse order in which you went up.

II. Variation procedure:

Many find it difficult in the beginning to raise the body up in this way, and to this extent, due to stiff neck vertebrae and general body weakness. Instead of keeping the legs stiff throughout the movement bend them at the knees and pull them in towards the chest. Then lift up the trunk with the palms on the back as shown in Fig. 12-2.

Keeping the legs bent push the buttocks forward toward the head. When the chest is fairly perpendicular to the floor straighten the legs vertically over head, Fig. 12-0.

If the neck is so stiff that you are unable to bring the body perpendicular to the floor, push the trunk toward the head as much as possible and then straighten the legs and hold with normal breathing for up to 5 minutes, Fig. 12-3.

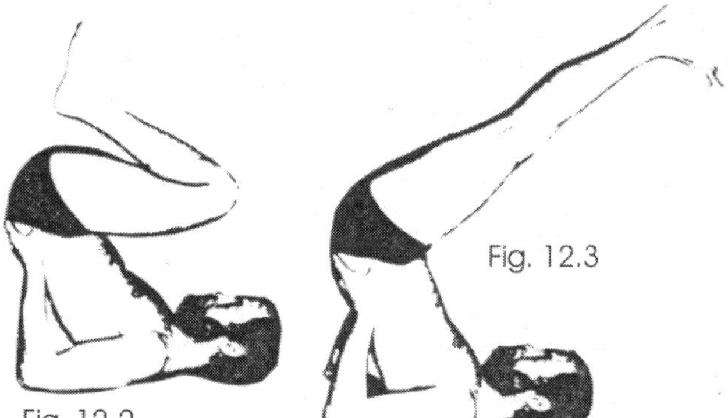

Fig. 12-2 Fig. 12.3

Those who are flexible enough to bring the body perpendicular to the floor may still be too weak to hold it vertical, but instead tend to drop the buttocks backward and swing the legs over the head similar to Fig. 12-2 only to a lesser degree. To counteract this and to make possible longer, more correct and thus more effective stays in this posture one may use a chair. Read the Teaching Procedure point below.

III. Perfecting procedure:

1. Raise the body up slowly and smoothly keeping the legs locked and feet touching throughout. Do all movements on an exhalation. After staying in the posture for 5-15 min. lower the body to the floor in the reverse order that you went up in. Do this extra slowly. From Fig. 12-0 slowly lower the body continuing to press the back of the neck as near to the floor as possible. This helps relieves any built up pressure on the neck vertebrae.

2. Place the hands on the back with the index finger pressing the lower rib of the back. From here, lift the trunk forward and upward until the sternum comes forward and presses into the chin firmly. Look at the center of the chest to aid your concentration on keeping the sternum flat and pressing into, or at least toward the chin.

3. To further open out the chest, concentrate on lifting the area between the navel and the sternum upward toward the ceiling. Simultaneously lift the lower back and hips, roll the buttocks in toward the anus, tighten the anus muscle and push the buttock and pubic area forward.

4. Remember to keep the ankles touching, knees locked, and the legs held in line with the rest of the trunk perpendicular to the floor. Extend the heels from the calves, as in the standing postures, as though you wanted to push them into the ceiling.

5. Aim at lifting the area between the shoulder blades (near the first thoracic vertebrae) inward towards the sternum and extend the floating side ribs on the back upward towards the hips, thus eventually the fingers of the hands may be placed, interlocked, behind the back with the index fingers pressing the lower ribs.

6. Keep the eyes open throughout this and all other Yoga postures for the first couple of years of regular practice for this directs the attention and helps overall watchfulness. Latter as one develops ability to gaze into the body and is keenly aware of what he is doing, he can practice asanas with eyes closed but with the "gaze" held either between the eyebrows or at nose level.

7. One may hold a broom handle in both hands and push the middle back area upward and forward with this. This effect is similar to using a chair and one is able to get maximum lift pushing the chest in towards the chin.

IV. Teaching procedure:

The main problem in this posture is getting the chest to open out flat and press the chin, while keeping the legs extended vertically. The teacher can help show the student what is aimed for by doing the following:

First adjust his chin, neck, and head so they are in line with the trunk. Approach the student from behind; grasp his legs near the feet with one hand and around the knees with the other such that his feet and calves extend past your right or left shoulder/ear. Then press your knee into his lower back and push this area forward towards his head while at the same time keeping his legs locked straight and leaned back slightly and pulled up toward the ceiling.

A chair may be used by those too weak still to hold their body perpendicular to the floor. Here the student holds the legs of the chair and pulls it toward him such that the edge of the seat pushes his buttocks forward. Simultaneously he slant his legs slightly back from vertical (and so away from the head) until his back is slightly concave.

The pressure from pushing the chest into the chin is often uncomfortable for beginners and breathing is difficult due to pressure on the throat. To relieve this, place one or two folded blankets under the shoulder/ elbow area, allowing the head and upper neck to rest off the blanket on the floor. Then perform the posture as usual.

Beginner's elbows will constantly drift apart wider than the shoulders, and the student looses important leverage. This can be countered by placing the upper arms (near the elbows) through a looped rope, which then holds the elbows to the required distance.

In order to get the student to lift the area between the shoulder blades at the first thoracic vertebrae try gently poking him in that region with the ball of your foot. You can also put the loop rope around him at this point and gently pull his upper chest toward you (and his head) while keeping his shoulders back by pressing them with your feet.

To get the proper heel extension as explained in point 4 on the preceding page, press a board or heavy weight momentarily down on his heels. He must then extend his heels from the calf to keep the weight up.

25. JANUSIRSASANA
    30 sec. each side with full breathing.
18. ADHO MUKHA SVANASANA
    SO sec. with full breathing
19. URDHVA MUKHA SVANASANA
    50 sec. with full breathing
21. SALABHASANA
    30—60 sec. with normal breathing.
22. USTRASANA
    30 sec. with normal breathing
23. 24. VIRASANA
    Stay as long as you like with normal or pranayama breathing.
23. 24. VIRASANA
    60 sec. each with full even breathing.
15. PARIPOORNA NAVASANA
    60sec. with normal even breathing
16. ARDHA NAVASANA
    10-60 sec. with shallow breathing
26. BHARADVAJASANA I.
    10 sec. each side with full breathing.
11. UTTANASANA
    1 to 5 min. with full breathing. This can be done any time during your Yoga practice that you feel fatigue.
13. SAVASANA
    5-15 minutes with normal breathing or Pranayama.

LESSON VI

3. UTTHITA TRIKONASANA,
   10 sec. each side with full breathing.
4. PARIVRTTA TRIKONASANA
   30 sec. each side with normal even breathing.
5. UTTHITA PARSVAKONASANA
   10 sec. each side with full breathing.
6. VIRABHADRASANA I.
   Stay fro 30 sec. each side with full breathing.
8. VIRABHADRASANA III.
   30 sec. each side with full breathing.

43. ARDHA CHANDRASANA

(Half moon posture)

This along with the other standing postures helps relieve gastric problems. It tones the lower spine and the nerves of the legs. It also greatly improves ones sense of balance.

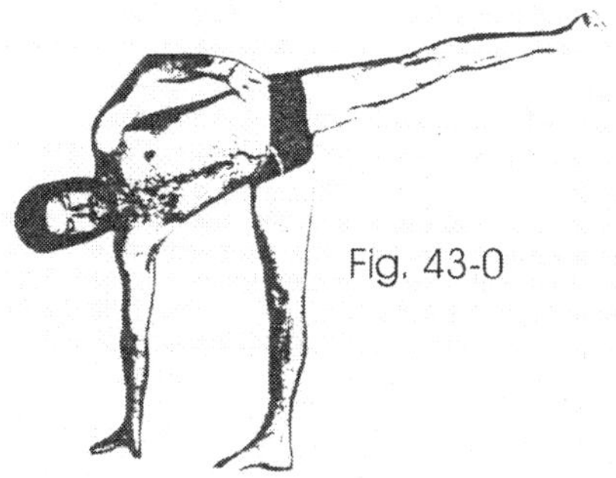

Fig. 43-0

I. Basic procedure:

1. Move into Trikonasana [3] on the right side momentarily. Then place the left hand on the hip. Bend the right knee and place the right hand 1 ft. directly in front of the right foot: Simultaneously slide the left foot about one foot in towards the right one, Fig. 43-1.

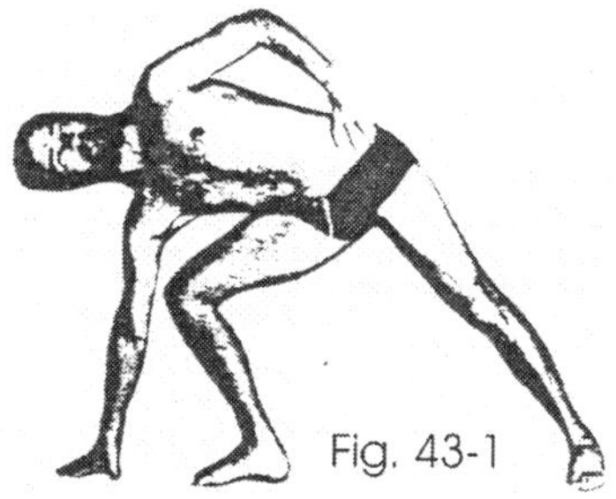

Fig. 43-1

2. After several breaths, exhale and raise the left leg while simultaneously straightening and locking the right one. Roll the left side of the trunk backward until the nipples are perpendicular to the floor (as in Fig. 3-7).

3. Balance in this posture for 30 sec. with full breathing. Gaze should be directed toward the feet, Fig. 43-0. Use the right hand for controlling the balance only and not as a support for body weight.

II. Variation procedure:

If you have trouble reaching the floor due to undeveloped frontal flexibility place the right hand on some stacked books or low table to raise the trunk up slightly. Balance and frontal flexibility should be developed before laying too much emphasis on rolling the left side of the body backward. Balance is made more difficult by gazing toward the feet but this should be pursued to develop your sense of balance.

III. Perfecting procedures:

1. While in Trikonasana [1] roll the left shoulder back and lift the abdomen/chest area. Then maintaining this space between the right leg and chest, move forward and then lift the left leg. Keep the nipples in a perpendicular line to the floor throughout the movement by pulling the left shoulder backward and extending the chest. This counters the tendency to slant the trunk off center.

2. The lift of the left leg can be increased by further tightening of the right thigh. Simultaneously concentrate on rolling the left hip and leg upward away from the groin. This is the opposite from the hip movement aimed for in Virabhadrasana

3. Spreading the fingers of the right hand and resting only them on the floor helps to maintain balance. Concentrate on maintaining a firm right ankle so it doesn't wobble and throw you off balance.

Simultaneously keep the extended rear foot in line with the left leg and with its toes curling inward toward the shin bone. Push the heel to the rear stretching it from the calf.

IV. Teaching procedure:

Roll (push) the student's upper left side trunk backward to make him more aware of the extent of the shoulder/hip movement. You can do this by having the student perform the posture with his back a few centimeters from the wall. Then press his back to the wall with both hands.

You can first have the student extend his left hand towards the ceiling as in Trikonasana [3] instead of placing it on the hip. Then, or when the hand is placed on the hip, let him use it as a guide indicating the position of the hip and the extent of backward rotation.

9. PARSVOTTANASANA
   10 sec. on each side with full breathing.
10. PRASARITA PADOTTANASANA
   10 sec. each with full breathing.
12. SARVANGASANA
   3-15 min. with normal breathing.

29. HALASANA

(Plough posture)

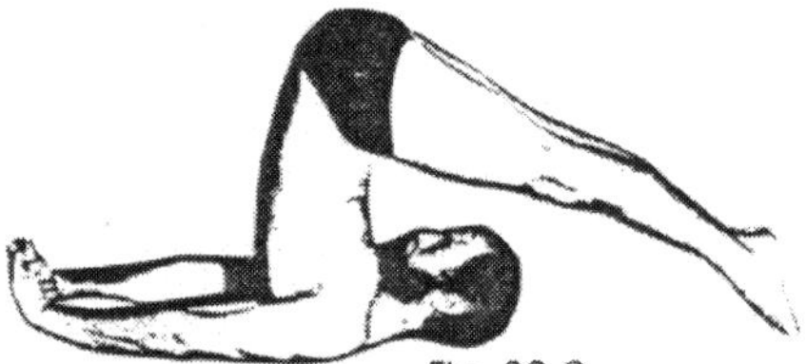

Fig. 29-0

The effects of Halasana are the same as Sarvangasana [12] above in many respects. Backaches are relieved benefiting sufferers of lumbago and arthritis. This posture also develops forward flexibility and thus prepares you for Paschimottanasana [31]. The interlocking of the fingers relieves stiffness in the finger, wrists, elbows, and shoulders.

I. Basic procedure:

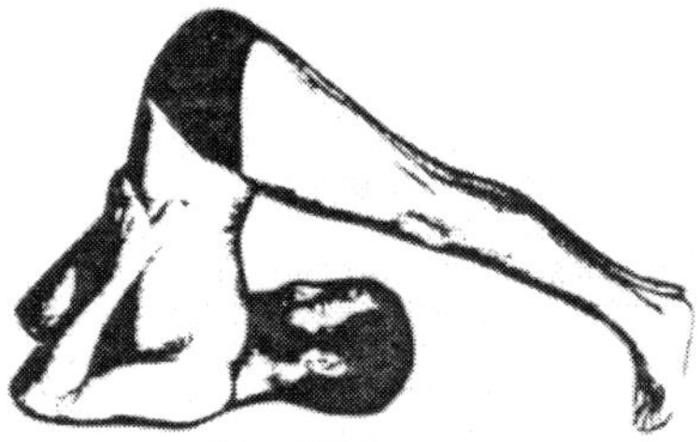

Fig. 29-1

1. From Sarvangasana [12], lower the legs beyond the head until the balls of the feet rest on the floor. Then tighten the knees by pulling up on the hamstring muscles at the back of the thigh. With the palms, press the trunk upward towards the ceiling and forward towards your chin until the trunk is perpendicular to the floor as show in Fig. 29-1.

2. Release the hands from the back and lay them flat on the floor behind you. Extend the arms from the shoulders and interlock the fingers so that the right hand interlocks the left with the right thumb pressing on top of the left one. Turn the wrist until the thumbs rest on the floor.

3. Stay in this position for 1-2 min. with normal breathing, with the balls of the feet or the toes resting on the floor. Hole the gaze at nose level.

4. Change the interlocking fingers so the left hand interlocks the right with the left thumb pressing the right one. Extend the arms again locking the elbows, and pressing the thumbs and arms to the floor. Stretch the toes out this time so that the upper part of the toes rests on the floor. Stay in this position for 1-2 min. with normal breathing, Fig. 29-0. Release the interlocking fingers and return to Sarvangasana [12], then lower yourself slowly to the floor.

II. Variation procedure:

Instead of doing Sarvangasana in step 1. of the Basic procedure, follow the Variation procedure for Sarvangasana. Then proceed normally.

Beginners with stiff hamstring muscles and necks may not be able to touch the feet to the floor. They can instead place the feet on a low table or chair placed several feet beyond the head. A long stay in Sarvangasana [12] enables you to bring the toes closer to the floor than otherwise possible.

Those who have too much difficulty interlocking the fingers and pressing the arms to the floor may perform the entire posture with the palms on the back, Fig. 29-1. Allow the flexibility of the wrists and fingers to developed through Virasana [23. 24.] for several months and then try Halasana again with interlocked fingers.

III. Perfecting procedure:

1. The important thing in this posture is to extend the back upward toward the ceiling and, simultaneously, forward toward your chin, pressing the sternum into the chin as in Sarvangasana [12].

2. Pull the hamstring muscles tight to lock the knees, until you feel the skin on the back of the knee stretched flat. Simultaneously roll the buttock muscle out from the anus/ groin area as in Adho Mukha Svanasana [18], making this area feel open and lifted.

3. In the first movement of Halasana (point #3 above) the heels should be extended as was done for the left heel in Ardha Chandrasana [44]. The toes curl slightly making the feet perpendicular to the calf. Then, in the second movement, point #4 above, the toes are extended as far as possible to the rear beyond the head, while the trunk is still kept perpendicular to the floor. The ankles touch throughout both movements.

4. Push the shoulders away from the neck until most of the body weight is on the lower neck and the upper most part of the shoulders. Then curl the arms away from the shoulders, stretching them as far as possible to the rear. Lock the elbows and stretch the palms and fingers, rolling the little finger in towards the trunk as far as it will go.

IV. Teaching procedure:

Those doing the posture with the palms on the back must be encouraged to keep the distance between the elbows the same or less than the distance between the shoulders. This may be aided temporarily by placing the upper arms through a looped rope as was done in Sarvangasana [12]. With this aid, most students should be able to interlock the fingers while having the palms flat on the back.

This teaching aid as well as many others should not be relied on for too long as one must develop the will and the muscle to maintain the proper positions voluntarily. Trying to do the posture correctly with maximum effort to whatever degree possible will usually lead to true improvement faster and safer than any learning "tool".

25. JANUSIRSASANA
10 sec. each side with full breathing.

18. ADHO MUKHA SVANASANA
60 sec. with full breathing

19. URDHVA MUKHA SVANASANA
80 sec. with full breathing

22. USTRASANA
30 sec. with normal breathing.

23. 24. VIRASANA
50 sec. each with full breathing

26. BHARADVAJASANA I.
30 sec. on each side with full breathing

33. BADDHA KONASANA I

(Bound angle posture)

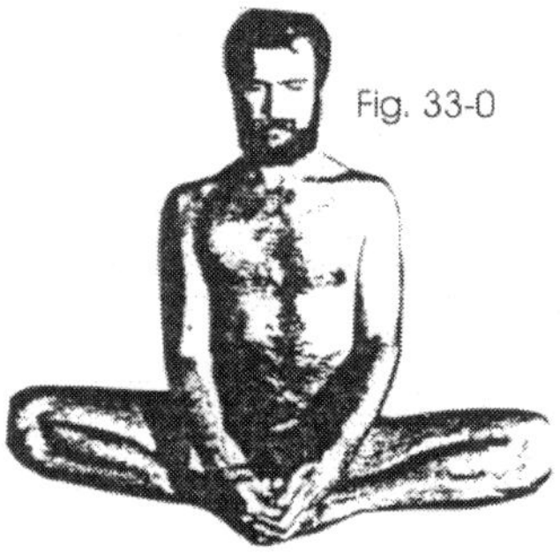

Fig. 33-0

This posture brings flexibility to the hip joints, relieves sciatic pain and helps cure varicose veins. For women, if done regularly for some time, it can result in painless childbirth, relieve menstruation pains and menstrual irregularity. It also prevents hernia and relieves urinary disorders.

I. Basic procedure:

1. Sit on the floor in Dandasana Fig. 15-1. Bend the knees and catching the toes, bring the heels in near the groin. Join the soles of the feet together.

2. Interlock the fingers firmly and grip the feet between the palms. Stretch the spine upward and keep the back slightly concave (Fig.9-3, 10-2).

3. Holding the feet as close to the groin as possible, press the thighs down as close to the floor as you can. Hold this position for 10 sec. with full breathing, and gaze a nose level focusing the eyes 3-5 feet in front of you.

II: Variation procedure:

The main difficulty in this posture is the placing of the legs (knees) flat to the floor. For some though, usually women, this comes fairly easily, whereas for others this may take years to accomplish well. On the other hand, other postures will came easily to those who find this one so difficult. Each of us has natural ability in some postures and natural inability in others ones. Above all else you must avoid the common tendency to skip or "do lightly" those posture which give you trouble. Just the opposite, put your greatest effort in them, for in them is where you are facing your core weaknesses. One must be patient and remember that progress comes only step by step to those who strive regularly, and not to those who practice lazily and irregularly.

Be satisfied with your progress however slowly it comes; at the same time give more of yourself, working in and surrendering to the posture.

III. Perfecting procedure:

1. Raise the sternum, extend the chest outward and upward. Roll the shoulders backward and keep the back concave.

2. While pushing the thighs down to the floor lift up on the feet slightly, pulling them in toward the groin. Make sure the feet are touching each other on the total area of the sole and heel of each foot and not just on the outer lower edges.

IV: Teaching procedure:

You can gently press the student's knees down towards the floor or alternatively place weight on them (10-20 lbs). Encourage him to relax the hip/groin region and "open up". Students unconsciously tense this area which prevents their knees going as far down as they might otherwise.

11. UTTANASANA
    1-5 minutes with-full breathing
13. SAVASANA
    5-15 min. with normal breathing or Pranayama.

LESSON VII

3. UTTHITA TRIKONASANA
    30 sec. each side with full breathing
4. PARIVRTTA TRIKONASANA
    10 sec. each side with normal breathing
5. UTTHITA PARSVAKONASANA
    30 sec. each side with full breathing
6. VIRABHADRASANA I.
    30 sec. each side with full breathing
8. VIRABHADRASANA III.
    10 sec each side with full breathing
43. ARDHA CHANDRASANA
    10 sec. each side with full breathing
9. PARSVOTTANASANA
    10 sec. on each side with cull breathing.

27. SIRSASANA

(Head posture)

Fig. 27-0

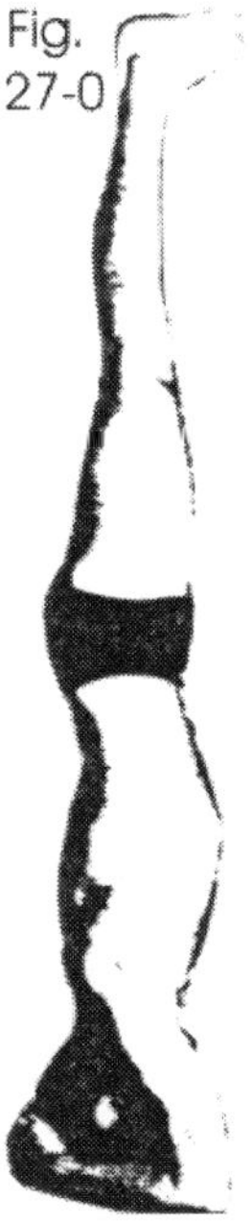

This, the father of Yogic postures, brings increased circulation to the head, benefiting the organs there: eyes, sinuses, brain, etc. Thus, memory and reason may be improved. It insures that the master gland, the pituitary and pineal glands in the head receives vital blood supply. In those who are anemic it increases hemoglobin bringing back youthful vitality. It relieves insomnia and benefits the throat and sinuses reducing the chance of colds, coughs, halitosis, and tonsillitis. Due to the inversion of the abdominal area, constipation seldom occurs.

I. Basic procedure:

1. With the elbows placed on the floor the same distance apart as the shoulders, interlock the fingers firmly and then place the head on the floor at the point shown by the arrow in Fig. 27-1.

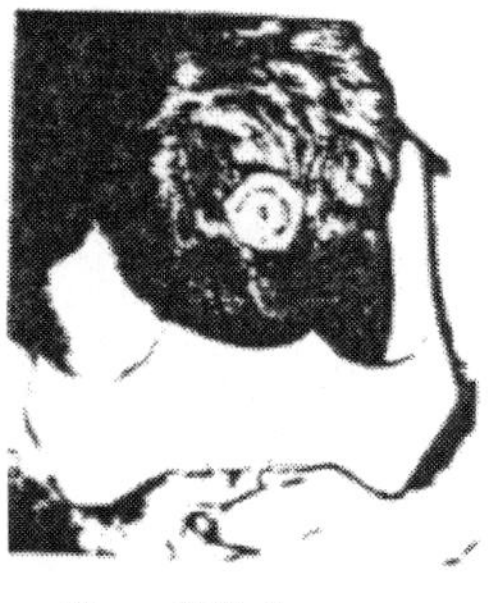

Fig. 27-1

2. Without moving the head or elbows, raise the trunk by straightening the legs. Slowly walk in towards the head with legs locked straight and

heels pressing into the floor. Stretch the spine upwards from the buttocks, pulling the middle back in slightly toward the feet to make the back as perpendicular to the floor as possible. Stay in this position and take a few full breaths, Fig. 27-2.

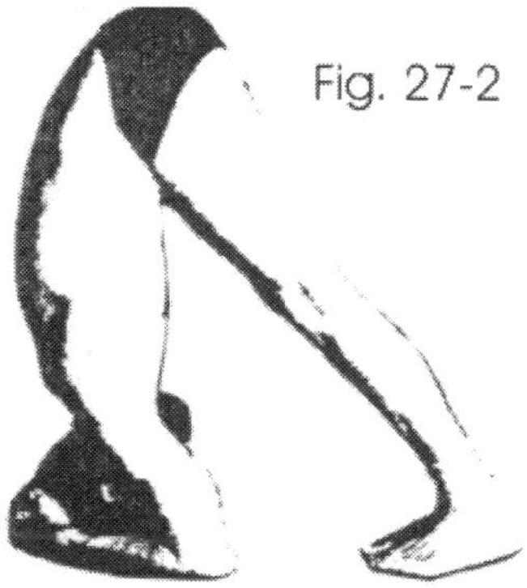
Fig. 27-2

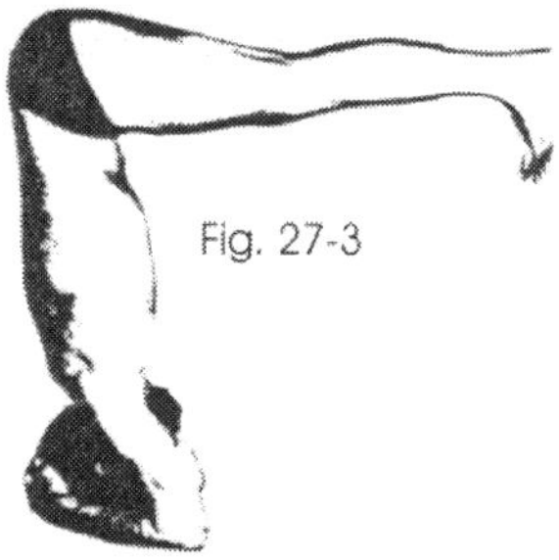
Fig. 27-3

3. On an exhalation, raise the heels off the floor and simultaneously rock the trunk slightly backward. Keeping the legs straight, lift them until they are parallel to the floor, Fig. 27-3. The trunk and buttocks are moved a little further backward to offset the weight of the legs, thus balance is easily maintained. Stay in this position for several full breaths.

4. Then, on an exhalation, raise the legs into the final position, Fig. 27-0. Stay in this position for 1-5 min. or longer with even breathing. Balance all of the body weight on the head and use the elbows only for maintaining balance. Keep the distance between them equal to or less than the distance between the shoulders. The fingers should be firmly interlocked and the knee caps pulled into the thigh throughout the posture. You can release finger lock and raise hands to touch the shoulders to check.

5. Slowly return in the reverse order that you went up into the posture, keeping the legs locked straight throughout. Stop in position shown in Fig. 27-3, for 60 sec. with normal breathing, then lower the feet to the floor.

6. Sirsasana [27] is basically the same as Tadasana [1] only upside down. Review the Basic and Perfecting procedures for Tadasana [1] and see how they apply here. After one can do Sarvangasana [12] and the standing posture well, Sirsasana [27] usually comes much easier.

II. Variation procedure:

You may begin learning this posture by placing the head a few inches away from the wall or for even more stability do it in a corner. Walk the legs in toward the head as explained above only this time bend them as much as you need to get the feet near the head. Raise the bent legs into the position in Fig. 27-4. Take a few full breaths and then slowly raise the bent legs higher and straighten them out until they are vertical, Fig. 27-0. Drop the feet or some other part of your body back-wards slightly to touch the wall to get more stability. Then work towards slowly bringing that part of the body off the wall until the whole body is vertical.

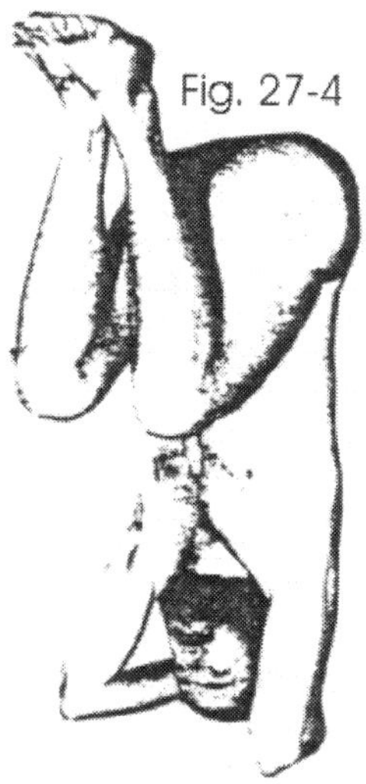
Fig. 27-4

You can just practice up to the position in Fig. 27-4, for awhile in order to develop confidence and balance. Then raising the legs vertically will come easier.

III. Perfecting procedure:

1. Hands should be held firmly interlocked and such that the thumbs touch each other at the tips only, and only the little finger touching the floor. Don't let the wrist twist so the ring finger touches the floor. Elbows always tend to be wider than the shoulders so keep the elbows in. Feet should always touch at the ankles and be held more or less parallel to the floor and not pointing to the ceiling.

2. Raising the shoulders upward and forward brings lightness and control to the posture. Stretch the shoulders apart sideways and open up the armpits making the angle formed by the arm/armpit/chest more obtuse. Think of pushing the chest side of the armpit outward and then think of raising the arm side of the armpit upward and sideways Fig. 27-5.

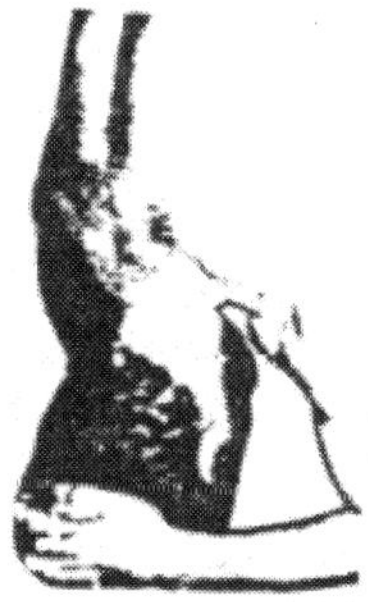
Fig. 27-5

Compare this with the sagging shoulder area shown in Fig. 27-6. This deadens the whole posture, making it heavy and uncomfortable.

3. Extend the back of the neck as in Tadasana [1], creating space between the 3rd. and last neck vertebrae. This lifting and straightening of the neck helps one balance on the right part of the head. "Feel" the ears rolling back slightly towards the clasped hands. These movements also help keep the shoulder blades pressed inward as in Fig. 27-5 and not hanging down as shown in Fig. 27-6.

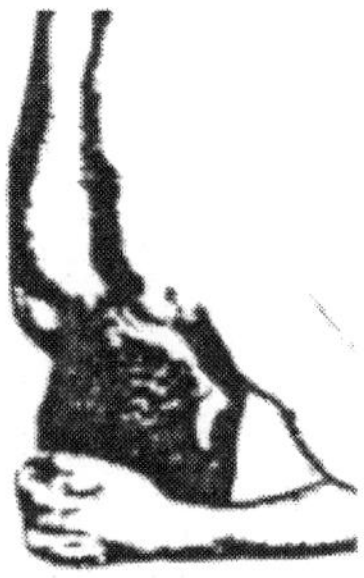

Fig. 27-6

4. Keep the upper back area pressed as flat as possible, and push the chest out slightly. Draw the stomach in flat and stretch the legs up from the abdomen and the side ribs. Pull the knee caps tight and thrust the heels upward towards the ceiling. This helps keep the lower spine lifted.

5. Spread the legs about a foot apart every minute or two and pull the buttock muscles in towards the anus and squeeze them tightly together. This together with tightening the anus muscle itself causes an opening and spreading apart of the pubic area.

Then holding the above contractions, move the legs together again and stretch the opened pubic area and abdomen upward towards the feet. When you loose this contraction, as you will, spread the legs and repeat.

6. The legs are held in the same manner as in Tadasana [1]. Turn the thighs in towards each other, extending the inner leg muscles. This movement will help keep the ankles touching.

7. Don't put too much padding under the head, for this adversely affects your balance. An average blanket folded four times is more than enough. In any case learn to get by with less and less. Doing the head stand on a firm, even hard surface isn't uncomfortable if you're balancing on the right part of the head and doing the rest of the posture correctly.

IV. Teaching procedure:

The teacher can lift the student into the vertical position from the position shown if Fig. 27-2. First adjust the distance between the elbows, head position, and the neck and shoulder lift. Then with your right hand under his ankles and your left lower arm under his thigh lift the student into position. If doing it next to the wall, place his feet to the wall.

In order to get the correct extension upward of the spine, legs, heels, etc., press a weight or board on the heels and have the student try to push this upward toward the foot. Have the student place his head next to the wall and perform the posture shown in Fig. 27-4. He then presses as much of his back to the wall as possible, until the body weight is borne by the back rubbing the wall, and the heels pressing into the floor.

12. SARVANGASANA
    5-15 min. with normal breathing.
29. HALASANA
    4-6 min. with normal breathing.
25. JANUSIRSASANA
    10 sec. each side with full breathing.

31. PASCHIMOTTANASANA

(West stretch posture)

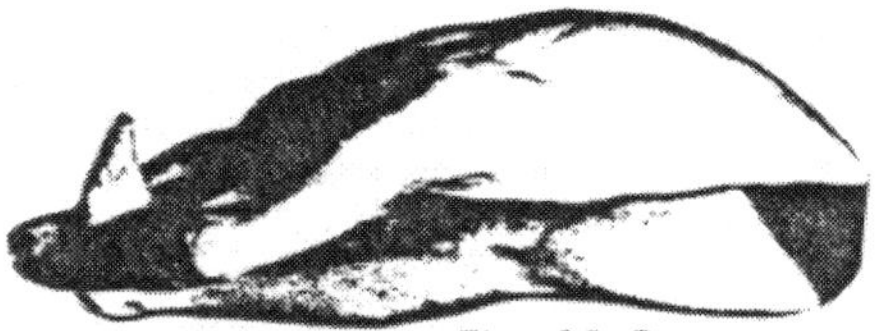

Fig. 31-0

In this posture, the spinal column gets massaged, as does the abdominal organs which improves digestion. It increases blood circulation in the sacral region, and by stretching out cramped vertebrae, helps to clear up lower back problems. It also benefits sufferers of both high and low blood pressure.

I. Basic procedure:

1. Sit in Dandasana, Fig.15-1, and take a deep inhalation. With an exhalation catch the toes while keeping the back as concave as possible. Extend the spine upward and lift the back of the neck. Fig. 31-1

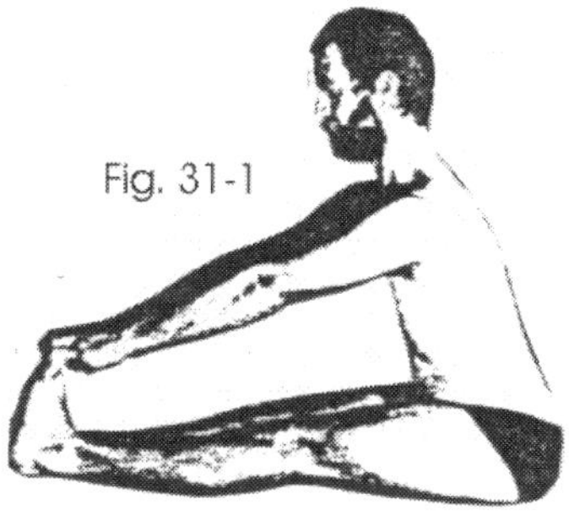
Fig. 31-1

2. Take several full breaths and keep extending upward and simultaneously making the back as concave as possible. Then on an exhalation bend forward slowly from the pelvic region keeping the neck lifted, the back concave as possible, and the arms stretched out from the shoulder sockets.

3. Keep the legs locked straight throughout the movement. Tighten the thighs stretching the skin on the back of the knees. On each exhalation extended the body a little further forward, pulling the trunk forward with the arms.

4. Grasping the toes firmly, widen the elbows as you bend, Fig. 31-2, then if possible clasp the hands beyond the feet, inhale, and then on an exhalation extend further and clasp the wrist of the left hand with the right hand. Fig. 31-0. Finally release the wrist lock and extend the hands straight out past the ankles, resting the hands, palms down, on the floor with the thumbs touching lightly. The bend here must come from the lower back muscles and high flexibility as there is no leverage to pull the trunk forward.

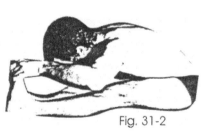
Fig. 31-2

5. Which ever position you can achieve should be held for 1-5 min. with even normal breathing and with the gaze between the eyebrows. Then on an inhalation raise the head and trunk partially off the leg. Straighten the arms and extend the chest. Then on the exhalation raise up to position in Fig. 31-1 and release.

6. Always strive to press the chest to the thighs and not of just touching the head to the legs. When the trunk is flexible enough, rest the chin and forehead on the legs and extend the chin down along the shin.

II. Variation procedure:

If the toes can't be reached do as with Janusirsasana [25] Fig.25-2 and grasp which ever part of the leg you can, or loop a towel or rope around the feet and use this as leverage in pulling yourself forward. NEVER BEND the legs to get further down.

III. Perfecting procedure:

1. Pull the thigh muscles in towards each other and roll the buttock muscles outward, opening up the anus/groin area. Always bend forward on an exhalation, slowly and effort-fully. Keep the ankles touching and the toes in a line

2. Don't just bend forward bringing the head nearer the legs and/or dropping the elbows towards the floor with sagging shoulders as shown in Fig. 31-3. Try instead to keep the back as flat as possible bending only from the lower lumbar region. Stretch the arms and shoulders upward and outward towards the feet and lift the elbows off the floor. Also raise the sternum and extend the chest and abdominal area towards the feet. Fig. 31-2.

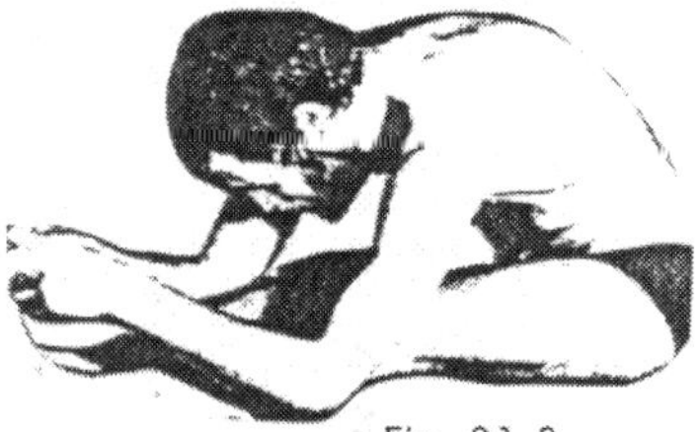
Fig. 31-3

3. In forward bends the back of the body tends to be elongated (stretched) more than the front of the body, so concentrate on the front. Roll the abdomen/chest area forward on an inhalation, then sink it into the legs on an exhalation, repeating this through-out the movement. On the inhalations roll the shoulders backward and rub the diaphragm along the thigh.

4. The head should not be lowered to the legs until you have enough flexibility to rest your abdomen on your thighs. Until then, practice the posture with the head raised and extended toward the feet. When flexibility is sufficient to press the trunk to the thigh, press the head firmly into the shin. The whole abdominal area should rub the legs, and on each inhalation the trunk should move forward slightly with a stretching of the side ribs towards the feet.

5. Those who can grasp the wrists or the palms should change the grip half way through the posture time so as to develop evenly. First you grasp the left wrist with the right hand then grasp the right wrist with the left hand.

IV. Teaching procedure:

Press down on the student's lower back with your palms and simultaneously gently press his knees flat to the floor with your feet. You can place a heavy weight (30-50 lbs.) on the back and instruct the student to "relax into it", to open up his lower back.

To get the proper extension towards the feet and not just a downward sinking motion, have the student run his arm along the top of his toes keeping his arms straight, of course. Alternately you can place a 5-8in. high block of wood for the elbows to rest on. This will keep the shoulders and elbows up as they should be. Then press down on the students back.

It's important that the student begin the posture correctly. Have him hold the posture shown in Fig. 31-1, for several full breaths, raising the back of the neck, rolling the shoulders back and extending the chest forward. Don't let the chin rise. Keep the toes in line, feet perpendicular to the shins and the knees locked.

32. ARDHA BADDHA PASCHIMOTTANASANA

(Half bound west stretch posture).

You can work at developing leg and ankle flexibility by doing Ardha Baddha Paschimottanasana [32], Fig. 32-0, for several minutes on each leg. Push the knee in towards the straight leg and down towards the floor as much as possible. Apply the same procedures as before for Paschimottanasana [31] Fig. 31-0.

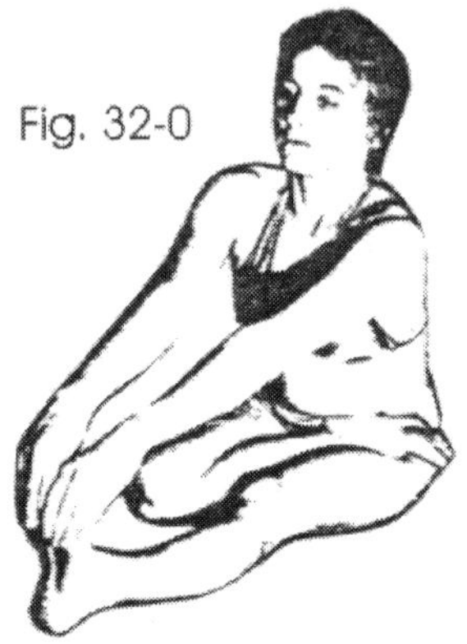
Fig. 32-0

22. USTRASANA
    Stay fro 10.sec. with normal breathing.
23. VIRASNANA
    Stay in first movement with normal breathing
24. VIRASNANA
    Stay in the nest two movements or SO sec. each with full breathing
26. BHARADVAJASANA I.
    10 sec. each side with full breathing
33. BADDHA KONASANA
    30 sec. with normal breathing.

39. SIDDHASANA

(Semi divine posture)

This is one of the most relaxing sitting postures and probably the easiest also as far as developing the flexibility goes. It develops the legs at the ankles, knees, and hips and prepares them for Padamasana [40] later. Circulation is increased in the lower spine making it excellent for meditation and Pranayama, or just plain sitting as it helps keep the mind alert while the body is at ease.

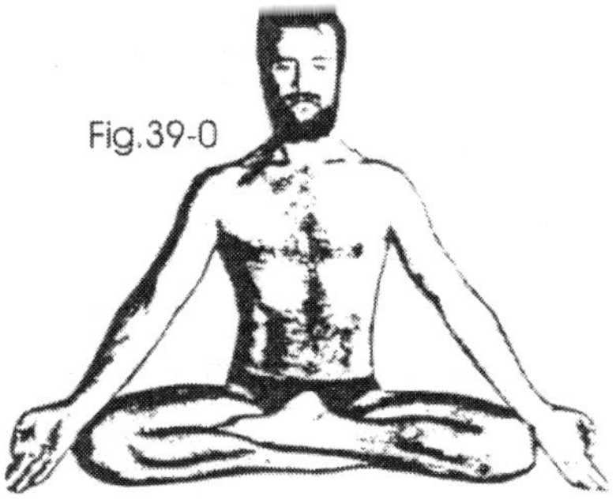
Fig.39-0

I. Basic procedure:

1. Place the left heel near the groin, resting its sole against the thigh. Then bend the right leg and push the sole and the toes of the right foot between the thigh and the calf of

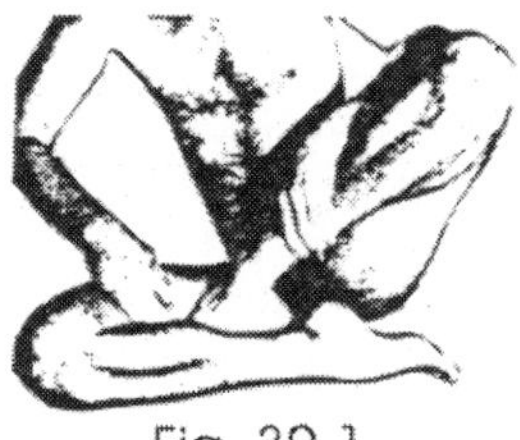
Fig. 39-1

the left leg as shown in Fig. 39-1. The right foot then rests on the left ankle with the right heel pressing against the pubic area.

2. Stretch the arms straight out to the sides resting the backs of the wrists on the knee. Keep the back concave, head and spine erect, and the neck extending upward as in Tadasana [1]. Keep the gaze at nose level and focus 1-5 feet in front of you with either eyes closed or half open.

3. Sit in this posture as long as you like when ever you like, for what ever reason you like. It is especially good for Meditation and Pranayama. Remember to change the legs the next time you sit in Siddhasana so you develop the legs evenly. Usually, one side will be more difficult than the other so spend longer in the difficult side until it is as developed and comfortable.

II. Variation procedure:

Beginners may find it easier to rest the right leg on top the left thigh instead of inserting it between the left thigh and calf. Another possibility is to lay both feet on the floor, the right foot in front of the left, and as near to it as possible.

Warm up the leg for some minutes with Ardha Baddha Paschimottanasana [32] Fig. 32-0. Also, doing Siddhasana [39] after a hot bath will be a lot easier and the mind and body will be more relaxed for meditation.

III. Perfecting procedure:

1. Extend the spine inwards and upwards. This is made easier by sitting on the low hard part of the buttock. To do this, lean forward slightly and keep the back concave. Then with your hands, pull the buttock muscle and flesh to the rear out from under the buttocks bone.

Some people sit with the buttocks on a folded blanket a few inches high. This raises the buttocks and helps you keep the back erect. It's best to dispense with this though as soon as strength and flexibility are fairly developed.

2. Maintain "life" in the spine by stretching it and the neck upwards towards the ceiling as in Tadasana [1]. The chin should be held in towards the throat slightly so that the ears are directly over the shoulders.

3. The shoulders are rolled back slightly but not at all strenuously. Make sure you don't unconsciously tense them or lift them; instead let them sink and feel heavy.

Extend the arms, locked at the elbows, to the knees. One may place the arms other ways too, as seen on statues of Buddha, with one palm resting on the other, and the thumbs just touching at the tips. See Meditation [48]. Maintain attentive finger positions in Meditation [48] and Pranayama [47] to help steady and focus the mind. In Fig. 39-0, the thumb and forefinger are joined just enough to barely touch. The other fingers extend straight out (mostly relaxed) towards the floor.

4. Both knees should touch the floor with the same degree of pressure. If one rises off the floor you can let the extended wrist push it down at the knee gently. It can take some years before the knees will touch the floor evenly.

IV. Teaching procedure:

If the student's knee rises, place a weight on it for a few minutes, or have the student himself push it down and hold it there.

Have the students do the posture with the buttocks touching the wall. Swivel the hip back until the upper half of the buttock touches the wall; the student sits on the lower half. Next, he presses his shoulders and the back of his neck to the wall. After he is flat to the wall have him lean forward away from the wall a few inches, but maintain the same back, shoulder, and head position as formed at the wall.

13. SAVASANA
5-15 min. with normal breathing or Pranayama.

LESSON VIII

3. UTTHITA TRIKONASANA
   30 sec. each side with full breathing
4. PARIVRTTA TRIKONASANA
   10 sec. each side with normal breathing
9. PARSVOTTANASANA
   10 sec. each side with full breathing
6. VIRABHADRASANA I.
   30 sec. each side with full breathing
8. VIRABHADRASANA III.
   10 sec. each side with full breathing
27. SIRSASANA
   1-5 min. with normal breathing
12. SARVANGASANA
   5-15 min with normal breathing
29. HALASANA
   4-6 min. with normal breathing
25. JANUSIRSASANA
   30 sec. each side with full breathing
31. PASCHIMOTTANASANA
   Stay fart-5 min. with normal breathing
19. URDHVA MUKHA SVANASANA
   SD sec. with full breathing
22. USTRASANA
   10 sec. with normal breathing

37. DHANURASANA

(Bow posture)

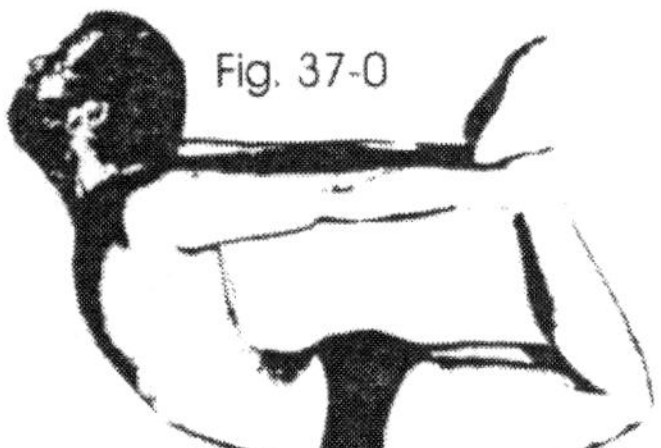
Fig. 37-0

This posture brings elasticity to the spine and massages the abdominal organs. The shoulders and arms are strengthened and the shoulder joints made more flexible. Minor muscles of the hip and thigh are awakened and toned.

<u>I. Basic procedure:</u>

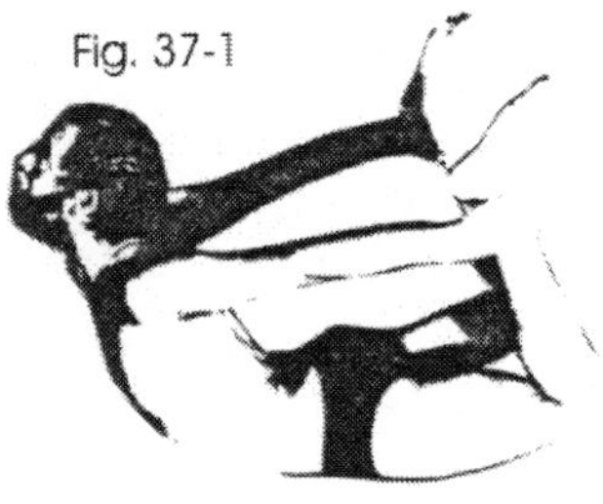
Fig. 37-1

1. Lie face down on the floor and with an exhalation bend the legs at the knees 90° or more, then with the hands reach back and catch the ankles. On the next exhalation pull the legs and trunk off the floor and lift and stretch the head back, Fig. 37-1.

2. The bend and lift of the trunk, and the legs should be great enough so that neither the ribs nor the pelvic bone touch the floor. All the body weight is carried on the abdomen.

3. With an exhalation, bring the legs together while maintaining the same degree of back bend and lift. Join the thighs, knees, and ankles, Fig. 37-0. Stay for 20-60 sec. with rapid even breathing and gaze between the eyebrows. Then return to the floor on an exhalation and relax.

<u>II. Variation procedure:</u>

Until enough flexibility is developed you can remain at Fig. 37-1. Also, forget about having the ribs and pelvis completely off the floor. Just bend the legs at the knees, hold the ankles, or grasp the toes and the balls of the feet. Then pull yourself into a bow to whatever degree possible.

<u>III. Perfecting procedure:</u>

1. Let the shoulders roll back towards the ankles as far as they will go, pressing the shoulder blades in towards each other. Grasp the ankles firmly and let the legs pull the arms back. Stretch the feet and the legs upward towards the ceiling and then use the power of the legs to lift up the trunk even further.

2. After reaching the maximum possible leg lift and back bend possible (Fig. 37-1) bring the legs together and try to stretch back and upward even further.

3. Pull the hips into the trunk, making the angle between them as acute as possible. Pull the buttock muscle in towards the anus. Tighten the anus and curl the tail bone into it. Then open out and stretch the area where the thighs join the pubic area.

4. Extend the sternum to open out the chest and simultaneously move the floating ribs downward towards the floor and stretch the head back towards the feet as

far as it will go. Be sure not to hold the breath in this or any other posture.

IV. Teaching procedure:

Stand behind the student and grasp his hands where they grasp his ankles (or toes). Pull the students legs backward and upward which draws his trunk into the maximum bend possible. Simultaneously join his feet and then rock him forward on his inhalations and rock him back and upward on his exhalation.

23. VIRASANA I.
Stay in the first movement with normal breathing
23. 24. VIRASANA II. III.
Stay for 60 sec. each with full breathing

38. VIRASANA IV

(Hero)

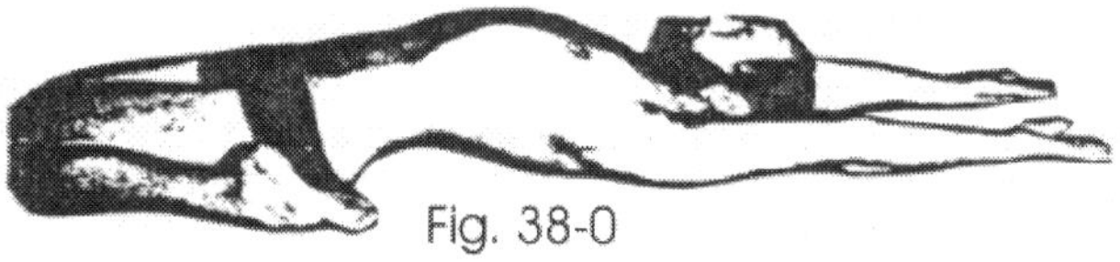

Fig. 38-0

This posture develops the knees and can alleviate rheumatism in them. It is especially beneficial for people whose legs ache or those who must stand or walk for long hours, if held for 10—14 min. at a stretch. In this movement the lower spine receives a good stretch.

I. Basic procedure:

1. Sit in the basic Virasana [23], and on an exhalation recline the trunk backward and rest on the elbows.

2. Then lower the trunk to the floor and stretch the arms out past the head. Keep the knees touching each other and the floor. Hold this posture for several minutes with full and even breathing and gaze at the nose level.

II. Variation procedure:

Just do step #1 above, eliminate step #2, and merely aim at keeping the knees pressed to the floor and pushed in towards each other as much as possible.

If you are too stiff to lay the back on the floor place a pillow or a folded blanket behind you to raise the trunk up as needed.

III. Perfecting procedure:

1. When you recline the trunk and rest the elbow on the floor as explained above, try lifting up the pelvic slightly, roll the buttock muscle into the anus and stretch the pubic region upward toward the abdomen as pointed out in Trikonasana [3], Fig. 3-4.

2. The arms and the shoulders are stretched out beyond the head intensely with the palms up and the thumbs slightly touching each other. This intense extension of the arms tends to affect the facial muscles and they automatically tense up. To counter this, aim at relaxing the face and letting it sag to the floor as you learned in Savasana[13] and simultaneously stretch arms out from the shoulder sockets. One must learn the coordination of being able to work ambitiously in one place and be totally relaxed in another at the same time. This ability will help you relax and release stress in life before they build up too much.

3. The lower part of the spine should be brought as close to the floor as possible. This can be done by pulling the thigh muscles tight which presses the knees to the floor. This pushes the back closer to the floor. It also helps to rotate the pelvis some until you have the higher part of the buttocks near the waste on the floor.

IV. Teaching procedure:

Pull the shoulders and arms of the student beyond the head and then pull on his hip to bring more of the lower back near the floor. Push his knees to the floor, or place a heavy weight there (20-40 lbs.) and leave it for 1-5 min. Pull the flesh on the buttock down towards the knees/thighs.

26. BHARADVAJASANA I.
Stay for 10 sec. each side with full breathing.

34. BHARADVAJASANA II

(Father of a warrior posture)

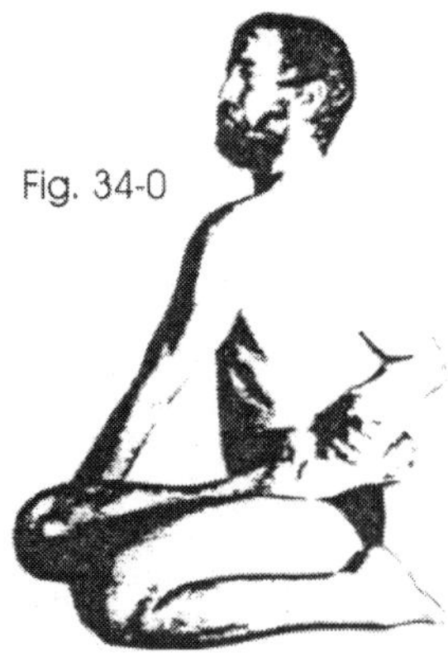
Fig. 34-0

This posture is especially beneficial for those with arthritis. It limbers up the knees and shoulders and increases spinal elasticity making the back supple. It also prepares the legs for Padmasana [40].

I. Basic procedure:

1. Bending the right leg, bring the right foot back and place it on the floor next to the right hip. The calf should press the thighs and the toes point straight to the rear. Next, bend the left leg and place the left foot high up on the right thigh.

2. Move the left knee closer toward the right knee and with a full exhalation, swing the left arm behind the back and grab the left foot. Then on the next exhalation move the right arm to the left knee and insert the fingers of the right hand, palm down, under the left thigh. Fig. 34-0

3. With several full exhalations, move the trunk to the left as far as possible using the arms for leverage. Gaze over the right shoulder and stay for 30-60 sec. with normal or full breathing. Then repeat on the other side,

II. Variation procedure:

Placing the left foot high enough up on the right thigh and grasping it with the left hand may be difficult in the beginning. Knee/ankle flexibility can be developed by doing Ardha Baddha Paschimottanasana [32], first. If the problem is in the shoulders and elbows you can loop a cloth or rope around the left ankle and grasp as far up on this as you can with your left hand. Use the right hand to first put your left hand and foot into position, then proceed as usual.

You can also perform the posture as usual but instead of grasping the foot, place the left hand flat on the floor (see Fig. 26-1).

III. Perfecting procedure:

1. Firmly grasp as much of the left foot as possible and insert the fingers of the right hands as far under the thigh as you can, bringing the left knee as close to the right knee as possible.

2. Raise the sternum and extend the chest as in Bharadvajasana I. Keep the lower back concave, the neck raising and the head erect. Accentuate these movements on the inhalations and hold them on the exhalations.

3. Screw the right shoulder, arm and side of chest to the left, and pull the left shoulder and trunk backward.

IV. Teaching procedure:

If the student is fairly flexible you can help him by pulling his arm around his back until he can grasp his left foot firmly. Press his lower hack concave and simultaneously twist him to the left by his shoulders. Press his left knee to the floor and see to it that his fingers of his right hand are well under the left thigh.

33. BADDHA KONASANA
    30 sec. with normal breathing.
39. SIDDHASANA
    as you like with normal or pranayama breathing.
13. SAVASANA
    5-15 min. with normal breathing or pranayama

LESSON IX

27. SIRSASANA
    1-5 min. with normal breathing
12. SARVANGASANA,
    5-15 min. with normal breathing
29. HALASANA
    4-6 min. with normal breathing
25. JANUSIRSASANA
    30 sec. each side with full breathing
31. PASCHIMOTTANASANA
    2-1 min with normal breathing
18. ADHO MUKHA SVANASANA,
    60 sec. with full breathing
19. URDHVA MUKHA SVANASANA
    60 sec. with full breathing
21. SALABHASANA
    30-60 sec. with normal breathing
22. USTRASANA
    10 sec. with normal breathing
37. DHANURASANA
    30 sec. with rapid breathing
23. VIRASANA
    Stay with normal breathing
23. 24. 38. VIRASANA II. III. IV.
    60 sec. each with full breathing
15. PARIPOORNA NAVASANA
    60 sec. with normal breathing
16. ARDHA NAVASANA
    30-60 sec. with shallow breathing
26. BHARADVAJASANA I.
    10 sec. each side with full breathing
34. BHARADVAJASANA II.
    10-60 sec. with normal or full breathing

36. ARDHA MATSYENDRASANA I

(The founder of Yoga posture)

Regular practice of this posture benefits the prostate gland and the bladder due to the squeeze pressure on the lower abdomen. Lumbago and other back and hip pains are relieved and the shoulder movements made freer. Ankles and knee flexibility is developed.

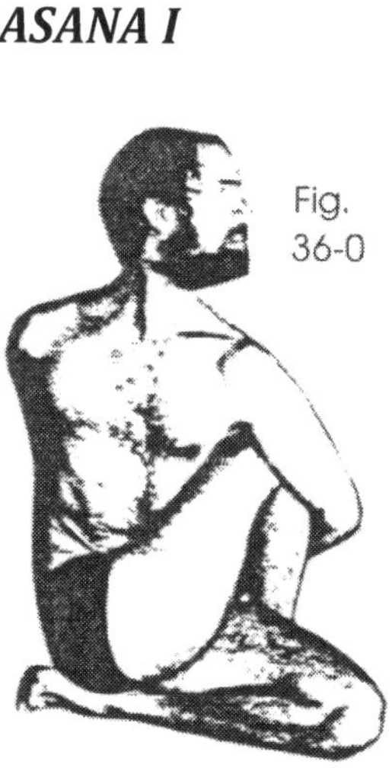

Fig. 36-0

I. Basic procedure:

1. Sit on the left foot and place the right calf next to the outer side of the left thigh and perpendicular to the floor, .

2. Turn the trunk as far to the right as possible and then, with an exhalation, wrap the left arm around the right knee and place its wrist near the back hip. Exhale again and swing the right arm from the shoulder around the back and grasp the left hand with the right one. Thus you lock the bent right knee tightly with the bent left arm.

3. Work the right hand up the left one until you can grasp the left wrist with the right hand, Fig. 36-1. Turn the head to the left and gaze over the left shoulder with the gaze either at nose level or between the eyebrows. Stay in this position for 30 sec. with normal breathing, and then repeat on the other side. Fig. 36-0

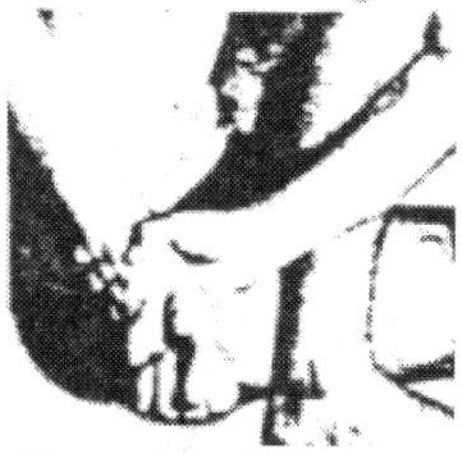

Fig. 36-1

II. Variation procedures:

If the ankles (and knees) are too stiff to make sitting on them impossible, place the left foot beside the right hip, on the floor.

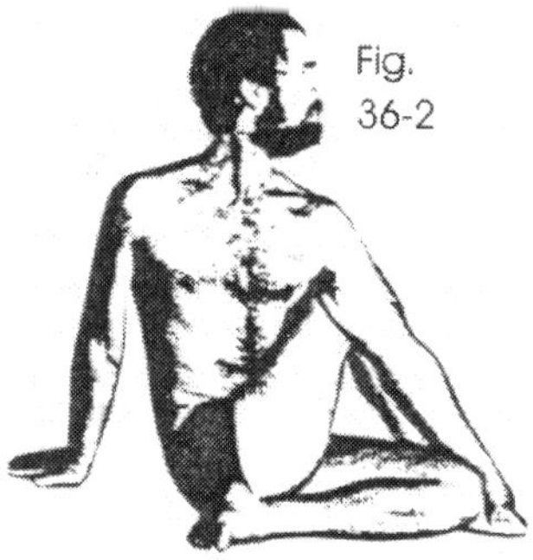

Fig. 36-2

Next, extend the left arm straight down towards the right foot, and grasp the right loot with the left hand. The right hand is then placed palms down directly behind the buttocks. Fig. 36-2.

As flexibility improves move your right hand further round the body but keep the elbow locked. One can also wrap this arm around the back and extend it as far as possible, bending at the elbow.

III. Perfecting procedure:

1. The foot you sit on should be kept as perpendicular as possible to its calf, with the toes curled in and the outer side of this foot

pressing the floor, Fig. 36-3. Compare this with a less correct placing shown in Fig. 36-4.

2. Before you wrap the left arm around the right knee, work the upper left arm down along the outer side of the right thigh towards the hip. Then with as exhalation, push the left shoulder away from the right knee, pressing the upper left arm into the right thigh and pushing the right shoulder to the rear. Inhale and lift the chest and abdomen upward and outward. Then on the exhalation pull them free from the bent right knee as much as possible.

Fig. 36-3

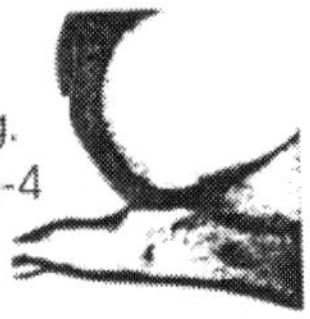
Fig. 36-4

3. Repeat the movement above several times to achieve a maximum twisting of the trunk. Then exhaling, wrap the left elbow around the right knee and press the left hand next to the hip.

4. On the next exhalation swing the right hand around the back and grasp the fingers of the left hand. Practice the posture with this finger grip until you can grasp the palms and then finally the wrists. At this point, grasp as far up on the wrists as possible. When doing the posture on the other side change the grip hands such that the left hand grips the right wrist.

5. Extend the spine upwards and aim for a flat back. Simultaneously lift the area from the navel to the sternum and extend it straight outward and upward. Lift the back of the neck and hold the head erect, turning the neck as far as it will go so that the chin eventually is directly over the left (forward) shoulder.

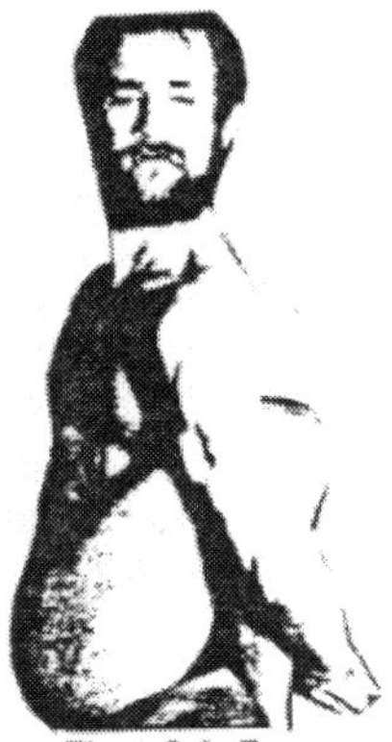
Fig. 36-5

Now extend the left shoulder forward and simultaneously pull the right shoulder to the rear, Fig. 36-5. Compare this with that shown in Fig. 36-6, where the chest is sunken, the back bowed, the head slanted, and the shoulders drooping.

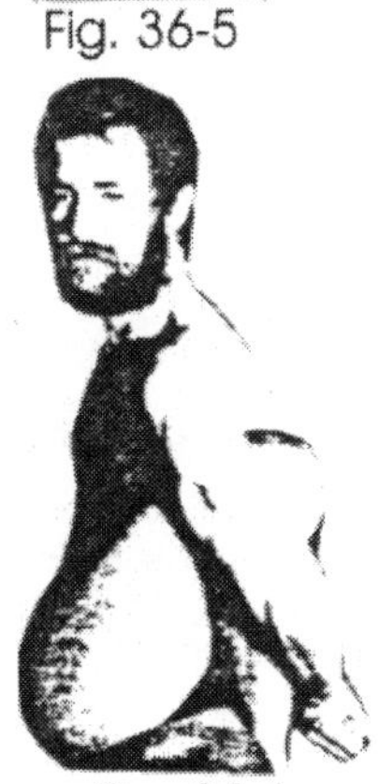

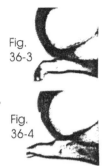
Fig. 36-6

IV. Teaching procedure:

If the student is doing the posture according to Fig. 36-2, he may place a folded blanket under his buttocks for an easier bend. Those who can't turn the trunk enough to grasp the foot in this variation may do the posture facing a bench or a wall and use that as leverage to push and pull themselves into a twist.

Students may also loop a rope around the right wrist and swinging the arm behind the back grasp this rope with the left hand and pull the right arm toward the left.

You can give the student a helping turn. Press your knee into his back to push his chest and abdomen outward and simultaneously pull his rear shoulder back and push his forward left shoulder to the front.

33. BADDHA KONASANA II

(Bound angle posture)

This posture brings even further flexibility to the hip joints. The effects are the same as for the simpler version of the first movement but more intense.

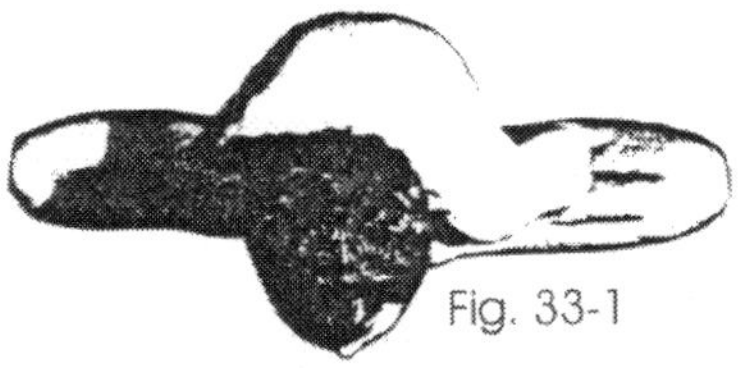
Fig. 33-1

I. Basic procedure:

I. Stay in the first movement, Baddha Konasana (I) Fig. 33-0, for 30 sec., then with an exhalation bend the trunk forward as far as it will go, until eventually the chest and chin touch the floor in front of you.

2. When you have bent as far forward as possible, hold this position for 10 sec. with normal breathing and with the gaze at nose level, Fig. 33-1

II. Variation procedure:

Practicing this more advanced version will help you in developing the more basic version of Bhaddha Konasana that you learned earlier, Fig. 33-0. This holds true for many Yoga postures: Working on a more advanced and difficult posture can improve postures previously learned.

III. Perfecting procedure:

1. The forward bend here is essentially the same as the other forward bends; one tries to keep the lower back concave as far into the bend as possible. You aim at pressing the extended chest into the floor and not at simply touching the chin to the floor. Bending to touch the chin, results in less correctly bending the upper back area instead of in the vital lower back area.

2. Widen the elbows when you bend forward and placing them on the thighs. Use them for leverage to keep your legs flat to the floor. Be sure to maintain a firm grip on the feet and press them together flat, sole to sole and heal to heel.

3. Bend slowly forward from the base of the spine. Breathe normally, and on each exhalation try to bend forward a little further. The hips take time to relax and open up, so spend 30-60 sec. going into the bend. Continuing to thrust the trunk forward on each exhalation, you will find that you are able to go much further than you could initially.

4. Concentrate on extending the chest forward, lifting the sternum, and keeping the shoulders back. The bending movement is the same as in Parsvottanasana [9], only here the abdomen presses flat on the feet instead of on the thigh, and the chin rest finally on the floor instead of on the shin.

IV. Teaching procedure:

Insist on the student keeping his back as straight as possible into the bend. He must aim at touching the abdomen to the feet and not the head to the feet or the floor.

40. PADMASANA

(Lotus posture)

This is the most relaxing and stable sitting posture after you achieve the required flexibility. This however may take years to develop. It is a very good posture for pranayama [47] and meditation [48] because of the ease with which the back is kept upright. It alleviates stiffness in the ankles and knees.

I. Basic procedure:

1. Bend the left leg and place the left foot high up on the right thigh with the heel pressing the abdomen. Then bring the right foot over the left calf and place it high up on the left thigh.

2. Hold the spine erect with the lower back slightly concave. Place the wrists on the knees, palms up, or in the Buddhist meditation position. Hold this posture for 30-60 sec. each side with normal breathing, or do it as long as you like later or earlier in the day with Pranayama or in meditation. Gaze at nose level with the focus 1-5 ft. in front and with eyelids half open or closed. Fig. 40-0

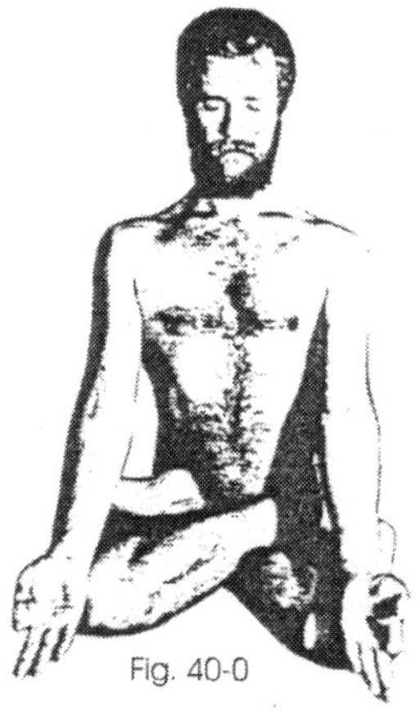

Fig. 40-0

3. Be sure to change the legs the next time you do the posture, so as to develop them evenly. Devote more time to the stiffest side.

II. Variation procedure:

In the beginning one will barely be able to get the feet into position on the legs let alone pulled up so far onto the thighs as shown in Fig. 40-0. This is nothing to worry about as improvement will come if you work at it conscientiously. Another problem faced by the beginner is that his legs may soon 'go to sleep', and though this is uncomfortable, it is not at all dangerous. This will stop after some years of practice.

One leg may rise higher off the floor than the other, as in Siddhasana [39], only more so. Keep pressing the knees as close to the floor as possible, while practicing and training Padmasana. If you wish to do meditation or Pranayama in this posture you may sit on a folded blanket 1-3 inches thick which stabilizes the posture by helping you keep your back erect and your knees on the floor. Be sure to dispense with this "aid" as soon as your strength and flexibility allow. If the legs are too stiff to do the posture at all then do Ardha Baddha Paschimottanasana [32] on both sides and Siddhasana [39].

III. Perfecting procedure:

1. Pull the feet as high up on the thighs as they will go until the ankles rest on the thighs with the feet extending beyond them. Keep pushing the knees in towards each other until the distance between them is about the same as the distance between the shoulders.

2. Extend the thigh muscle and push the knees down into the floor. Press as much of the knee and leg down to the floor as possible to give maximum stability and strength to the posture.

3. Rest on the lower part of the buttocks as you did in Siddhasana [39], keeping the lower back slightly concave. Raise the sternum, and stretch and hold the spine upward. Simultaneously keep the shoulders and chin down and rolled back.

4. The head is extended upward and backward enough so that the chin is perpendicular and inline with the navel and the floor. The arms should extend straight out and lock at the elbows.

5. This posture may be done for meditation or pranayama just before you go to bed or just after you get up in the morning. It will be easier to perform and be less painful if you try it after taking a hot bath. The same applies to the other postures as well, and is especially helpful for those who have arthritis.

IV. Teaching procedure:

Have the student do this posture against the wall with as much of the buttock pulled up onto the wall as possible as detailed in Siddhasana [39]. You can also place weights on the student's knees to bring them closer to the floor.

13. SAVASANA
   5-15 min. with normal breathing or pranayama.

LESSON X

27. SIRSASANA
   1-5 min. with normal breathing
12. SARVANGASANA
   5-15 min. with normal breathing
29. HALASANA
   4-6 min. each side with normal breathing
25. JANUSIRSASANA
   10 sec. each side with full breathing
31. PASCHIMOTTANASANA
   2-5 min with normal breathing
18. ADHO MUKHA SVANASANA
   50 sec. with full breathing
19. URDHVA MUKHA SVANASANA
   60 sec. with full breathing
21. SALABHASANA
   10-60 sec. with normal breathing
22. USTRASANA
   30 sec. with normal breathing.
37. DHANURASANA
   30 sec. with rapid even breathing
23. 24. 38. VIRASANA II, III and IV.
   S0 sec. each in the last three movements with full breathing
15. PARIPOORNA NAVASANA
   S0 sec. with normal breathing
16. ARDHA NAVASANA
   30-60 sec with shallow breathing
26. BHARADVAJASANA I.
   10 sec. with full breathing
34. BHARADVAJASANA II.
   10-60 sec. with normal or full breathing

35. MARICHYASANA III

(Son of Brahman posture)

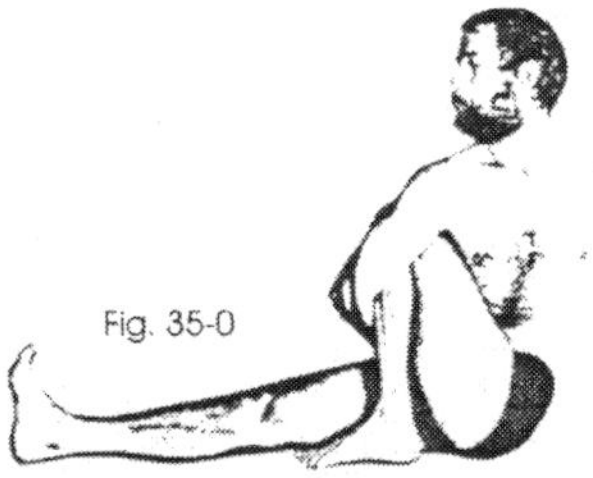
Fig. 35-0

The liver and spleen are contracted which helps reduce sluggishness. The posture massages the intestines so they function better. Neck muscles are strengthened and the shoulders made to move freely. It works on the lower spine relieving backaches there and lumbago, and it reduces fat around the waste.

I. Basic procedure:

1. Sit in Dandasana Fig. 15-1. Place the left foot next to the inner side of the right thigh with the calf perpendicular to the floor and the left heel close to the groin. Keep the right leg locked at the knee.

2. On an exhalation turn the trunk to the left as far as you can, bringing the right shoulder passed and outside the bent left knee. With an exhalation again, press the outer side of the right shoulder against the outer side of the bent left knee which helps turn the trunk further to the left.

3. Inhale fully, raising the chest from the sternum to the navel upward, and extend it outward and backward away from the bent left knee. Then work the right arm father down the bent left leg, and with an exhalation turn the trunk further to the left. Bring as much of the abdominal and chest area free of the bent leg as possible.

4. Repeat step 2 and 3 above several times until you have turned the trunk fully. Then exhale and wrap the right arm around the left knee and place the right wrist at the back of the waste.

Exhaling fully swing the left arm behind the back and grasp it with the right hand. Grasp firmly and turn the spine further by tugging at the clasped hands, Fig. 35-1. This action locks the bent leg tightly to the right side of the chest. Repeat the steps 2 and 3 above to free the chest a little more from this frontal lock.

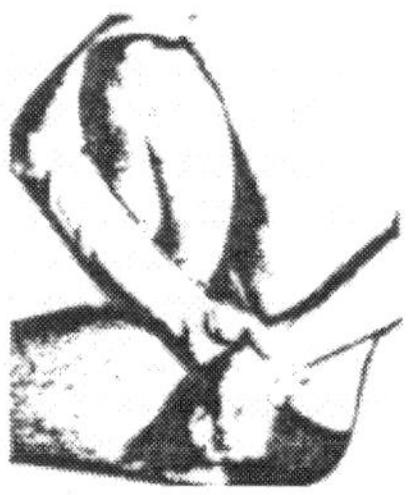

Fig. 35-1

5. Elongate the spine and stretch it upwards toward the ceiling. Turn the neck to the right and gaze over the right shoulder at nose level, holding the chin directly over and above the shoulder. Stay in this posture for 10 sec. with normal breathing, and then repeat on the other side.

II. Variation procedure:

Until you develop enough flexibility to grab your fingers or hands behind you, you can do this posture as shown in Fig. 35-2. Lock the right arm and grasp the outer side of the right knee with the right hand. Lock the left arm and use it to support and turn your trunk from behind. You may also use a towel or a rope to connect the hands and use as leverage to pull you, as detailed in Ardha Matsyendrasana [36].

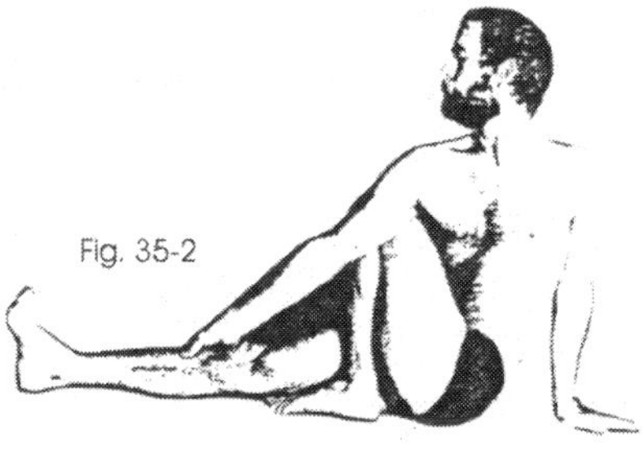

Fig. 35-2

III. Perfecting procedure:

1. When doing the basic procedure steps 2 and 3 above, lift and extend the chest and get as much of the lower abdominal area clear of the upright leg. The action here is basically the same as a forward bend, i.e., Paschimottanasana [31]. The movement comes from the front center chest to navel area. If the chest and floating ribs are extended forward and raised, the twisting of the lower trunk will follow correctly and naturaly.

2. Don't let the shoulders and sternum sink forward as shown in Fig. 35-3. Instead draw the left shoulder back. The left shoulder is drawn further back by extending the left arm down towards the floor, using as leverage the firm grip of the right hand on its wrist. The right shoulder is pushed out and away from the body slightly, Fig. 35-4

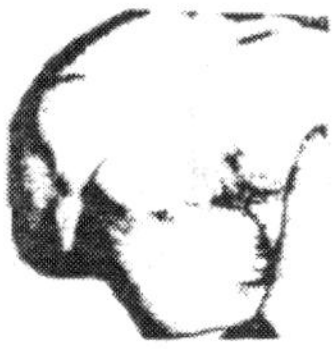

Fig. 35-3

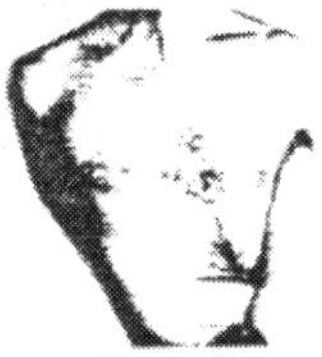

Fig. 35-4

3. The trunk should be thrust forward towards the straight right foot by using the lower abdominal and hip muscles. This maintains balance and poise in the posture. If you do the posture as shown in Fig. 35-2, the left arm also helps push the trunk forward.

4. Extend the straight leg from the heel, lifting the knee cap up into the thigh and drawing the right foot perpendicular to the floor. This

extension done correctly will lift the right heel a half inch or more off the floor as shown in Fig. 35-5. Otherwise the ankle and the foot become dead areas of the posture as shown in Fig. 35-6 with the heel on the floor.

Fig. 35-5
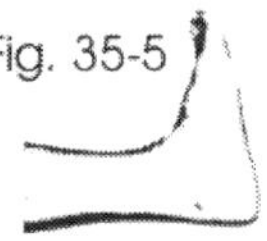

Fig. 35-6
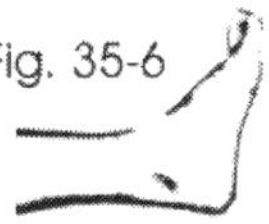

Besides keeping this foot off the floor slightly, also keep it from slanting to one side or the other. The toes should be in line and parallel to the forehead.

IV. Teaching procedure:

Place the folded blanket under the student's buttocks to aid him in making a more complete straight leg lock. As the trunk is raised, the heel will be on the floor. Lifting the trunk up on the blanket also helps balance and makes wrapping the arm around the upright leg a little easier.

You can help the student draw his arm around his knee. Use your heed, feet, legs, for leverage while you use your hand to push and pull the students shoulders back, head erect, chest out, etc

Have him do the posture next to a wall, with his back to the wall. You then gently press his shoulders, back, neck to the wall.

36. ARDHA MATSYENDRASANA I.
    10 sec. each side with normal breathing
33. BADDHA KONASANA
    3Q sec. in each movement with normal breathing
40. PADMASANA
    30-60 sec. on each side with normal breathing

42. MATSYASANA

(Fish posture)

The dorsal region gets fully extended, and the chest is expanded, which develops full breathing. The pelvic joints become elastic and inflamed piles are relieved.

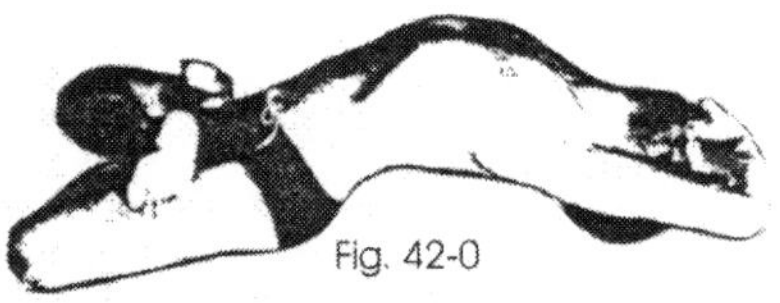
Fig. 42-0

The shoulder joints are made more flexible and the extension of the chin backwards benefits the thyroid and parathyroid glands.

I. Basic procedure:

1. Perform Padmasana [40], placing the left ankle on the right thigh first. Then exhale and recline the trunk backwards, resting first on the elbows. On the next exhalation recline the trunk further until the trunk and head rest on the floor.

2. Grab the toes and the balls of the feet and, pulling on them, drag the trunk into an arch. Only the crown of the head, the buttocks, and the legs will rest on the floor.

3. Release the toes grip and bring the arms beyond the head and cross them. Now stretch the crossed arms away from the head and shoulders and push them down to the floor.

4. Stretch the neck and extend the chin outward towards the crossed arms. Stay in this position for 10-60 sec. with full breathing and gaze between the eyebrows. Then repeat the posture with the arms and legs folded the opposite way.

II. Variation procedure:

Those who can't do Padmasana [40] yet may instead perform this variation of Virasana [38] as shown in the Fig. 42-1. Don't worry about the elbows not touching the floor at first, as this may take a long time to develop the required shoulder flexibility.

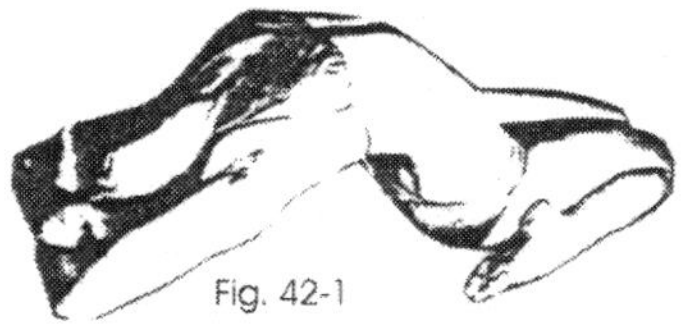
Fig. 42-1

III. Perfecting procedure:

1. When dragging the trunk into an arch extend the lower abdomen upward making the lower back as concave as possible. Don't let the knees rise off the floor as shown in Fig. 42-2. Press them into the floor by stretching the upper thigh muscle towards

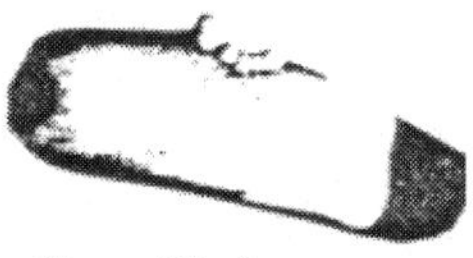
Fig. 42-2

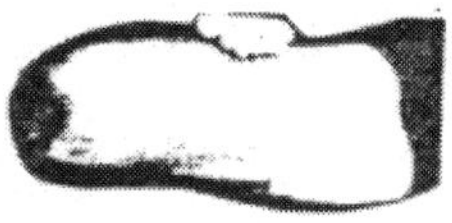
Fig. 42-3

the knees, and by contracting the buttock and anus muscle and opening cut the groin area.

2. After the arms are folded beyond the head extend the chest upward and outward from the sternum to the navel and draw the shoulders and arms down towards the floor. Feel the shoulder blades pressing in towards each other.

IV. Teaching procedure:

You can lay weights, if available, on the students crossed legs and crossed arms. Then place your hand under his waste and lift him upward from the lower back.

13. SAVASANA
5-15 min. with normal breathing.
PRANAYAMA
Do pranayama [47] either 30 minutes before or after Yoga posture practice, or at another time of the day. Its best though in the early morning just after you get up or just before bed in the evening. Practice Pranayama for 5-15 minutes while sitting in Siddhasana [39]. Virasana [23], Baddha Konasana [33], or in Padmasana [40].

For more information on pranayama, read posture dynamics page for Pranayama (in Savasana) [14] and Pranayama (upright) [47].

Note: I prefer *sui Zen* (blowing Zen) for doing the pranayama side of yoga. This is done using a shakuhachi (end blown Japanese bamboo flute). I personally feel this to be a safer, more effective method long term for anyone serious about this aspect of yoga.

There is a tendency for people to stick with one path, which probably accounts for why there are so few Christian-Buddhist-pagans. That is understandable; sticking with one path is challenge enough. Nevertheless, I felt it important to introduce this. For more see, **www.centertao.org/essays/blowingzen**

LESSON XI

3. UTTHITA TRIKONASANA
30 sec. each site with full breathing
4. PARIVRTTA TRIKONASANA
30 sec. each side with normal breathing
5. UTTHITA PARSVAKONASANA
30 sec. each side with full breathing

44. PARIVRTTA PARSVAKONASANA

(Side angle posture revolved)

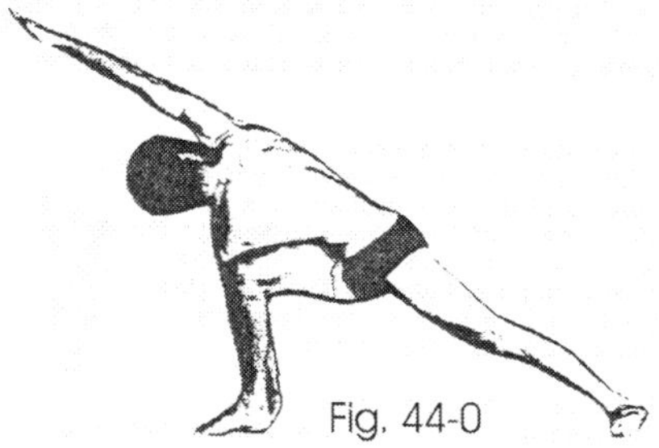
Fig. 44-0

This posture intensifies the effects of Parivrtta Trikonasana [4] except for the hamstring muscles.
The circulation is increased around the abdomen and spine improving the digestion and countering any tendency towards constipation. It strengthens the whole body from fingers to toes and is one of the most difficult postures to perform well.

I. Basic procedure:

1. From Tadasana [1], jump on the exhalation, spreading the legs 4 feet apart. Turn the right foot 90° to the right and the left 60° to the right.

2. Bend the right leg and bring the right thigh parallel to the floor as in Utthita Parsvakonasana [5], only this time twist the trunk to the right and rest the back of the left arm/shoulder on the outer side of the bent right knee.

3. Draw the right shoulder upward and backward to bring it into a perpendicular line with the other shoulder and the floor.

4. Stretch the right arm out beyond the head directly over the ear. Turn the face upwards and gaze passed this outstretched arm. Stretch the entire body from outstretched fingertips to heels of the rear left foot. Stay in the posture for 30-60 sec. with full breathing. Then on an inhalation return and repeat on the other side.

II. Variation procedure:

This is a very difficult and strenuous posture to do correctly, but don't let that discourage you. Do it the best you can, be patient and you will succeed.

In attempting to place the rear left foot flat on the floor you can either keep working at it, or raise the heel of that foot so that the left leg rest on the tall and toes of the left foot only. This foot should be held perpendicular to the calf. Ankle flexibility will improve through practice of the other standing posture, after which time you can perform this posture in the standard way.

III. Perfecting procedure:

1. Its important to get the greatest twist possible so treat this posture as a twisting posture and follow the same techniques as for the other twisting postures. Use the left arm to push its shoulder away from the bent right leg. Extend the area from the chest to the navel and work as much of this area as possible free from the right thigh. Use the right hand to push thigh.

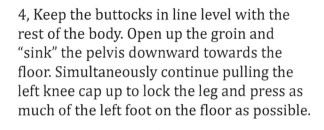

Repeat this action a few times as was done in the Basic procedure 2 and 3 in Marichyasana [35], in order to obtain the maximum possible twisting of the trunk. Eventually the medial line of the left side of the chest/ribs should be in line with the median line of the right thigh.

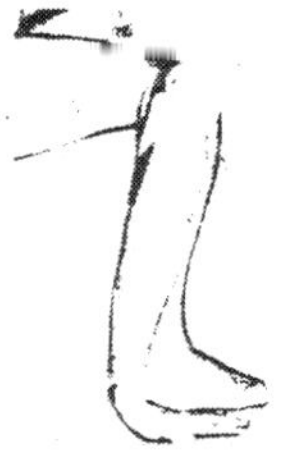

Fig. 44-1

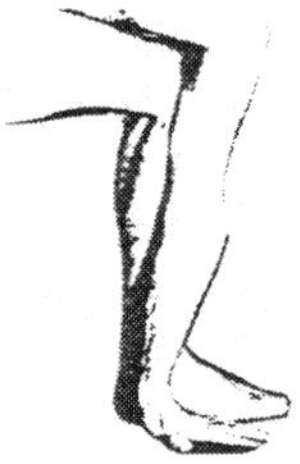

Fig. 44-2

2. Place the left arm well inside the right calf as shown in Fig. 44-1. Placing it less than this as shown in Fig. 44-2, decreases the twisting potential of the posture.

3. Roll the right side of the trunk backward and stretch it until you feel the skin stretched tight from the out-stretched arm to rear left heel. The trunk should be twisted around enough for the nipples and shoulders to be in a perpendicular line to the floor similar to that shown for Parivrtta Trikonasana, Fig. 4-1.

4, Keep the buttocks in line level with the rest of the body. Open up the groin and "sink" the pelvis downward towards the floor. Simultaneously continue pulling the left knee cap up to lock the leg and press as much of the left foot on the floor as possible.

5. Extend the right arm out, locked firmly at the elbow with the hand locked into a bow at the knuckles, Fig. 44-1. Gaze upward with the head/neck turned enough so that you can see the arm full with the right eye closed.

IV. Teaching procedure:

For a little easier variation that allows the student to concentrate more on the twisting movement, you can have the student stretch the right arm straight up toward the ceiling similar to Parivrtta Trikonasana [4], or put hand on hip.

You may drop the insistence on looking up passed the arm in the beginning as this can be an added distracting strain. Instead have him look ahead.

You can have the student perform the posture with his back to the wall and then have him press as much of his back to the wall (and touch it) as possible.

6. VIRABHADRASANA I.
 30 sec. each side with full breathing
8. VIRABHADRASANA III.
 Stay fro 30 sec. each side with full breathing
43. ARDHA CHANDRASANA
 30 sec. each side with full breathing
9. PARSVOTTANASANA,
 30 sec. each side with full breathing
10. PRASARITA PADOTTANASANAI.
 Do version I or the one below.

10. PRASARITA PADOTTANASANA II

Fig. 10-0

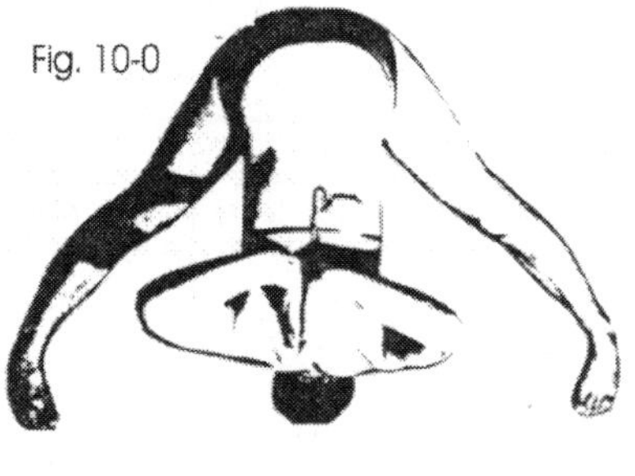

Stay for 10 sec. in each position with full breathing. The only difference between the two versions is in the placing of the hands. If your wrists are flexible enough replace the easier version with this one. Join the hands behind the back and jump spreading the legs 4 ft. apart and perform as detailed earlier.

11. UTTANASANA
    1-5 min. with full breathing
27. SIRSASANA
    3-5 min with normal breathing
12. SARVANGASANA
    Stay 10 min. with normal breathing
29. HALASANA
    Stay 5 min. with normal breathing
31. PASCHIMOTTANASANA
    Stay 3 min. with normal breathing
22. USTRASANA
    Stay 10 sec. with normal breathing
37. DHANURASANA
    10 sec. with rapid breathing

MARICHYASANA
    10 sec. each side with normal breathing

ARDHA MATSYENDRASANA
    10 sec. each side with normal breathing

40. PADMASANA
    30 sec. on each side with normal breathing.

67. BADDHA PADMASANA

When if you have the flexibility, perform the following variation of Padmasana [40], which will further improve leg and hip flexibility and make the standard Padmasana [40] more comfortable.

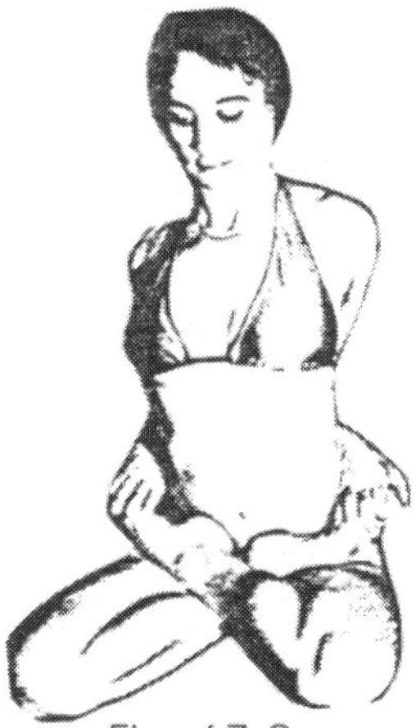
Fig. 67-0

1. Draw the feet further up on the thigh, and then on an exhalation swing the arms behind the back and grasp the big toe-ball of feet with the hand from the opposite side of body. Extend the chest and roll the shoulders back, Fig. 67-0.

2. Hold this position for 30 sec. with full breathing with the gaze at nose level. Then with a full exhalation bend the trunk forward until the chest touched the thighs and the chin extends beyond the knee.

Follow the same principles of movement as other forward bends. Maintain the finger/ toes grip firmly throughout the bend. Stay in this position with normal breathing for 30 sec., then on inhalation raise the trunk up. Now, repeat on the other side.

13. SAVASANA
    5- 15 min. with normal breathing

48. MEDITATION:

Meditation [48] can be done after Savasana [13], in morning after you get up, in the evening just before bed, or at any time during the day. And of course informal meditation in action can be done throughout the waking hours. For formal meditation sit in any of the postures recommended for Pranayama already. The usual minimum time for meditation should be 5 min. and increase this time as you like or need.

FINALLY, VIDEO YOURSELF!

As I mentioned earlier, one very useful 21st century advance has been the ability of anyone to video their yoga practice. Do this sporadically to can reveal 'blind spots', i.e., general errors and ways you may be cheating yourself. This endows you with a teacher's eye. (Using a mirror can help too.)

OTHER CONSIDERATIONS

The disclaimer made on page 177 applies here even more. I went through this and deleted the more redundant. over-the-top, or otherwise irrelevant parts. I'm also a much better writer than I was 30+ years ago, but I've decided to rework the contents of this book as little as possible. Only the first few pages, Principles (from an older and perhaps wiser point of view) are 100% freshly written.

As I said earlier, my views have softened and changed over the intervening 30+ years. Nevertheless, some of this may serves a purpose for some. That is perhaps why I've chosen not to rewrite it from scratch; I'd end up changing too much, or perhaps not even write anything at all. So, I just leave it be. After all, "For everything there is a season, and a time for every purpose under heaven". (Ecclesiastes 3:1)

Moving Forward

By now you will probably have proven for yourself that yoga can help ward off illness, increase alertness, and improve overall well being. After you have studied and practiced the postures given under programs 1 and 2, or have completed the Step by Step Lesson you are ready to begin program three. The Step by Step Lessons along with the dynamic illustrations and some of the points covered in this chapter should be enough to take on and complete all the postures in this book.

If you wish to realize the maximum benefit for mind and body through Hatha Yoga, however, you best proceed to the more advance postures as you are able. As the basic postures become easy to do you proceed to intermediate ones, which then become your "basic" postures of development. As these in turn become "easy" you go on to more advanced ones and make them your "basic" postures. By continuing to advance in this way you remain a beginner of sorts, and benefit by the growth and challenge of being a beginner.

The Yoga sessions set up the condition for learning and feeling the whole body. The nature of the action in Yoga allow you to get to know your body and mind as few other techniques can. The various parts of the body are made to live - in a sense, to have their own awareness linked to your awareness.

This is similar to learning a musical instrument: If you learn only a few simple melodies, like "Ba Ba Black Sheep" and never learn more challenging music you will never really get to know the instrument well, and may never realize its full potential.

By pushing at the limits of ability, then the limits of ability extend further and further.

Here, in Yoga, your body is the instrument, and you are learning to fine tune it and play it. In fact the sensations you feel during advanced Yoga session are very similar to playing of music - even though you are relatively still and there is no sound present.

Questions will arise as to when you are ready for the next program. This is totally relative to how hard you work and how confident you are. Generally speaking, you can advance to the next program as soon as you are able to perform most of the postures in your present program fairly well. Of course there is no question about perfecting postures before going on. Indeed, only through going on to more advance postures can you bring increasing understanding of the more basic postures you have already 'mastered'. It is through doing advanced postures that you actually learn how to master the basic ones.

Injuries

As you advance to more difficult postures you may be more likely to injure yourself slightly in one way or another. Those who work extra hard can stumble right from the beginning programs. Here are several possible reasons for this:

1) First, you have not achieve much awareness of your body and so when you attempt to do something physically challenging you may easily overdo it, or forget something, stumble and stub your toes.

2) Some people get "greedy" in the postures, overworking a muscle or a tendons; ambition overtakes prudence.

3) There are certain areas of the body which are "hereditarily" weak, and through Yoga you discover these - sometimes painfully - and work for some years strengthening them. These areas left to themselves as is the case in most people, show up in latter years. Here you are essentially performing preventive maintenance.

The 12 Cycles

All the 138 Yoga postures presented in this book are arranged into 12 cycles, each specializing in one or more areas of the body. It takes a number of years of daily practice to develop the mind and the body to the point where you can do them all, and still longer before you truly know what you are doing. Over time (decades really) these cycles do give you excellent health and a heightened sense of well being. They are well worth the time and effort. However, considering the decades involved you do need a certain degree of faith that yoga will deliver on this promise.

Here are some of the main areas of the body which the cycles work on, to learn which postures are in which cycles refer to the Programs 3-9.

Cycles

Basic: for; stomach, arms, back, hips, knee.

Standing: for; whole body, increasing basic flexibility in neck, spine, legs, arms, trunk, ankles, nips, etc.

Forward bend: for lower back, hips, legs,

Twist: for spinal twist, lower back.

Shoulder stand: for neck abdomen, brain, sinuses, thyroid and parathyroid glands.

Head stand: for; neck, shoulders, balance, brain, pituitary gland.

Lotus: for; hips and knees.

Backward: for lower spine, shoulder,

Basic arm: for; arms, wrists, shoulders, stomach, legs

Advanced arm: for stomach, spine, arms shoulder, wrists, legs, hits, back muscles, side abdominal

Leg head: for neck, lower back, pelvis, abdomen.

Knee-hip: for knee, ankles, hips

Stages of Development

I will attempt here to give a rough idea of the steps you may pass through, and the time needed, for a serious student of Yoga.

For the first year of two the beginner should work on programs 1, 2, and 3. He should be able at the end of that time to be able to do Pranayama in Savasana, do a mantra meditation (OM or SA-HA), have a partial knowledge of anatomy and the Bhagavad Gita, He should be able to run a mile in under- 10 minute, understand what is involved in choosing a healthy diet, be able to recognize his inappropriate habits, and be capable of fasting for 24 hours.

An intermediate student should be able to complete programs 4, 5, 6, in two to four more years of regular practice. He should be able to do Pranayama in Padmasana, sit in "silent" meditation (formal), and have a solid knowledge of the Bhagavad Gita anatomy. He should be able to prepare food in the healthy manner, jog a mile in under 8 minute, and begin moving past extremes of one's more self destructive habits. He should have kept a reflection chart for at least six months, and experienced the different kinds of fasts, i.e., food for 3 days, speech for a few days, no make up, meat, beer... whatever you feel you can't do without.

An advanced student should be able to complete most programs in four to nine-years or more. He will be able to perform pranayama in all the asanas, practice meditation in daily activity. He should find the reflection chart unnecessary for he continually remembers what, why, how. He will be highly consistent in matters of diet, detached from habits, be concerned to aid his fellow man in whatever way come natural to him, be able to jog the mile in under 7 minutes, be deeply familiar with passages of the humankind's major scripture.

Of course this is just an ideal view of the journey. You will find that advancement is-not uniform. You may be able to do all the posture perfectly bit still not have fulfilled other subtler aspects and visa versa. There is also the question of backsliding - This can be a very good thing, especially after a few steady years of conscientious practice, for it gives humility and greater perspective, and helps to counteract the tendency to cling to Yoga.

Tips for Perfecting Your Practice

1) As you continue on with more advanced Yoga postures and attitude, you will awaken kundalini, or "cosmic" intelligence or energy. Put more simply this Indian word symbolizes a "watchful" universe where all its parts are, at a certain point, in sync. By awakening our mind we become more conscious of this cosmic watchfulness, or intelligence, the human, passive attention or watchfulness is the energy of Kundalini. In man the nervous system is the source of human watchfulness. It is, through it that we perceive the nature of the universe. The nervous system is centered in the spine and head. The spine is awakened through Yoga practice. This spinal 'intelligence' is what maintains watchfulness in our conscious minds. In Indian mythology this is depicted as a snake rising in the spine to the brain and out to the universe. Thus awakening of Kundalini is awakening of watchfulness, which is facilitated by spinal extension - especially the back of the neck. (See Tadasana, also Eka Pada Sirsasana helps greatly to train

2) Slight improvements in extension may seem trivial. Such slight, improvements, however, represent major improvements in coordination and awareness of -the path .of perfection in action.

3) The absolute time spent on a posture is generally not less than 30 sec. More important is the evenness and rhythm, which make each posture seem timeless though you spent a short time only in it. On the other hand spending long time 5-10 minute in posture can be developing these "timings" are done at a lower intensity than the usual practice of course.

4) In Hatha Yoga a posture is perfected not by forceful effort, but by relaxing under appropriate effort. Through the attitude of surrender you can find the greatest level of relaxation in any posture (or other action for that matter) while simultaneously striving for the greatest perfection of that action.

Perfection in action leads to perfection in emotion and thought and attitude. Perfection in the easy actions is vitally important for a continuous life of self harmony. Striving for perfection in "difficult" action trains this. Confronting the easy is usually easy. When confronting the difficult becomes easy then self harmony comes more naturally.

So learn not to resist or avoid the difficult, but instead flow with it. Surrender to it, for with surrender comes real peace and joy. What is the difficult aspect in Yoga you must surrender to? Part is the muscular effort-energy demand, but re difficult is achieving the perfection of use of that energy: the right amount in the right place at the right time with the right attitude.

5) The two poles of nature + and - , work and rest, life and death, etc., should be the focal point of your attention. When one is "ruling", let the other serve as the root. Never loose sight of the other, from compulsive attachment to one. The mountain has its valley, the long has short, and the in has out. The subtler your awareness becomes the less difference there appears to be between these two seemingly opposite poles. Within this subtlety lies the innermost secret of existence, which words fail to convey.

In Hatha Yoga you strive to join these two poles, the active and the passive, in harmony. Thus in your practice look or calmness in the activity and activity in the calmness. Then the wholeness of creation is experienced fully.

Teaching the Asanas

"Let not the wise disturb the mind of the unwise in their selfish Work. Let him, working with devotion; show them the joy of good work." Bhagavad-Gita 3-26

People constantly either expect or try to teach others to do "right", without really doing "right themselves. In fact we do this to such an extent that we aren't even aware of it half the time, and the other times we quickly rationalize it.

A teacher of Yoga should consider all viewpoints, contemplate the condition of life, etc., and thus in time determine certain priorities which are essential for self harmony. The wise teacher then aims at living in harmony with these priorities and thus eliminates the extremes of self hypocrisy.

How much you' live in accordance with you priorities (your wisdom) is relative to your nature, and degree of interest, and always imperfect, We are ALL human, caught up in the works of nature, evolving and evolving, and so you should never feel guilty for having weakness and giving into "temptations". However, if you are to be a competent teacher of this subject you must be a conscientious student of yourself. As a chain is only as strong as its weakest link, try to always look for those weak links in your life!

"Among thousands of men perhaps one strives for perfection; and among thousands of those who strive perhaps one knows in truth." Bhagavad-Gita 7-3

Much has already been said about the special teaching considerations for each posture. These suggestions and anything said here should be considered loosely and then adjusted to your particular needs and the needs of the student.

Style

There are two basic and slightly different teaching styles to use according to the teaching conditions, and your own personality. One is the strict "Zen" training approach with which you can start beginners out with, and the other is the "brotherly" approach where you share greater contact with the student. Any blend of the two styles or even alternating between them could be useful.

1) The "Zen" approach is especially effective for larger classes. It cuts down on daydreaming and the resulting boredom and waste of time for both you and the students. It instills discipline and perfection in action - alertness. It gets the student to work harder on himself which of course brings results. During the lesson you insist on silence, and accept questions .only at certain times. You insist on quick movement and careful listening and berate those who daydream or are sloppy. Pattern your approach to that of the marine drill sergeant. Shout a bit, bark instructions .at times, and be ruthless. Never, never, however get personally angry or cling to expectations. Keep your humor.

2) The brotherly style is better with private students, small groups, and in groups where they have "learned" the ropes and so respond efficiently and with attention (where there is class discipline established already). Here you will be able to relate to the students more directly and personally.

You will soon notice a tendency among students to daydream, and neglect to do those things which you know they know they should be doing but aren't due to inattentiveness. An assortment of "aggressive" techniques can be used: sharp shout, push, pull, slap, kick, etc. This may seam objectionable at first to "peace loving" people, but is really a very valuable teaching aid. You use this "shock" treatment on those students who are past the beginning stage and so should know better. A slap-on the area ("dead area") which they are forgetting is the most effective way to reinforce their memory and focus their attention to that area. Verbal correction on the other hand often goes in one ear and out the other and rob the rest of the class of time and your attention.

Use touch as the main medium of instruction. Besides the "shock" form detailed above, you should use 'a gentler touch as well. Touch students face (especially one that appears relaxed) and tell him to relax his tongue, eyeballs, throat, and brain. There is always too much tension, if he is doing the posture correctly with full energy, even if you don't notice it. Use gentler pull and push or touch dead area instead of tapping or slapping them. Also touch areas where you want them to use more energy, or be more aware of, or relax. Combine techniques: touch, then slap, then shout, then reason, then show!

Teach with the question. Through questions you open up students mind and make him more receptive, stimulate his reasoning power, and motivate him to discover the "answer" in himself. Also encourage them to ask questions of you. Ask question's about the posture, how to do it, its effects, mistakes most often made, etc. Ask students to point out mistakes in others, themselves, or in the mistakes you imitate in a demonstration posture.

Demonstrate posture in different ways:

1) You can do it in a very perfect symmetrical way, and then with "relaxed" perfection not necessarily symmetrical. You ask, "Which was more watchfully done?" They both were, thus watchfulness isn't necessarily only present with perfect symmetry! But striving for symmetry on the other hand is very useful in training attention and care. So you must first learn posture in a very symmetrical way and then perhaps in a perfectly asymmetrical way.

2) First do the posture wrong and ask the student to point out mistakes in it. If they can't, you do so. Then do posture correctly and ask them to point out differences.

3) Merely perform the posture as it should be done, before they do it, especially with new postures. Then as they repeat it you give verbal instruction and go around and correct them.

You can't make people know that which is beyond their present need, ability or willingness to know. But if they are motivated and want to know and have patience, they can be taught step by step through example and reason. After a conceptual understanding is awakened, the next step is to arrive at true knowing which comes through application on the student's part. A very effective way to teach the conceptual understanding is through questions.

In the lesson, let the students experience the extremes of movement, which are possible in the posture. First he does the posture in a "dead" way and then with full "Life". Thus, he will know the posture through contrast.

You can also help a student to experience the limit of his movement or strength in' a posture. You push or pull or twist him into the perfect position. Of course considerable care must be exercised. This is very useful especially for those who don't go anywhere near there limit. To do this, first notice the students breathing sequence. Instruct him to inhale and then with the next exhalation to surrender into the movement. You apply force to his movement during his exhalation, and move as one with him.

Class vs. Home Practice:

In class there will be some weaker and some stronger students. Pace the holding times of each posture such that weaker students can do them, then demand the most perfection in the posture from the stronger students (perfection of all aspects) and go easy on the weaker ones. It's also possible to have longer holing times, and just allow the weaker students to release the posture earlier so they get more rest.

It's very important for students to learn the spinal lift - raising of the back of the neck especially. This is the fundamental root to all posture, even all action. You can have them stand against the wall, and (1) they relax completely, allowing chin to rise and shoulders to droop. (2) You place your hand on top of their head and then instruct them to push your hand up to the ceiling, as you simultaneously push downwards. Thus they have to extend upward against the downward pressure you are applying by extending the spine. You can do this while they are in a posture as well.

When teaching the postures use the different parts of the room for reference, i.e., "turn the chest towards the wall, raise sternum to the ceiling, push heal into floor, raise calf and ankle toward wall,"

Students will need a rest after performing the standing postures, or other strenuous postures. Have them do Uttanasana for a minute or so as explained in *IV. Teaching Procedure of Uttanasana*. They need not lean against the wall if this is inconvenient at the time. At this time, or in a less formal break you can spend a few moments explaining Yoga principles, effects, or practical tips. At these times too you can accept questions from the student. Be careful not to let the break, explanation, or question and answer period last too long. Some people especially love much more to discuss Yoga than to do it, and every one gets cooled down.

Variations: There is a variety of different ways to give a lesson, or team a posture. Using variations can broaden understanding of the posture:

1) A cycle of pastures can be-done very quickly with short but intense holding times and no breaks between. Here you try for smooth transition from posture to posture. This challenges endurance, and even breathing, and your real knowledge of the posture.

2) Even some lessons can be at a fast pace, and so very strict and exhausting, then the next time gives a more relaxed lesson with timings, or using different variations of the posture and using tools.

3) Some times give one or more postures in the lesson for long hold time "timings" in fact this can just be one posture for the whole lesson. With timings the intensity is much less of course. You strive for much greater relaxation in the posture, while applying as much effort as might seam appropriate, using watchfulness and surrender to the utmost.

4) A cycle can be done slow, with use of tools and variations, and examples and repetitions (good for new postures), and then the next cycle can be fast and intense (good for basic postures).

5) Can do postures moderate pace as one would do at home practice session. You can even tell students the lesson before that they will have to do a certain cycle for the next lesson at their vim pace. Then while they are doing this you can go around and correct. You can have one student go up to the front of the class to set the pace or have them all go at their own pace (such review at home to prepare them for the next lesson gets them to become more familiar with the cycle)

6) Students will be of different levels. You can give the advance students more advanced postures to do while the other students are doing the basic variations. Only start doing this once the whole class knows the basics of the basic postures.

7) For one whole lesson, or even just one posture, concentrate on one aspect of Yoga practice, i.e., counting the breaths, extending the chest, or keeping the legs straight, or maintaining spinal extension, or keeping the face relaxed, or doing long timings or short ones with even flow from posture to posture.

8) Use the various tools to broaden and deepen students understanding of the posture. One very good tool is a pole about 4 feet long. Use this, especially in the standing and other basic postures, to show the student what straight is! Also use pole to push here or there, or place it such that student tries, to extend toward it. Experiment with it in your own practice and you will discover many used. Another tool is the rope. This is most handy in forward bends, allowing student to get the right shoulder and chest movement while still "touching" his toes.

9) Occasionally you can put the, students through a fast paced Yoga warm-up cycles. Many people who don't have the motivation to practice Yoga seriously at least find the time to do these. They can provide a new dimension to the lesson.

If they are to be done at a very fast pace then the movements are to be done on the exhalation, and even on the inhalation, which means that the posture is only heir for half a breath cycle or even just during the pause between the exhalation and the inhalation - thus giving only a moment of intense extension in the posture before moving on to the next posture. The cycle can of course be done much slower, allowing to stay in each posture for a number of breaths - it's all up to you!

To get the even flow to fast paced cycle you should practice it on your own first and work it out.

A) Beginner cycle: (done at a fast pace)

1) Begin in Tadasana, and on the exhalation move to...

2) Uttanasana. Inhale deeply and then on the exhalation jump back to...

3) Adho Mukha Svanasana. On the inhalation move forward into...

4) Urdhva Mukha Svanasana. Extend into this posture on the exhalation and then on the inhalation move down into...

5) Chaturanga Dandasana extend forward in this on the exhalation and then on the inhalation move upward into...

6) Urdhva Mukha Svanasana again. On the next exhalation move back to...

7) Adho Mukha Svanasana. Inhale and then jump back to...

8) Uttanasana. Now repeat this cycle as many times as you wish.

B) Advanced cycle;

1) From point 5 above, instead of moving upward back to Svanasana you hop forward a number of times, one foot each time, this is...

2) Nakrasana. Now inhale and lower your self into...

3) Salabhasana, and extend into this on the exhalation. Inhale and reach back and grasp the ankles and on the exhalation extend into...

4) Dhanurasana. Inhale and return to step 5 above and then go to step 6, 7, and 8.

You can try some other movements as well, for example; from step four above (Dhanurasana) you can do Bhekasana, the movements of Virasana (three positions), then Ustrasana, Mayurasara, and back to Adho Mukha Svanasana. From Adho Mukha Svanasana go to Chakorasana, then Navasana, Paschimottanasana, Halasana, and Parsvottanasana (of course you will have to work out the smoothest breathing sequence etc., before this can be done well)

Teaching Pranayama

First, I have found attempting to 'control' one's breath can sometimes lead to over control which is no fun. Fortunately there is Blowing Zen, a better alternative, even when one encounters no problems in pranayama.

To learn more about this, visit http://www.centertao.org/essays/blowingzen. Blowing Zen is a form of Buddhist meditation and breath training that employs an end blown bamboo flute known in Japan as the Shakuhachi.

That said, I've found that many folks dislike mixing paradigms. So, I offer these pointers for those who wish to teach and learn pranayama. Note, I suppose it should be apparent by now that I don't see much distinction between a student and a teacher. Anything you do seriously in life makes you both.

In teaching Pranayama it is especially important to ask questions, and encourage students to ask question, because it is very hard to detect whether a student is really understanding or misunderstanding. This holds true for meditation too.

Make sure that they understand that Pranayama should only be done as a practice and not to think about or control breath during the day because this can cause troublesome breathing rhythms. If fact, "full" normal breathing will come naturally with good posture.

First have the student lie in Savasana, and make sure he can do this correctly (see Savasana [13]). The next thing to do is explain the basic process of breathing (diaphragm, intercostal muscle, etc.). Then have them examine their own breathing as follows:

1) First they take a normal full inhalation with the belly muscles completely relaxed, they should notice their belly bulging.

2) Now they take a normal full inhalation with the abdominal muscles "toned" flat. They would feel the downward pressure of the organs as they are pushed into the pelvic cavity. (The inhalation is as full as possible in these two cases without using the chest so chest is kept flat)

3) Now let them repeat, #2, and at the peak of inhalation, have them extend the chest fully. This, they will notice, reduces the pressure (the push) in the pelvic area away.

In Pranayama, as in all activity, they should maintain the tone of the abdominal muscles Let them tap there own belly to see it this is firm (maintaining muscle tone not forcefully contracted).

Have all the students exhale at once and then begin the Pranayama on the next inhalation. After a number of rounds the Pranayama will end at the end of the exhalation - just as with the asanas. You should begin with the simplest Pranayama: just breathing, and use SA – HA. Observe each student to see if they are maintaining an even respiration rhythm. If not they must concentrate on even rhythm before going on. Tell them so and instruct them to practice SA - HA at home.

For the procedures for the different stages of Pranayama cheek the chapter on this. You can teach normal inhalation followed by longer exhalation to begin with, and then progress from there the different method which takes prolonged inhalations, pauses, and prolonged exhalations may need to be timed so you keep an accurate rhythm. This can easily be done by silently spacing the breaths in your mind.

For example: in complete Savasana Pranayama where student uses both the diaphragm and costal muscles you say, "everyone inhale" I - 2 - 3 - 4 - 5 - 6 - 7 "extend and pause" 8 - 9 -"exhale" 1 - 2 - etc., thus counting the spaces silently .in your head. Set this pace such that all the students can keep up.

Keep a close eye on each student notice the movement of their belly, chest, and encourage them to search within for the last bit of air in the inhalations and exhalations and the last bit of relaxation too. Look for tension, daydreaming, sleeping, other actions. Remember pranayama takes a long time to perfect.

Teaching Meditation

There are different ways to practice meditation, but they are all basically aiming at training watchfulness, through directing the attention. Until the student is able to focus on 'just being', let him use a verbal mantra, like OM or SA-HA, or SO-HAM etc. This can be repeated out loud or in the mind silently. It's important to encourage student to learn correct posture 'alive', especially the lift covered in Tadasana [1] Fig. 1-1. This is the meditation's foundation.

Encourage student to practice real world meditation (simply being watchful) when walking, driving, or in the asanas, or any other activity. One way to describe this is the attempt to see what has yet to be seen. One is looking for the invisible, in a kind of 'peeking outside the box' sort of way.

Visualization - During Savasana, Pranayama, meditation, or the Asana practice you can encourage the students by trying to bring the vision of Yoga to them verbally. Through certain concepts you can set up images of Yoga they are aiming for.

Work, Watch, Flow

Later on less is said, and much of what is said is redundant—a repetition of information given earlier. That should come as no surprise really. Yoga is simply applying a basic principle to a range of body position. The advance postures are really just a way of keeping you "at the beginning", where keeping the balance of Ha and Tha is most alive.

Below is a list of wordsunder three categories which relate to the three main aspects of Yoga: Watching, Working, and Flowing. Watching is close to stillness, Working is close to action, and Flowing is like the bridge between the other two - when Work evolves to Watching and Watching revolves to Working.[1]

WORK:	WATCH:	FLOW
rule	observe	surrender
support	discern	submit
live	listen	abandon
fight	touch	sink
determine	feel	yield
serve	alive to	let go
challenge	awake to	give
extend	see	drop
free will	penetrate	spread
discover	witness	accept
steer	care	immerse
volunteer	attend to	open up
command	consider	fall
explore	devote	silence
do battle	notice	still
summon	sensitize	cooperate
take	presence (mind)	offer up

Conclusion

It takes a student a long time to really assimilate and apply the various technique aspects of any Yoga practice, so you must

review often and try to insure that their is a minimum of misunderstanding.

1 This - Work, Watch, Flow – word list is a precursor to a process I later developed in 1982, a few years after writing this book. "Using Yin and Yang to Pop Preconceptions" is an introduction to this work and can be found at, http://www.centertao.org/essays/correlations.

I'll admit this "correlations" work may not serve most folks any better. Its counterpart is simpler and somewhat poetic, and so may be more palatable. This is posted as "Couplets and the Co-generating Principle", at http://www.centertao.org/essays/couplets-and-the-co-generating-principle/ might be helpful. The couplets portray an essential dynamic of Ha-Tha.

Postscript

The Tao Te Ching, chapter 36, speaks to something important... perhaps the most important of all.

If you would have a thing shrink,
You must first stretch it;
If you would have a thing weakened,
You must first strengthen it;
If you would have a thing laid aside,
You must first set it up;
If you would take from a thing,
You must first give to it.
This is called subtle discernment:
The submissive and weak will
overcome the hard and strong.

Why is this so significant? It has given me confirmation of how life happens, which is not usually the ideal we hold of how life 'should' happen. The view that you must first strengthen something before weakening it helps, for example, put selfishness and selflessness in perspective. Meaning, one must first be selfish before one can be selfless. You can't take from something that which it has not first been given.

For years I believed I had free will and the power to control my destiny. I finally realized that was more wishful thinking than reality. Over the years I've gone on to 'just let it be'. Yet, I strive on diligently. Striving on diligently parallels the Tao Te Ching's "*He who perseveres is a man of purpose*". Let go, yet persevere. Let it be, yet strive on diligently. That's it, the Yin and the Yang, the Tha and the Ha of life.

Hatha Yoga, I expect, has been very instrumental in helping me taste and test this process. To the extent possible, have this be your guiding ideal. It won't be realized on your time-table, but it can be a beacon to guide you as you 'strive on diligently'.[2]

1 Those are reportedly Buddha' final words bidding farewell to his disciples before the moment of death. At the end of the day what else can one do but strive on diligently.

Proof

11361745R00136

Made in the USA
Charleston, SC
18 February 2012